Protein Purification and Analysis II

Methods and Applications

Protein Purification and Analysis II – Methods and Applications

Publisher: iConcept Press Ltd.
Cover design: Pineapple Design Ltd.
Interior design: iConcept Press Ltd.
Typesetting and copy editing: iConcept Press Ltd. and Pineapple Design Ltd.

ISBN: 978-1-922227-63-8

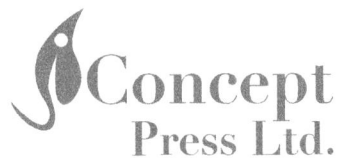

iConcept
Press Ltd.

www.iconceptpress.com

Contents

Preface

Proteins are biochemical compounds consisting of one or more polypeptides typically folded into a globular or fibrous form, facilitating a biological function. A polypeptide is a single linear polymer chain of amino acids bonded together by peptide bonds between the carboxyl and amino groups of adjacent amino acid residues. The sequence of amino acids in a protein is defined by the sequence of a gene, which is encoded in the genetic code. The complexity and sheer number of proteins in a cell are impediments to identifying proteins of interest or purifying proteins for function and structure analysis. Thus, reducing the complexity of a protein sample or in some cases purifying a protein to homogeneity is necessary. *Protein Purification and Analysis* discusses varies aspect related to protein analysis. There are totally three volumes. This book is the second volume.

There are totally 12 chapters in this book. Chapter 1 describes protein-based methods for the analysis of plant alcohol dehydrogenases. The described methods comprise crude protein extraction from different tissues, photometric activity assays, isoenzyme separation/detection by native-PAGE and histochemical ADH staining. Chapter 2 demonstrates production of recombinant fungal cell wall-degrading enzymes and their tag-affinity purification and biochemical analyses. Cell wall-degrading enzymes act on cleaving glycosidic bonds of polysaccharides and oligosaccharides, affecting morphological changes, plant-microbe interactions and nutrient acquisition. Chapter 3 contains a number of methodologies including recombinant protein purification and analysis, enzymatic reporter assays and fluorescent tag detection. Contents are formalized to demonstrate how these methods can be used in physiological, biochemical, molecular and cell biology research fields. Chapter 4 allows the reader to become acquainted with methods of recombinant expression, purification and determination of the level of activity of staphylococcal epidermolytic toxins. Biological activity, structure and function of those exotoxins are also briefly discussed in the chapter so as to allow the understanding of the unique properties of the described toxins.

Chapter 5 discussed the recombinant expression, purification and biochemical analysis of a variety of extremophilic enzymes with potential industrial application. Chapter 6 discusses tellurite, which is highly toxic for most living organisms. The chapter describes how the mechanism by which this oxyanion exerts its toxicity can be assessed by studying the effect of some metabolic enzymes which seem to help in detoxifying the toxicant. Chapter 7 describes the principle of, devices used for, protocol for, and mechanism underlying gene introduction. Gene introduction is a basic biotechnology technique that is essential for protein production and analysis. Chapter 8 outlines a SELEX method for the discovery of a target-specific aptamer. The aptamer is then used to purify the target (SEB) from a mixture of closely related enterotoxins using non-fat dry milk as a representative food matrix.

Chapter 9 proposes an overview of the methodologies employed for the manipulation of membrane protein transporters, from their purification to their reconstitution into proteoliposomes. The authors presented an original approach they developed for the functional study of a multidrug efflux pump responsible for the active transport of antibiotics in bacteria. Chapter 10 is about the versatility of substrate analogues containing unnatural amino acids in the challenging study of peptidyl-aminoacyl-L/D-isomerases. Enzymes of this class catalyze an exciting post-translational reaction, namely the change of chirality of amino acids within peptide linkage whereby an L-amino acid is converted to the D-isomer. Chapter 11 investigates the the effects of combined heat and pressure on whole beef muscle proteins and isolated myofibril solubility and protein electrophoretic pattern. It attempts to understand the relative effects of heat and pressure treatments on the proteins of beef muscle. Chapter 12 reviews the normal synovium including it's microscopic structure, cell origins and recruitment, function and its clinical relevance as a target of immunologic disease.

Editing and publishing a book is never an easy task. Each chapter in this book has gone through a peer review, a selection and an editing process so as to guarantee its quality. Without the supports and contributions of the authors and reviewers, this book can never be able to complete. We would like to thank all of the authors in this book and all of the reviewers who participated in the reviewing process: Sebastiana Angelaccio, Puran S. Bora, Silvia Buroni, Marcin Drag, Julia M Foght, Makoto Fujimaki, Monika K Grudzinska, James F. Holden, Vesa P. Hytönen, Jean-Michel Jault, Glenn W. Kaatz, Shigeru Kotake, Sachin S. Kunde, Suzie Lavoie, Timothy J. O'Leary, Evgeny Petrov, Mohammad A. Qasim, Gary Sawers, Herbert P. Schweizer, Giuseppe Spano, Bianka Steffens, Steven W. Suljak, Bas G. J. Surewaard, Kamilla Swiech, Bryan Swingle, S. M. Tietz, Juliette K. Tinker and Claudio Vásquez. We hope that you, the reader, will find this book interesting and useful. Any advices please feel free and are always welcome to tell us.

iConcept Press Ltd
May 2014

Basic Protein-based Methods for the Analysis of Plant Alcohol Dehydrogenases

Reinhard K. Proels
Lehrstuhl für Phytopathologie
Technische Universität München, Germany

Ralph Hückelhoven
Lehrstuhl für Phytopathologie
Technische Universität München, Germany

1   Introduction

As early as 1860, Pasteur showed that yeast is essential for the formation of alcohol from sugars in the widely applied biotechnological application of ethanolic fermentation. Later, in 1896, Buchner and Hahn observed that cell-free yeast extracts retained the ability to convert sugar to ethanol and CO_2, this event is regarded as the onset of biochemistry. Since then, much of attention focused on alcohol dehydrogenase (ADH) throughout different areas of research in microbes, animals and plants. Consequently, there is ample knowledge on diverse aspects of ADHs, reaching from protein structures, to catalytic mechanisms, the physiological functions and biotechnological applications.

Plants are obligate aerobic organisms. Under hypoxic conditions pyruvate decarboxylase and ADH, central enzymes in the fermentative metabolism, are induced (Fukao & Bailey-Serres, 2004). By the sequential activity of those enzymes pyruvate is eventually converted to ethanol and the concomitant regeneration of NAD^+ is essential for maintaining glycolysis and ATP production. ADH is critical for plant survival under flooding-induced hypoxic stress conditions (Kennedy *et al.*, 1992; Bailey-Serres & Voesenek, 2008), during the seed development (Hanson *et al.*, 1984; Macnicol & Jacobsen, 2001) and in aerobic metabolism in pollen (Bucher *et al.*, 1995). Furthermore, ADH was found to hold an important role in the production of aromatic volatiles (reviewed by Strommer, 2011). Recently, a role of ADH in course of plant-pathogen interactions is described (Wildermuth, 2010; Pathuri *et al.*, 2011), highlighting the diverse functions of ADH in plant physiology.

In plants it is a common theme that genes are organized in small gene families, which comprise several members with distinct functions. In most plants the ADH gene family consists of two or three ADH genes (Strommer, 2011), members of the medium-length dehydrogenase/reductase superfamily. The barley ADH gene family consists of three members, ADH1, ADH2 and ADH3 (Genebank accession X07774.1, X12733.1 and X12734.1, respectively) (Harberd & Edwards, 1983; Hanson & Brown, 1984; Trick *et al.*, 1988). Compared to horse liver ADH (Genebank accession NP_001075414.1), the "type specimen" of alcohol dehydrogenases, the sequence identity on the amino acid level is 50% for HvADH1, 49% for HvADH2 and 51% for HvADH3. Plant ADHs are active as dimers and all six combinations of homo- and heterodimers have been shown for barley ADHs (Hanson & Brown, 1984; Hanson *et al.*, 1984). ADH1 is expressed in different tissues and amounts to almost all of the activity detected during aerobic growth, whereas expression of ADH2 and ADH3 requires hypoxic induction (Good & Crosby, 1989; Hanson & Brown, 1984; Hanson *et al.*, 1984). Interestingly, ADH2 is strongly induced in course of pathogen attack (Proels *et al.*, 2011).

In this article we describe basic protein-based methods used to analyze ADH in barley. Methods described are crude protein extraction from different plant organs, photometric ADH activity assays, isozyme separation by native-poly-acrylamide gel electrophoresis (PAGE) and histochemical ADH staining. Described methods allow for characterization of plant ADHs in different plant tissues, as an example of cytosolic plant proteins. Background information is provided on how to optimize and troubleshoot the methods.

2   Crude Protein Extraction

ADH is a cytosolic protein, which allows for a straight forward crude protein extraction method. Therefore, plant tissue was harvested, immediately frozen in liquid nitrogen and stored at -80°C prior further analysis. Using a mortar and pistil the plant tissue was ground to a fine powder in presence of liquid nitrogen. At this stage it is important to ensure proper homogenization of the material, in particular root tissue requires more time of grinding to reach homogenization. It is recommended to aliquot appropriate amounts, here 500 μl of homogenized material in 2 ml reaction tubes, for subsequent protein extraction. The reaction tubes have to be pre-cooled in liquid nitrogen to avoid thawing of the tissue powder. Ground material can be kept for further analysis at -80°C. To start the extraction, 400 μl of ice-cold breakage buffer containing 50 mM HEPES pH 7.5, 15% (v/v) glycerol, 1 mM EDTA, 3 mM MgCl$_2$, 10 mM Dithiotreitol (DTT) and 2 mM PMSF was added to the tissue powder. The reaction tube was vortexed vigorously till all the material was solubilized. Hereby the breakage buffer might initially freeze as the ground material is pre-cooled in liquid nitrogen. Samples were kept on ice and were repeatedly vortexed for 3 seconds with 1 min intervals till all samples were extracted. It is recommended to process a maximum of 30 samples per analysis, in order to keep overall processing time short. Samples were centrifuged at 13000 rpm and 4 °C for 10 min and the supernatant was transferred to a new reaction tube. This centrifugation step was repeated at least one more time, till the supernatant was clear and all debris were removed. This crude protein extract was used to determine enzymatic ADH activity and perform native-PAGE, as detailed below. First, the protein amount in the crude extract was determined according to Bradford (1976). Therefore, 2 μl (leaf samples) to 10 μl (root samples) of crude extract were supplied in corresponding wells of a 96-well-plate (Elisa-Plate, 96K, F-form; Greiner, Solingen, Germany) and Bradford solution (BioRad Protein Assay, diluted 1:4 with distilled water according to the manufacturer`s instructions; BioRad, München, Germany) was added to yield a total volume of 200 μl. For better accuracy the mean of two to three technical replications for each sample was used. Total protein amounts were determined according to the Bovine serum albumin (BSA) standard curve with an increasing amount of 0, 1, 2, 4, 6 μg BSA protein. Right after addition of Bradford solution to BSA standards and samples the absorbance was measured in a multi titer spectrophotometer (Infinite M200, Tecan, Crailsheim, Germany) at 595 nm.

Crude protein extracts were attained from different tissues of 3-week-old soil-grown barley plants (Figure 1A). Different plant tissues result in greatly varied protein amounts in the crude extract. As shown in one representative experiment (Figure 1B), the protein concentration in root extracts amounts to 0.3 μg/μl and in stem tissue to 1.2 μg/μl. The highest amount of protein was achieved in leaf tissues (4.5 μg/μl). To modify the protein concentration in the crude extract, the ratio of ground material to extraction buffer can be varied. There are limitations however, as a certain minimum volume of buffer is required to solubilize the tissue powder.

Background information: Crude extracts from plant tissues may contain considerable amounts of sugars and/or other metabolites, which might interfere with activity assays. These compounds can be removed from the extract by dialysis. Therefore, dialysis tubes (Visking dialysis tubing 8/32, SERVA, Heidelberg, Germany) are supplied with 500 μl protein extracts and up to 12 samples are dialyzed in 2 liters of dialysis buffer (12.5 mM potassium phosphate pH 7.5, 10% (v/v) glycerol, 125 μM DTT). It is important to pre-cool the dialysis buffer to 4 °C before adding the samples. Samples are dialyzed at 4 °C for 20 h with permanent stirring.

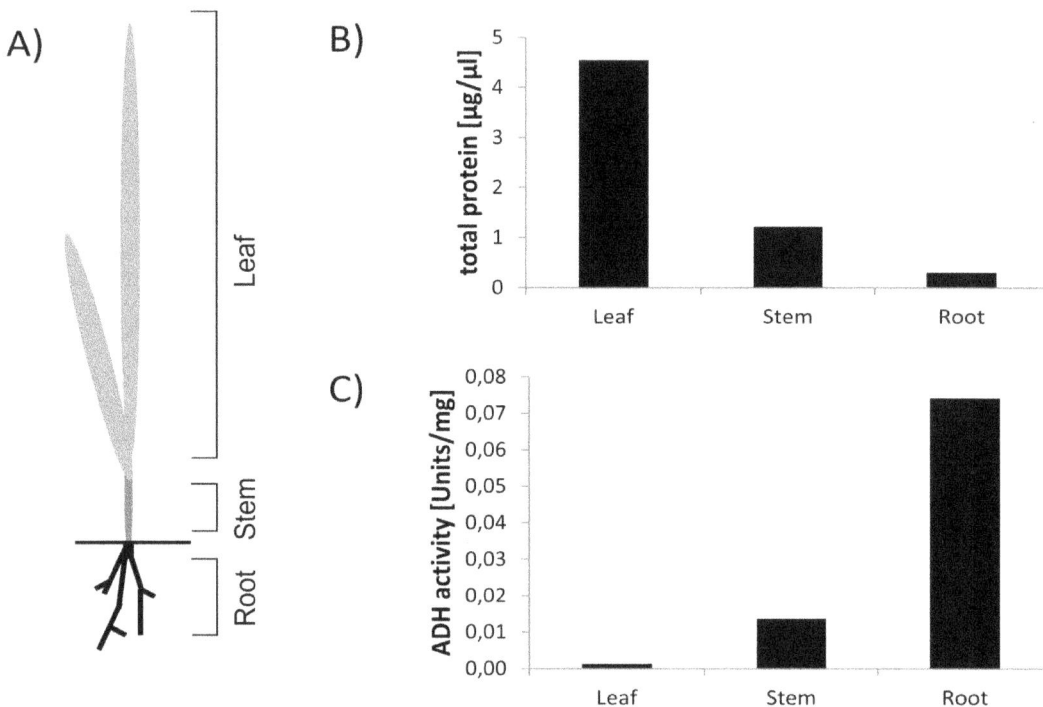

Figure 1: ADH activity recovered from different barley tissues. (A) Scheme of different barley tissues used for the analysis. (B) Different tissues of 3-week-old barley plants (cultivar "Golden Promise") were harvested and ground in presence of liquid nitrogen to a fine powder. Soluble proteins were isolated from 500 μl of ground tissue. Therefore, 400 μl of ice-cold breakage buffer (50 mM HEPES pH 7.5, 15% (v/v) glycerol, 1 mM EDTA, 3 mM $MgCl_2$, 1 mM DTT, 2 mM PMSF) was added to the tissue powder and the samples were vortexed vigorously till all material was solubilized. The debris was removed by centrifugation at 13000 rpm and 4 °C for 10 min. The total protein amount of the crude extracts was determined using the Bradford method. Leaves show the highest amount of soluble protein in the extracts. Compared to leaf samples the concentration of total protein in stem and root samples is 4 or 15 time less, respectively. (C) Specific ADH activity in crude protein extracts was measured by photometric assays. Therefore, 5 μg (root samples) to up to 300 μg (leaf samples) of total protein were supplied with the assay solution (50 mM sodium phosphate buffer pH 8.0, 300 μM NAD^+, 150 mM ethanol) in a total volume of 1 ml. The reaction was followed by measuring the increase in absorbance at 340 nm using a spectrophotometer. The specific ADH activity was calculated as Units/mg protein, that is, μmol NADH formed per min and mg total protein, with an extinction coefficient for NADH of $\varepsilon = 6200 \ l*mol^{-1}*cm^{-1}$. Specific ADH activity in leaves is close to detection limit. Stems show about 10 times and roots more than 50 times higher specific ADH activity compared to leaves.

3   Photometric ADH Activity Assay

To quantify the ADH activity in crude protein extracts, the conversion of ethanol to acetaldehyde and the simultaneous reduction of NAD^+ to NADH were followed by photometric measurements at 340 nm. The assay solution contained 50 mM sodium phosphate pH 8.0, 300 μM NAD^+ and 150 mM ethanol. For the measurement different volumes of crude extract were used depending on the ADH activity to ensure that the initial linear increase in absorption could be evaluated. Thereby, the range of total protein in the assay varied between 150 - 300 μg in leaf samples and 5 - 20 μg in root samples. Corresponding volumes of crude extract were provided in a 1 ml cuvette and a premix of the assay solution was added to yield a total volume of 1 ml. Samples were quickly mixed and the kinetics of the increase in absorbance at 340 nm was measured in a spectrophotometer (UVIKON Spectrophotometer 922 A, Kontron Instruments, UK). The specific ADH activity was calculated as Units/mg protein, that is, μmol NADH formed per min and mg total protein, with an extinction coefficient for NADH of $\varepsilon = 6200$ l*mol^{-1}*cm^{-1}. For high throughput analysis, the assay can be scaled down and performed in 96-well-plates in a total volume of 200 μl using a multi titer spectrophotometer. However, in non-induced leaf samples the ADH activity is too low to be detected in this experimental setup. The reason is probably the smaller light path, which is 1 cm for the cuvettes, but just 0.6 cm in the titer plates, which results in a lower sensitivity.

As shown in Figure 1C, the specific ADH activity of crude protein extracts from different plant tissues (Figure 1B) varies considerably. Roots have a very high specific activity of 0.074 U/mg. Compared to that, stems have about five times less activity (0.014 U/mg). In leaf tissues the ADH activity is very low, more than 50 times less compared to roots, and with 0.001 U/mg it is close to the detection limit.

Background information: ADH activity may also be measured in the reverse direction, that is, the reduction of acetaldehyde to ethanol, with the concomitant oxidation of NADH to NAD$^+$. Substrate concentrations are 0.9 mM NADH and 5 mM acetaldehyde in 85 mM MES pH 6.5 (Kato-Noguchi, 2000). However, there is substantial unspecific background activity for NADH oxidation in plant extracts and proper controls have to be included.

To analyze the effect of metabolites or inhibitors on ADH activity the use of young seedlings grown on agar plates or hydroponically grown seedlings have been reported. In those systems inhibitors, hormones or sugars can easily be applied by adding those substances into the agar or growth medium. In 7-day-old Arabidopsis seedlings Baxter-Burrell *et al*. (2002) showed the impact of inhibitors on ADH activity. Pathuri *et al*. (2011) analyzed how exogenously applied sucrose to hydroponically grown barley seedlings effect ADH activity. Kato-Noguchi (2000) treated 6-day-old alfalfa seedlings with plant hormones and observed an induction of ADH activity with distinct hormone treatments.

4   ADH Isozyme Separation by Native-PAGE

The ADH gene family in barley comprises three members, *HvADH1*, *HvADH2* und *HvADH3* with distinct functions, as outlined in the introduction. Moreover, plant ADHs are active as dimers and all six combinations of homo- und heterodimers have been shown to be active in barley (isozyme identification according to Good & Crosby (1989) and references therein). Therefore, to analyze particular functions of the different isozymes it is indispensable to separate and detect the corresponding isoforms. One straight forward method to achieve this goal is native-PAGE and subsequent in-gel activity staining. To minimize work load it is recommended to run native-PAGE gels from the same extracts as used for photometric activity assays (as described in the previous chapter), in this way, enzyme activity and isozyme composition can be determined from the same samples within one working day. Native gels are prepared essentially as described for lactate dehydrogenase (Hanson & Jacobsen, 1984) with modifications. Native-PAGE can be performed conveniently with standard equipment (Mini-PROTEAN, Bio-Rad, München, Germany) using 1.0 mm thick gels. An effective separation of all six ADH isozyms can be achieved in separating gels with an effective length as small as 6 cm. The components of the running and stacking gel are given in table 1. Gels were cast the day before use and stored at 15 °C to ensure complete polymerization. Prior sample loading, the gels are mounted to the electrophoresis apparatus, the upper and lower tank are filled with pre-cooled running buffer (25 mM Tris pH 8.5, 190 mM glycine) and the gels are pre-run for 30 min at 70 V. In our experience it is sufficient to run the gels in a 4 °C cold room without further cooling of the gel tank, given that the running buffer was pre-cooled to 4 °C. Loading dye (3 % w/v glycerol, 0.003 % w/v bromphenol blue) was added to 150-300 μg of total protein extracts prior sample loading. Gels were run at 75 V for 1 h and then the voltage was increased to 90 V for further 4 h. Following electrophoresis, the stacking gel was disposed and the separating gel was stained for ADH activity (stain solution according Brown et al., 1978, with modifications). Therefore, 10 ml of stain solution (Table 1), without phenazine methosulfate (PMS) added, was supplied in glass-petri dishes of 9 cm diameter and the gel was floated in the stain solution with gentle shaking at 20 rpm on a rotary shaker for 5 min. Then 10 μl of PMS (5 mg/ml) was added, after 5 min of incubation further 10 μl of PMS (5 mg/ml) was added to reach a final concentration of 0.01 mg/ml PMS in the stain solution. Staining proceeded for a total of 30 min. Thereby, the reduction of the nitro blue tetrazolium (NBT) results in the formation of the insoluble and deep blue colored NBT-formazan. For flooding induced samples bands appeared after a few minutes of staining, non-induced leaf-samples required much longer incubation times of up to 30 min till visible bands appeared. The staining was stopped by replacing the stain solution with distilled water. The gels can be stored for some days at 4 °C in water till evaluation. Gels can be either scanned or photographed for data analysis.

The described method has been applied to study isozyme composition in barley leaves after pathogen attack (Proels et al., 2011). Here, a typical native-PAGE of barley leaf extracts in course of flooding is shown (Figure 2A). Barley plants (cultivar "Golden Promise") were grown for three weeks on soil. Following, control leaf samples (0 h) were harvested and plants were completely submerged in tap water. Leaf samples were harvested after 4 h and 24 h of flooding. Before flooding (0 h) there is very little ADH activity present in the aereated leaf, just a weak band of the ADH1-ADH1 homodimer is detectable. Four hours of flooding does not induced ADH activity, but 24 h of full submergence of barley plants results in a strong induction of ADH1 and ADH2 homo- and heterodimers. To check for the specificity of the staining, the substrate ethanol was omitted from the stain solution. No bands were observed under those conditions. Figure 2B shows the specific ADH activity of corresponding samples with a very low basic level at 0 h and 4 h, but about 7 times induction after 24 h of flooding. As shown in figure 2C, ADH3 and corresponding homo-/ and heterodimers are slightly induced 48 h after flooding of 2-week-old barley plants (cultivar "Ingrid"). ADH3 has been described to be induced only under severe oxygen deprivation (Hanson & Brown, 1984; Good & Crosby, 1989). Longer running times (up to 20 h) at reduced voltage might improve separation of bands. However, in our hands 4 h of electrophoresis were sufficient to separate all six ADH isozymes. In summary, native-PAGE allows for detection of individual homo- und heterodimers of barley ADHs and is a straight forward method to characterize the functions of different isozymes. Based on such data targeted approaches can be performed, e.g. knock down of a specific ADH gene and analyzing its function under particular physiological conditions. Relative quantitation of band intensities in native-gels can be obtained using a high-resolution imaging system and corresponding analysis software. To this end, we applied the Fusion SL imaging system and Fusion-Capt software (Vilber Lourmat, Eberhardzell, Germany). Relative quantitation of isoenzyme-specific band intensities can give clear information on specific ADH isoenzyme functions. A specific ADH isoenzyme function was shown for the role of ADH2 in the interaction of barley with the powdery mildew (Proels et al., 2011). ADH2, which was not expressed in non-infected leaves, was considerably induced six days after infection, other than ADH1, which was expressed constitutively and showed just a moderate induction in response to powdery mildew infection.

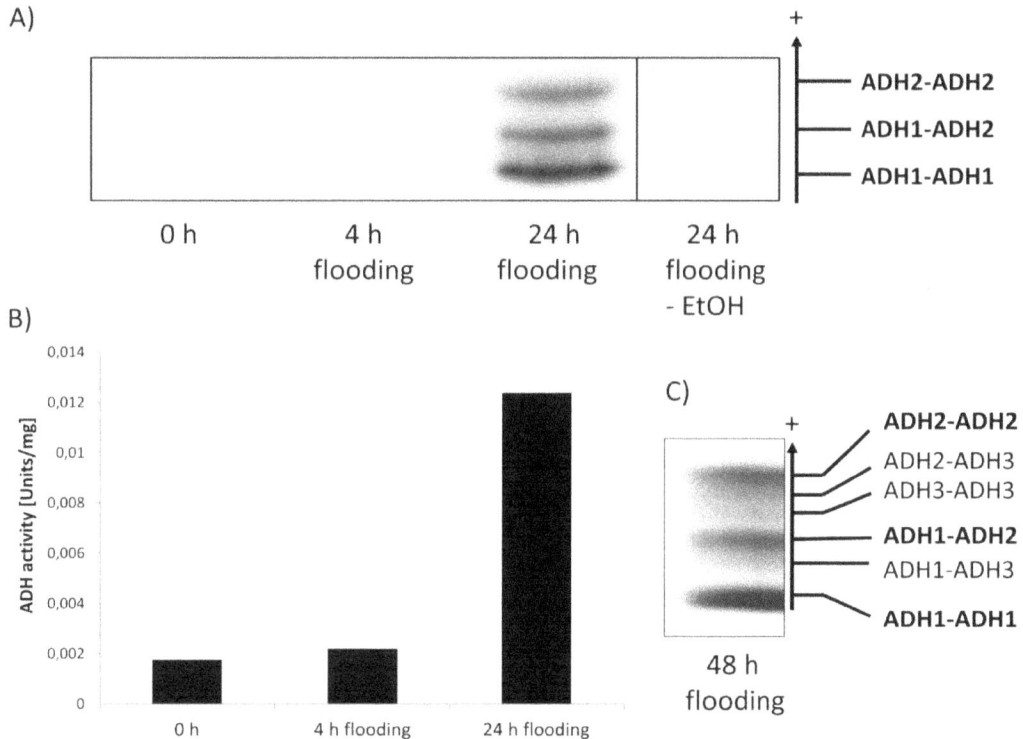

Figure 2: Isozyme composition of barley ADHs in response to flooding. (A) Barley plants (cultivar "Golden Promise") were grown for three weeks on soil. Following, control leaf samples (0 h) were harvested and plants were completely submerged in tap water. Leaf samples were harvested after 4 h and 24 h of flooding. Crude protein extracts were isolated and 300 μg of total protein were separated by native-PAGE (Acrylamide/Bis-acrylamide 7.5 %/ 0.2% (w/v) in the separating gel) at 90 V for 4 h. Following electrophoresis, the separating gel was floated in stain solution (40 mM sodium-phosphate pH 8.0, 400μM NAD$^+$, 100 μM NBT, 0.05 mg/ml PMS, 3 % (v/v) ethanol) at room temperature for up to 40 min. At sites of ADH activity dark NBT-formazane bands appeared. No bands appeared when ethanol was omitted from the stain solution. In the non-induced state and after 4 h of flooding only a very weak band of the ADH1-ADH1 homodimer is detectable. After 24 h of flooding a clear induction of ADH1-ADH1, ADH1-ADH2 and ADH2-ADH2 isozymes can be observed. (B) Specific ADH activity of the same protein extracts as used in (A) was evaluated by photometric assays. In line with the native-PAGE data in A, control leaves and leaves that were flooded for 4 h show a very basal ADH activity, whereas 24 h of flooding induces ADH activity about 7 times compared to non-flooded controls. (C) 2-week-old barley plants (cultivar "Ingrid") were flooded for 48 h and leaf material was harvested. 150 μg of total protein were analyzed for ADH isozyme composition by native-PAGE. After 48 h of flooding all 6 ADH isozymes are detectable. Isozymes containing ADH3 are significantly weaker compared to ADH1 and ADH2 containing isozymes. Isozymes were identified according to Good & Crosby (1989) and references therein.

Background information: To check for equal loading of native gels an aliquot of the extract may be kept to be analyzed by SDS-PAGE.

The separation of isozymes is enhanced when wide combs (1.2 cm pocket width, 5 pockets per gel) are used compared to standard combs (0.5 cm pocket width, 10 pockets per gel). Moreover, the use of wide combs allows for loading up to 100 μl of sample per lane, which is recommended for leaf samples that are characterized by a very low specific ADH activity.

Separating gel	Final concentration
Tris-HCl pH 8.8	380 mM
Acrylamide/Bis-acrylamide	7.5 % / 0.2% (w/v)
Ammonium peroxodisulfate (APS)	0.036 % (w/v)
TEMED	0.08 % (v/v)
Stacking gel	
Tris-HCl pH 6.7	63 mM
Sucrose	20 % (w/v)
Acrylamide/Bis-acrylamide	2.5 % / 0.07% (w/v)
APS	0.036 % (w/v)
TEMED	0.06 % (v/v)
In-gel stain solution	
Na-Phosphate pH 8.0	40 mM
NAD⁺	0.4 mM
NBT	0.1 mM
Phenazine methosulfate	0.01 mg/ml
Ethanol	3 % (v/v)

Table 1: Components of the separating/stacking gel and the in-gel stain solution. If not otherwise indicated chemicals were purchased from Sigma-Aldrich (Hamburg, Germany). Sucrose, ethanol, TEMED, APS and acrylamide (Rotiphorese Gel 30, Acrylamide/Bis-acrylamide 30 %/0.8 % w/v) were purchased from Roth (Karlsruhe, Germany). N,N,N′,N′-tetramethylene ethylene diamine (TEMED).

5   Histochemical ADH Staining

To localize ADH activity within different tissues histochemical staining of ADH activity was performed (essentially as described by Papdi *et al.*, 2008). 3-week-old barley plants (cultivar "Golden Promise") were flooded for 24 h in tap water and root tips were harvested and immediately transferred to the reaction buffer containing 100 mM sodium phosphate pH 8.0, 400 μM NAD⁺, 100 μM NBT and 3% (v/v) ethanol. Samples were incubated at 30 °C for about 15 min in the dark until a dark NBT-formazane stain appeared. Subsequently, the reaction was stopped by removing the reaction buffer and rinsing the samples in distilled water. Pictures were taken immediately thereafter using a digital camera mounted on a stereomicroscope (Stemi 200-C, Zeiss, Germany). A NBT-formazane stain, which is indicative of ADH activity, appeared mostly at the central cylinder starting about 0.5 mm proximal the root tip and reaching up to 5 mm proximal the root tip (Figure 3 A/B). To check for ADH specificity, the substrate ethanol was omitted from the stain solution (Figure 3C). Omitting ethanol prevents staining, except for sites of mechanical wounding (indicated by arrows). In barley seedlings that were germinated on moistened filter-paper (the roots were submerged in tap water) a strong NBT-formazane staining locates over the full length of the roots (Figure 3D). To check for ADH specificity, the substrate ethanol was omitted from the stain solution (Figure 3E). We also tested leaf tissue, however the low ADH activity in leaves did not allow for histochemical ADH staining. Specific signals could be detected only when leaves were flooded for 24 h and the incubation time in the stain solution was raised to several hours (data not shown).

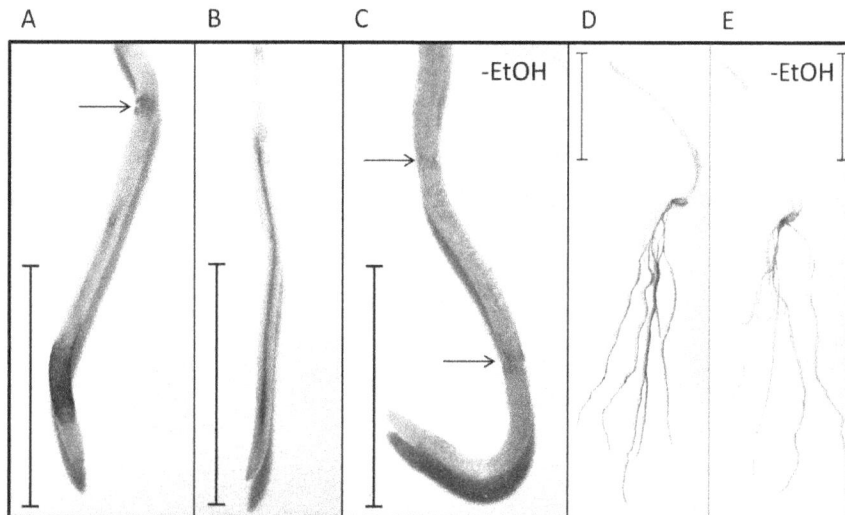

Figure 3: Histochemical ADH staining in barley. (A-C) Barley seedlings (cultivar "Golden Promise") were grown for three weeks on soil. Following, plants were completely submerged in tap water. Roots were harvested after 24 h of flooding and immediately transferred to the reaction buffer (100 mM sodium phosphate pH 8.0, 400 μM NAD$^+$, 100 μM NBT and 3% (v/v) ethanol). Roots were incubated in the reaction solution at 30 °C for about 15 min in the dark until a dark NBT-formazane stain appeared. For controls ethanol was omitted from the stain solution (C, -EtOH). Pictures were taken with a digital camera mounted on a stereomicroscope (Stemi 200-C, Zeiss, Germany). Bars represent 4 mm. Histochemical ADH staining, mostly at the central cylinder, appears about 0.5 mm proximal the root tip reaching up to 5 mm proximal the root tip. At sites of mechanical wounding, indicated by arrows, an unspecific signal can be detected. (D/E) Barley seedlings (cultivar "Golden Promise") were germinated for six days on moistened filter paper in the dark. Following, histochemical ADH staining was performed with whole seedlings (D). For control ethanol was omitted from the stain solution (E, -EtOH). After staining seedlings were rinsed with tap water and pictures were taken with a digital camera. Bars represent 5 cm. Dark NBT-formazane staining, indicating ADH activity, locates over the full length of the roots.

Background information: The strong unspecific signals at the wounding sites (Figure 3A/C, indicated by arrows) probably result from the release of reactive oxygen species. When leaves were stained for ADH activity, we observed a very strong unspecific signal along the cutting edge, reaching about 1 mm inwards (data not shown). Therefore, special care has to be taken to avoid wounding or application of mechanical stress to the tissue to be analyzed. Previously, histochemical ADH staining was successfully applied to maize pollen (Freeling, 1976).

6   Conclusions

Here basic protein-based methods for the analysis of ADH in barley are presented. The described methods comprise protein extraction from different tissues, photometric ADH assays, native-PAGE and histochemical ADH staining. These straight forward methods can be applied to analyze overall ADH activity in crude protein extracts, isozyme composition and histochemical localization within one working day. Isozyme separation via native-PAGE is of particular interest as with the help of this method certain isozymes can be linked to particular physiological functions. These protein-based methods can be complemented by analyzing the gene expression patterns of corresponding ADH genes. In a following step, certain ADH genes may be knocked down thereby modulating specific isozyme functions.

Acknowledgement

The authors are grateful to Angelika Muhr for excellent technical assistance.

References

Bailey-Serres, J. & Voesenek, L.A.C.J. (2008). Flooding Stress: Acclimations and Genetic Diversity. Annual Review of Plant Biology, 59, 313-339.

Baxter-Burrell, A., Yang, Z., Springer, P.S., Bailey-Serres, J. (2002). ROPGAP4-dependent Rop GTPase rheostat controls of Arabidopsis oxygen deprivation tolerance. Science, 296, 2026–2028.

Bradford, M.M. (1976). A rapid and sensitive method for the quantitation of microgram quantities of protein utilizing the principle of protein-dye binding. Analytical Biochemistry, 72, 248-254.

Brown, A.H.D., Nevo, E., Zohary, D., Dagan, O. (1978). Genetic variation in natural populations of wild barley (Hordeum spontaneum). Genetica, 49, 97-108.

Bucher, M., Brander, K.A., Sbicego, S., Mandel, T., Kuhlemeier, C. (1995). Aerobic fermentation in tobacco pollen. Plant Molecular Biology, 28, 739–750.

Freeling, M. (1976). Intragenic recombination in maize: Pollen analysis methods and the effect of parental Adh1+ Isolates. Genetics, 83, 701-717.

Fukao, T. & Bailey-Serres, J. (2004). Plant responses to hypoxia – is survival a balancing act? Trends in Plant Science, 9, 449-456.

Good, A.G. & Crosby, W.L. (1989). Induction of alcohol dehydrogenase and lactate dehydrogenase in hypoxically induced barley. Plant Physiology, 90, 860-866.

Hanson, A.D. & Brown, A.H.D. (1984). Three alcohol dehydrogenase genes in wild and cultivated barley: Characterization of the products of variant alleles. Biochemical Genetics, 22, 495-515.

Hanson, A.D. & Jacobsen, J.V. (1984). Control of lactate dehydrogenase, lactate glycolysis and a-amylase by O2 deficit in barley aleurone layers. Plant Physiology, 75, 566-572.

Hanson, A.D., Jacobsen, J.V., Zwar, J.A. (1984). Regulated expression of three alcohol dehydrogenase genes in barley aleurone layers. Plant Physiology, 75, 573-581.

Harberd, N.P. & Edwards, K.J.R. (1983). Further studies on the alcohol dehydrogenases of barley: evidence for a third alcohol dehydrogenase locus and data on the effect of an alcohol dehydrogenase-1 null mutation in homozygous and in heterozygous condition. Genetics Research, 41, 109-116.

Kato-Noguchi, H. (2000). Induction of alcohol dehydrogenase by plant hormones in alfalfa seedlings. Plant Growth Regulation, 30, 1-3.

Kennedy, R.A., Rumpho, M.E., Fox, T.C. (1992). Anaerobic metabolism in plants. Plant Physiology, 100, 1-6.

Macnicol, P.K. & Jacobsen, J.V. (2001). Regulation of alcohol dehydrogenase gene expression in barley aleurone by gibberellin and abscisic acid. Physiologia Plantarum, 111, 533-539.

Papdi, C., Abraham, E., Joseph, M.P., Popescu, C., Koncz, C., Szabados, L. (2008). Functional identification of Arabidopsis stress regulated genes using the controlled cDNA overexpression system. Plant Physiology, 147, 528-542.

Pathuri, I.P., Reitberger, I.E., Hückelhoven, R., Proels, R.K. (2011). Alcohol dehydrogenase 1 of barley modulates susceptibility to the parasitic fungus Blumeria graminis f.sp. hordei. Journal of Experimental Botany, 62, 3449-3457.

Proels, R.K., Westermeier, W., Hückelhoven, R. (2011). Infection of barley with the parasitic fungus Blumeria graminis f.sp. hordei results in the induction of HvADH1 and HvADH2. Plant Signaling and Behavior, 6, 1584-1587.

Strommer, J. (2011). The plant ADH gene family. The Plant Journal, 66, 128-142.

Trick, M., Dennis, E.S., Edwards, K.J.R., Peacock, W.J. (1988). Molecular analysis of the alcohol dehydrogenase gene family of barley. Plant Molecular Biology, 11, 147-60.

Wildermuth, M.C. (2010). Modulation of host nuclear ploidy: a common plant biotroph mechanism. Current Opinion in Plant Biology, 13, 1-10.

Production, Purification and Biochemical Analyses of Recombinant Cell-Wall-Degrading Enzymes

Takumi Takeda

Iwate Biotechnology Research Center, Japan

1   Introduction

Growing cells of plants are surrounded by primary cell walls that are composed of   polysaccharides, cellulose, hemicelluloses and pectins, and a small quantity of proteins. Cellulose is a linear polymer of β-1,4-linked glucose residues that form into bundles of cellulose fibers, called cellulose microfibrils. Hemicellulosic polysaccharides, xyloglucan in dicotyledonous plants and 1,3-1,4-β-glucan and xylan in monocotyledonous plants, are embedded and bound to the cellulose microfibrils by hydrogen bonds, resulting in the formation of tethers between cellulose microfibrils (Hayashi, 1989; Carpita & Gibeaut, 1993). Pectins such as rhamnogalacturonan are embedded in cell walls and the interface between cells. Such structural polysaccharides give rigidity and flexibility to the cell walls. During cell growth, the tethers formed by the hemicellulosic polysaccharides between the cellulose microfibrils are cleaved by enzymatic actions, leading to the loosening of the cell wall and a decrease in physical strength. Enzymes that degrade hemicellulosic polysaccharides such as xyloglucan endotransglucosylases, endo-1,4-β-glucanases, 1,3-1,4-β-glucanases and endoxylanases are thought to induce cell wall loosening by cleaving the hemicellulosic tethers (Hayashi, 1989; Takeda *et al.*, 2002). In addition, expansins, cell-wall associated proteins, are believed to loosen the wall by cleaving the hydrogen bonds formed between hemicellulosic polysaccharides and cellulose microfibrils (Cosgrove, 2000). Simultaneously, cells take up water, thereby enlarging the cells. After cell expansion ceases, polysaccharide and lignin polymers comprising the secondary wall are synthesized to increase the physical strength of the cell wall. Furthermore, cleavage of polysaccharides in the abscission layers releases leaves from the plant body, and degradation of pectic polysaccharides softens plant fruits. Thus, wall degradation and synthesis determine cell strength and cell shape.

Plant cell walls also play a significant role as a physical barrier to plant-pathogens; however, plant-pathogens secrete a battery of cell-wall-degrading enzymes (CWDEs) to break the wall barrier, which enhances pathogen invasion and nutrient acquisition. Against pathogen attack, plants secrete enzymes that can hydrolyze pathogen cell walls. For example, plants produce chitinases to hydrolyze chitin, a long-chain polymer of *N*-acetylglucosamine and a characteristic component of fungal, but not plant, cell walls (Kasprzewska, 2003).

Studies of plant cell wall degradation by fungal enzymes will enhance our fundamental knowledge of naturally occurring plant-microbe interactions and novel modifications of wall polysaccharides. In this chapter, the production of fungal CWDEs identified from genomic DNA databases and their purification and biochemical characterization are described.

2   *In silico* Identification of Fungal CWDEs from Genomic DNA Databases

Recent research has focused on the elucidation of genomic DNA sequences of various species including animals, plants and microbes, which will contribute to genetic healing, increases in crop yields, fermentation, production of valuable substances and many other proposed benefits. The amount of data in fungal DNA databases is increasing, but the databases are sufficiently detailed at present to be utilized. DNA and amino acid sequences of CWDEs are extractable from published genomic DNA sequences by *in silico* comparisons with identified DNA and amino acid sequences. The protein databases associated with cell wall modification, glycoside hydrolases (GHs), glycosyl transferases (GTs), polysaccharide lyases

(PLs) and carbohydrate esterases (CEs), are organized and can be accessed at the Carbohydrate-Active Enzymes database (CAZY) website (http://www.cazy.org/). Out of more than 100,000 non-redundant entries in the database, GHs are at present classified into 133 families based on amino acid similarity (Henrissat & Davies, 1997).

    Magnaporthe oryzae is the pathogen that causes rice blast, the most devastating fungal disease of rice. The complete genomic DNA sequences of *Magnaporthe grisea* and *M. oryzae* have been published (Dean *et al.*, 2004; Yoshida *et al.*, 2008). To investigate the significance of rice cell wall degradation by the *M. oryzae* enzymes during infection, biochemical analyses of native or recombinant CWDEs are needed. To produce recombinant proteins, DNAs encoding CWDEs are amplified by polymerase chain reaction (PCR) using DNA polymerase, dNTPs as substrates and DNA primers designed from the genomic DNA sequence. Amplified DNAs are cloned into plasmid vectors suitable for protein expression and transformed into host cells (Figure 1A). For protein expression, addition of DNA sequences encoding a secretion signal peptide and an epitope-tag peptide such as polyhistidine-tag (Figure 1B), human influenza hemagglutinin (HA)-tag, c-Myc-tag or FLAG-tag, enables proteins to be secreted extracellularly and easily purified. The production, purification and characterization of the *M. oryzae* recombinant CWDEs are described in more detail in the following sections.

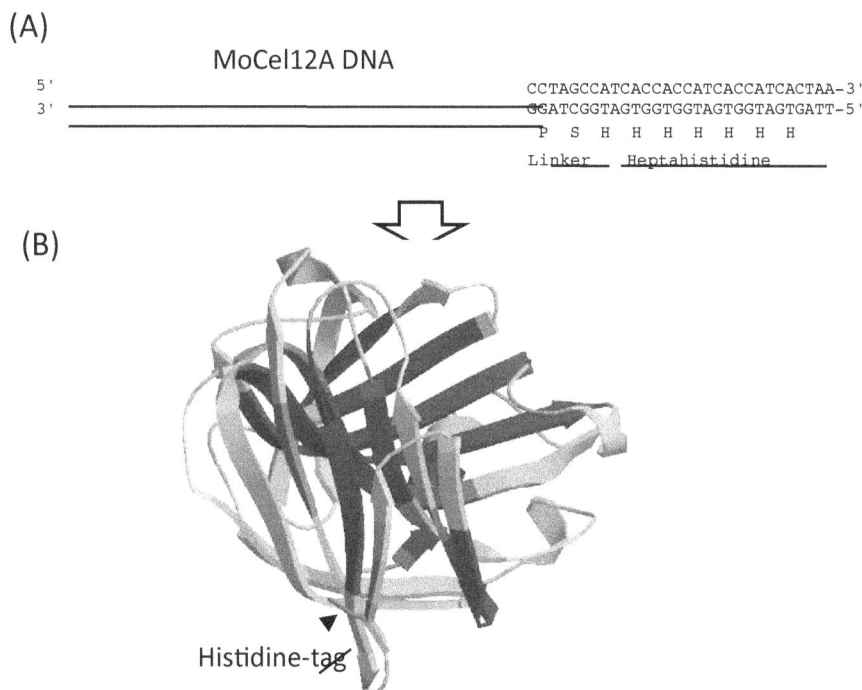

Figure 1: Production of recombinant MoCel12A. A gene for MoCel12A is obtained by PCR and fused with heptahistidine-tag sequence (A). A protein encoded by the gene with the heptahistidine-tag is produced in host cells and purified by polyhistidine affinity chromatography (B). A three-dimensional structure of MoCel12A was constructed by the Swiss-Model Program at http://swissmodel.expasy.org.

3   Production of Recombinant CWDEs

Productivity of recombinant proteins depends on the host cells, culture medium and culture conditions. Experiments determining the growth period, the levels of protein accumulation and enzymatic activity must be carried out. The principal CWDE of *M. oryzae* is a cellulase (MoCel12A) belonging to the GH 12 family (MoCel12A). A gene encoding MoCel12A was fused with a heptahistidine-tag for easy detection and purification and was expressed in *Brevibacillus choshinensis*. The protein was secreted into the culture medium and accumulated during growth as judged by immunoblotting using an antibody against the polyhistidine-tag (Figure 2A). Hydrolytic activity towards 1,3-1,4-β-glucan was determined by measuring the increase in reducing ends that were generated by cleavage of carbohydrate chains using *p*-hydroxybenzoic hydrazide-HCl (PAHBAH method, Lever, 1972). The activity of MoCel12A towards 1,3-1,4-β-glucan increased during growth of the culture (Figure 2B). Thus, enzymatically-active recombinant MoCel12A was produced and could be used for biochemical analyses.

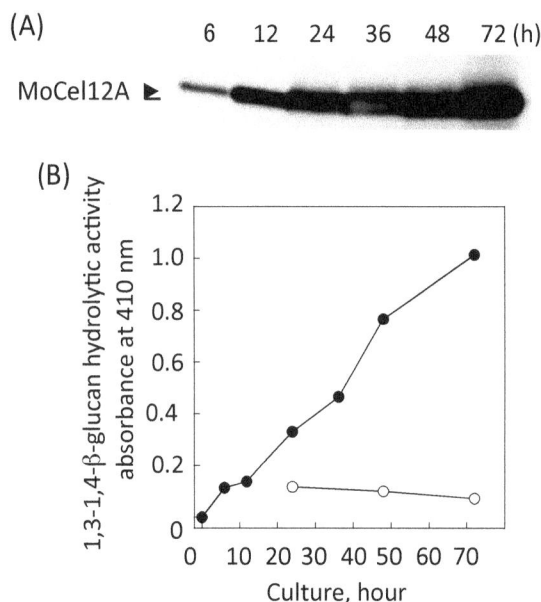

Figure 2: Expression of MoCel12A in *B. choshinensis*. A gene encoding MoCel12A with a heptahistidine-tag was cloned into an expression vector (pNCMO2) and transformed into *B. choshinensis*. A transformed cell was cultured at 30 °C for 6-72 h with vigorous shaking. Culture filtrates were subjected to SDS-PAGE and immunoblotting using an anti-polyhistidine as the primary antibody (A). Hydrolytic activity of the culture filtrates towards 1,3-1,4-β-glucan was determined by the PAHBAH method after incubation at 40 °C for 1 h (B).

4   Purification of His-tagged CWDEs

Heptahistidine-tagged *M. oryzae* enzymes, 1,3-1,4-β-glucanase (MoCel12A) from *B. choshinensis*, cellobiohydrolase (MoCel6A) from *Aspergillus oryzae* and two β-glucosidases (MoCel3A and MoCel3B) from *M. oryzae* were expressed as described above. Recombinant proteins should be purified before determining their enzymatic properties so as to remove the effects of contaminant proteins. Enzymes secreted to the culture medium were concentrated by ultrafiltration and applied to a polyhistidine-binding resin in order to obtain purified proteins. The resin contains bound cobalt ions that can bind to contiguous histidine residues. Therefore, the histidine-tagged enzymes bind to the resin. After the resin was washed to remove unbound and non-specifically bound proteins, the bound enzymes were eluted with an imidazol solution that displaces the enzymes bound to the resin. Purity of the eluates was judged by Coomassie Brilliant Blue (CBB) staining after separation by sodium dodecyl sulfate-polyacrylamide gel electerophoresis (SDS-PAGE). Using this method of purification, MoCel12A, MoCel6A, MoCel3A and MoCel3B were purified to electrophoretic homogeneity (Fig. 3). Thus, affinity chromatography using a polyhistidine-tag is an advantageous method to obtain highly purified proteins quickly.

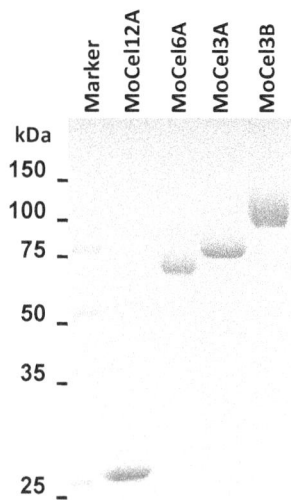

Figure 3: Visualization of purified proteins. Recombinant proteins, MoCel12A expressed in *B. choshinensis*, MoCel6A expressed in *A. oryzae*, MoCel3A and MoCel3B expressed in *M. oryzae*, were purified by polyhistidine affinity chromatography and subjected to SDS-PAGE followed by CBB staining.

5   Functional analyses of CWDEs

5.1   GH12 Family Enzymes Hydrolyzing Polysaccharides

In order to determine the proposed functions of hydrolytic enzymes in cell wall degradation, in physiological changes and as reagents for modifying cell-wall polymers, the enzymes must be characterized in detail. The GH12 family is a group of enzymes that degrade β-1,4-linked glucans such as cellulose, 1,3-1,4-β-glucan, xyloglucan and chemically modified carboxymethyl cellulose. MoCel12A preferentially hydrolyzes 1,3-1,4-β-glucan (Takeda *et al.*, 2010). Similarly, a *Cochliobolus carbonum* enzyme in the GH12 family also exhibited specific 1,3-1,4-β-glucan hydrolysis (Kim *et al.*, 2001). On the other hand, an *Aspergillus aculeatus* enzyme showed specificity toward xyloglucan hydrolysis (Pauly *et al.*, 1999). Hemicellulosic polysaccharides, 1,3-1,4-β-glucan and xyloglucan, are thought to play an important role in controlling plant cell wall strength by tethering cellulose microfibrils. These enzymes may function to loosen the cell wall by cleaving hemicellulosic tethers, thereby enhancing fungal invasion. Enzymes from *Trichoderma reesei* and *A. oryzae* and *Humicola insolence* hydrolyze a wide range of β-1,4-glucans such as crystalline cellulose, phosphoric acid swollen-cellulose, 1,3-1,4-β-glucan and carboxymethyl cellulose (Schülein, 1997; Takeda, 2012). Such fungal enzymes are proposed to degrade β-1,4-glucans randomly to acquire carbon sources for the fungus. Thus, the modes of action for enzymes can be predicted based on amino acid sequence similarity, but real action is defined based on the results from enzymatic analyses.

5.2   GH6 Family Enzymes Producing Oligosaccharides

Cellobiohydrolase II, belonging to the GH6 family, generates cellobiose by cleaving 1,4-β-linked cellulose derivatives. MoCel6A produced cellobiose from phosphoric acid swollen-cellulose and crystalline cellulose, and diverse oligosaccharides from 1,3-1,4-β-glucan as judged by HPLC analysis (Figure 4). CWDEs appear to be inhibited by their reaction products. For example, cellobiohydrolase I belonging to the GH7 family and β-glucosidases belonging to the GH1 and GH3 families are inhibited by the presence of cellobiose and glucose, respectively (Gruno *et al.*, 2004; Riou *et al.*, 1998; Takahashi *et al.*, 2010). These findings suggest that these enzymes have an affinity for their reaction products and are unable to proceed to the next reaction. As a result, the generation of reaction products is delayed. In contrast, the activity of MoCel6A was not inhibited, but rather enhanced, by the presence of cellobiose, a reaction product generated by MoCel6A. MoCel6A has 6 substitutions in 26 highly conserved amino acids among the GH6 family of cellobiohydrolases. Some of these substitutions might cause the enhanced activity by cellobiose.

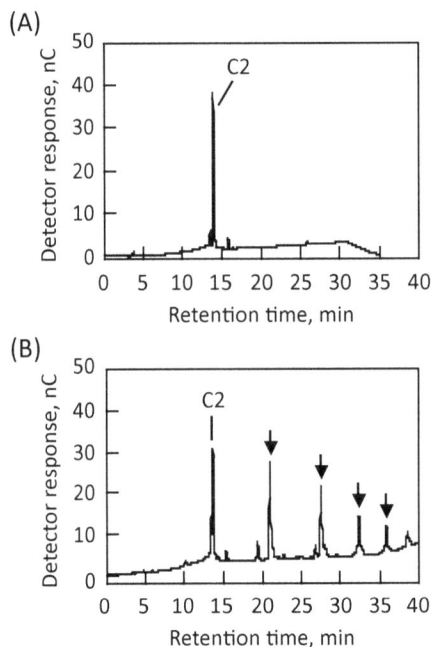

Figure 4: Product analyses by HPLC after digestion with MoCel6A. Phosphoric acidswollen-cellulose (A) and 1,3-1,4-β-glucan (B) were treated with MoCel6A at 40 °C overnight with vigorous agitation, and the mixture was analyzed by HPLC. C2 indicates the position where cellobiose eluted in this system. Arrows represent unidentified oligosaccharides.

Amino acid alteration by gene mutation is an important method for investigating the significance of individual amino acids for enzyme activity and for potentially increasing the activities. MoCel6A has substitutions at highly conserved amino acids that may have developed evolutionarily to degrade β-1,4-glucans.

5.3   GH3 Family Enzymes Producing Glucose

Glucose is an important carbon source that generates energy in living cells. Several wall polysaccharides, cellulose, 1,3-1,4-β-glucan, xyloglucan and β-1,3-glucan (called callose), contain a glucosyl backbone. Complete hydrolysis of such polysaccharides causes the production of glucose residues. Endoglucanase and cellobiohydrolase catalyze the depolymerization and oligomerization of polysaccharides, whereas β-glucosidase releases glucose residue from oligosaccharides. The activity of β-glucosidases can be determined colorimetrically using glucose oxidase. β-Glucosidases from *M. oryzae*, MoCel3A and MoCel3B were produced by overexpression in *M. oryzae* (Takahashi *et al.*, 2011). MoCel3A produced glucose from oligosaccharides linked by a β-1,4 bond (cellooligosaccharides), oligosaccharides linked by a β-1,3 bond (laminarioligosaccharides) and laminarin, a β-1,3-linked polymer. The results indicate that MoCel3A is significantly involved in glucose production from β-1,4- and β-1,3-linked polysaccharides. On the other hand, MoCel3B liberated glucose mainly from cellooligosaccharides. These two β-glucosidases are grouped into the GH3 family but their enzymatic properties are significantly diverse. Thus, β-glucosidases function in the final step to produce glucose from plant cell wall components. Although classification and amino acid similarity help predict the enzymatic functions, the precise knowledge of the enzymatic properties is gained only by detailed biochemical analyses.

6   Application of CWDEs

Plant-derived polysaccharides are used as structural materials, pulp, textile, and in many other commercial and industrial applications. Recent attention has been focused on converting polysaccharides into precious substances such as ethanol as an alternative to gasoline or nanofibers to increase the strength of cellulose-containing materials. A combination of CWDEs will enable the efficient production of glucose from cell wall polysaccharides. Cellulose, a major component of plant cell walls and the most abundant biopolymer on earth, is degraded into glucose by three steps: i) depolymerizatin by endoglucanases, ii) oligomerization by endoglucanases and cellobiohydrolases, and iii) monomerization by β-glucosidases. To efficiently produce glucose from polysaccharides, exploitation of enzymes with high activity and increases in enzyme productivity are required using biotechnological techniques. Selecting enzymes with high activity based on biochemical analyses is fundamentally important. The alteration of amino acids in enzymes, either by site-directed or random mutagenesis offers the possibility of improving enzymatic activity. Introduction of a foreign gene encoding a CWDE or a transcription factor to enhance transcript levels of CWDEs causes higher production of CWDEs in host cells.

Trichoderma reesei is a fungus that produces a high level of CWDEs extracellularly. Repeated mutagenesis and screening of *T. reesei* lines with high activity for a long period led to the selection of a line that produced high levels of CWDEs. In general, however, the *Trichoderma reesei* enzyme preparations have a relatively low ability to produce glucose due to their low level of β-glucosidase activity. Therefore, β-glucosidase activity must be reinforced to increase glucose production from cell wall polysaccharides. MoCel3A, an enzyme that releases glucose from β-1,3- and β-1,4-linked oligosaccharides, was expressed in *T. reesei* under the control of the cellobiohydrolase I (*cbh I*) promoter (Figure 5A). Expressed MoCel3A was secreted into the culture medium by the addition of cellulose, cellooligosaccharides and laminarioligosaccharides because the *cbh I* promoter was activated by these additives. The amount of glucose produced from phosphoric acid swollen-cellulose by the enzyme preparation from the *T. reesei* transformant overexpressing MoCel3A was greater than that by the enzyme preparation from *T. reesei* wild type (Figure 5B and C). Conversely, the level of accumulated cellobiose decreased using the enzyme preparation from the *T. reesei* transfomant. This result implies that the enhanced glucose production resulting from the introduction of the MoCel3A gene facilitates conversion of cellobiose into glucose.

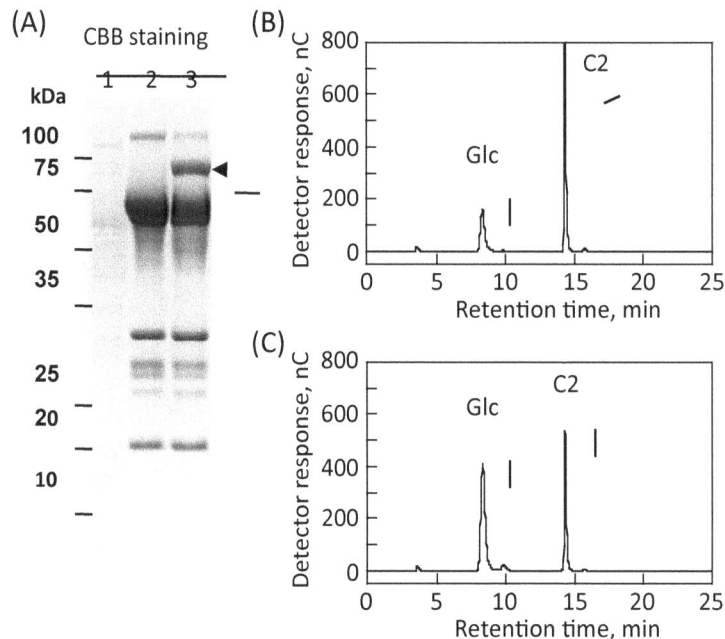

Figure 5: Production of MoCel3A in *T. reesei* and enhanced glucose production. *T. reesei* wild type was cultured for 3 days (1) and further cultured in the presence (2) or absence (3) of cellulose powder. Culture media were recovered by centrifugation and subjected to SDS-PAGE followed by CBB staining (A). The arrow indicates the location of the expressed MoCel3A. Culture media from *T. reesei* wild type (B) and a transformant overexpressing MoCel3A were incubated with phosphoric acid swollen-cellulose in 100 mM sodium acetate buffer (pH 4.5) for 1 h at 40 °C. Glucose (Glc) and cellobiose (C2) produced were detected by HPLC.

7   Other Aspects of CWDEs

Microorganisms use CWDEs to facilitate their invasion into host plants and to acquire nutrients. Plants also secrete enzymes to degrade the cell walls of invaders as a countermeasure. Hence, the actions of CWDEs are significantly involved in plant-microbe interactions. In addition, the CWDEs from *Ustilago esculenta* participates in gall formation of *Zizania latifolia* (Nakajima et al., 2012). Detailed mechanisms of how CWDEs function in plant-microbe interactions and in determining plant cell shape will be elucidated in the near future, and the efficient use of these enzymes will make our lives better.

References

Carpita, N. C. & Gibeaut, D. M. (1993). Structural models of primary cell walls in flowering plants: consistency of molecular structure with the physical properties of the walls during growth. Plant Journal, 3, 1-30.

Cosgrove, D. J. (2000). Loosening of plant cell walls by expansins. Nature, 407, 321-326.

Dean R. A. et al. (2005). The genome sequence of the rice blast fungus Magnaporthe grisea. Nature, 434, 980-986.

Gruno, M., Valjamae, P., Pettersson, G. & Johanssen, G. (2004). Inhibition of the Trichoderma reesei cellulases by cellobiose is strongly dependent on the nature of the substrate. Biotechnology and Bioengineering, 86, 503-511.

Hayashi, T. (1989). Xyloglucans in the primary cell wall. Annual Review Plant Physiology, Plant Molecular Biology, 40, 139–168.

Henrissat, B. & Davies, G. (1997). Structural and sequence-based classification of glycoside hydrolases. Current Opinion Structural Biology, 7, 637-644.

Kasprzewska, A. (2003). Plant chitinases--regulation and function. Cell Molecular Biology Letters, 8, 809-824.

Kim, H., Ahn, J., Görlach, J. M., Caprari, C., Scott-Craig, J. S. & Walton, J. D. (2001). Mutational analysis of β-glucanase genes from the plant-pathogenic fungus Cochliobolus carbonum. Molecular Plant-Microbe Interactions, 14, 1436-1443.

Lever, M. (1972). A new reaction for colorimetric determination of carbohydrates. Anaytical Biochemistry, 47, 273-279.

Nakajima, M., Yamashita, T., Takahashi, M., Nakano, Y. & Takeda, T. (2012). A novel glycosylphophatidylinositol-anchored glycoside hydrolase from Ustilago esculenta functions in β-1,3-glucan degradation. Applied Environmental Microbiology, 78, 5682-5689.

Pauly, M., Andersen, L. N., Kauppinen, S., Kofod, L. V., York, W. S., Albersheim, P. & Darvill, A. (1999). A xyloglucan-specific endo-β-1,4-glucanase from Aspergillus aculeatus: expression cloning in yeast, purification and characterization of the recombinant enzyme. Glycobiology, 9, 93-100.

Riou, C., Salmon, J., Vallier, M., Günata, Z. & Barre, P. (1998). Purification, characterization, and substrate specificity of a novel highly glucose-tolerant β-glucosidase from Aspergillus oryzae. Applied Environmental Microbiology, 64, 3607-3614.

Schülein, M. (1997). Enzymatic properties of cellulases from Humicola insolens. Journal of Biotechnology, 57, 71-81.

Takahashi, M., Takahashi, H., Nakano, Yuki., Konishi, T., Terauchi, R. & Takeda, T. (2010). Characterization of cellobiohydrolase (MoCel6A) produced by Magnaporthe oryzae. Applied Environmental Microbiology, 76, 6583-6590.

Takahashi, M., Konishi, T. & Takeda, T. (2011). Biochemical characterization of Magnaporthe oryzae β-glucosidases for efficient β-glucan hydrolysis. Applied Microbiology Biotechnology, 91, 1073-1082.

Takeda, T. (2012). Polyhistidine affinity chromatography for purification and biochemical analysis of fungal cell wall-degrading enzymes: Affinity chromatography, INTECH, chapter 10, 177-186.

Takeda, T., Furuta, Y., Awano, T., Mizuno, K. & Hayashi, T. (2002). Supression and acceleration of cell elongation by integration of xyloglucans in pea stem segments. Proceedings of the National Academy of Sciences of the United States of America, 99, 9055–9060.

Takeda, T., Takahashi, M., Nakanishi-Masuno, T., Nakano, Y., Saitoh, H., Hirabuchi, A., Fujisawa, S. & Terauchi, R. (2010). Characterization of endo-1,3-1,4-β-glucanases in GH family 12 from Magnaporthe oryzae. Applied Microbiology Biotechnology, 88, 1113-1123.

Yoshida, K., Saitoh, H., Fujisawa, S., Kanzaki, H., Matsumura, H., Yoshida, K., Tosa, Y., Chuma, I., Takano, Y., Win, J., Kamoun, S. & Terauchi, R. (2008). Association genetics reveals three novel avirulence genes from the rice blast fungal pathogen Magnaporthe oryzae. Plant Cell, 21, 1573-1591.

Application of Recombinant Technology in Protein Investigations

Yu Hua Wang

Biosciences Research Division, Department of Environment and Primary Industries
The Victorian State Government, Victoria, Australia

Victor Muleya

Monash Institute of Pharmaceutical Sciences
Monash University, Victoria, Australia

Helen R. Irving

Monash Institute of Pharmaceutical Sciences
Monash University, Victoria, Australia

1   General Introduction

Protein science is a rapidly expanding area of research in the biological sciences. It joins genomics, transcriptomics and metabolomics as an intact research subject termed proteomics employed to understand biological organisms in a systemic way. Proteomics deals with not only the end product of gene expression but also the functional mechanism of the product in an integrated pattern (Anderson & Anderson, 1998; Blackstock & Weir, 1999; Wilkins *et al.*, 1996). In protein science, one single analytical approach usually cannot generate sufficient information to clearly understand a research target, therefore multiple methodologies are needed for drawing a comprehensive and broader picture. Nowadays, many techniques such as X-ray crystallography, nuclear magnetic resonance spectroscopy, mass spectroscopy, various chromatographic techniques in conjunction with recombinant DNA technology and electrophoresis are being widely adopted for protein investigations (Alberts *et al.*, 2008; Lian & Roberts, 2012; Maurya *et al.*, 2009). Combined with the simultaneous development of bioinformatics and other novel techniques, these technologies have become powerful tools used in the characterization of protein structures and their functions, post-translational modifications, protein interactions, and purification of target proteins (Alberts *et al.*, 2008; Alterovitz *et al.*, 2008; Maron *et al.*, 2009; Ole, 2004).

Different research methodologies have distinct advantages that can be exploited for characterizing proteins. It is well known that there are two main barriers for studying proteins in more detail. One major challenge is that, obtaining a better understanding of how a target protein functions in a specified biological environment is complicated by the diverse and dynamic range of its living context. The other difficulty is that there are limitations associated with isolating large amounts of target protein from its natural environment. However, recombinant technology, which allows specific genes to be cloned and expressed in recombinant or chimeric forms, has proven helpful in mitigating such hindrances. Apart from aiding the successful isolation and purification of target proteins, recombinant technology also provides distinct and detectable means of tracking and monitoring protein activities *in vivo* (Alberts *et al.*, 2008; Brown, 2006).

For the above-mentioned reasons, this chapter describes various recombinant methodologies that are usually applied in protein science investigations. We selected five representative experiments from our two research themes: plant natriuretic peptides (PNPs) and receptor kinases. Plant natriuretic peptides are relatively newly identified signaling peptides in plants which are recognized by the antibody of human natriuretic peptide (a human hormone). Research findings indicate that PNPs play significant roles in regulating fluid homeostasis in plants, particularly under stressful conditions. There is general consensus amongst researchers that PNP possibly operates via a signaling pathway involving the second messenger guanosine 3', 5'-cyclic monophosphate (cGMP) (Gehring & Irving, 2003; Meier *et al.*, 2008; Wang *et al.*, 2010; Wang, Donaldson, *et al.*, 2011; Wang *et al.*, 2007; Wang, Gehring, *et al.*, 2011). Cyclic GMP production is catalyzed by a class of enzymes known as guanylate cyclases (GCs) that convert the nucleotide triphosphate, guanosine 5'-triphosphate (GTP) to cGMP. We have identified a group of leucine-rich repeat receptor like kinases that have a GC catalytic center that is embedded within the kinase domain (Kwezi *et al.*, 2007; Kwezi *et al.*, 2011). A lot of valuable information in these two research fields is obtained by employing recombinant protein technology.

The chapter contains a number of methodologies including recombinant protein purification and analysis, enzymatic reporter assays and fluorescent tag detection. Contents are formalized with various research aspects covering physiological, biochemical, molecular and cell biology fields.

2 Recombinant Protein Applied for Physiological & Biochemical Analyses

2.1 Experiment: Plant Natriuretic Peptide Induces Stomatal Opening

2.1.1 Introduction

Stomatal movements are used by plants in initiating adaptive responses to stressful environmental stimuli. PNP, a plant hormone which has been shown to significantly enhance guard cell opening in plants (Gehring & Irving, 2003) counteracts the action of abscisic acid (ABA), another plant hormone, which stimulates stomatal closure. Such a noteworthy antagonist reaction suggests that PNP and ABA are most likely to have a close interaction. Stomatal closure is necessary for the maintenance of plant water status during stressful environmental conditions that favor water loss. On the other hand, stomatal opening is influenced by a number of factors which include light, higher temperatures and low carbon dioxide concentrations. Therefore, sensitive regulation of stomatal movements is a pre-requisite for normal plant growth and development. In plants, there is a need to maintain this delicate balance between various survival demands particularly during stressful conditions. The interplay among plant hormones can reduce the dominance of any one molecule (Wang & Irving, 2011). Hence the final output of a physiological activity may be a combined result which is possibly favorable for the maintenance of plant homeostasis. This experiment shows the outcomes of AtPNP-A (a PNP identified from model plant *Arabidopsis thaliana*) and ABA acting on stomata simultaneously (Wang *et al.*, 2007).

In this experiment, recombinant protein AtPNP-A was expressed and purified from bacteria. A denaturing purification method was used because AtPNP-A was expressed as insoluble protein aggregates (inclusion bodies) in the bacteria. Then recombinant AtPNP-A was added to stomatal assay solution containing leaf sections of *Tradescantia multiflora* Sw. and different concentrations of ABA. After 1 or 2 hours of incubation, the results revealed that guard cell aperture was increased in response to AtPNP-A but closed by ABA (Figure 1A). In the presence of ABA and AtPNP-A together, the ABA effect on guard cell apertures was greatly reduced with higher stomatal opening rate (Figure 1B) and wider pore size (Figure 1C).

2.1.2 Materials

Buffers for denaturing protein purification

1. Buffer A: 100 mM NaH_2PO_4, 10 mM Tris, 8 M Urea, 0.2 mg/ml Lysozyme, 30 µg/ml DNase I, pH = 8.0

2. Buffer B: 100 mM NaH_2PO_4, 10 mM Tris, 8 M Urea, pH = 7.0

3. Buffer C: 20 mM Tris, 20 % (v/v) Glycerol, 500 mM NaCl, 8 M Urea, pH = 7.4

4. Buffer D: 20 mM Tris, 20 % (v/v) Glycerol, 500 mM NaCl, 6 M Urea, pH = 7.4

5. Buffer E: 20 mM Tris, 20 % (v/v) Glycerol, 500 mM NaCl, 1 M Urea, pH = 7.4

6. Buffer F: 50 mM NaH_2PO_4, 300 mM NaCl, 250 mM Imidazole, pH = 7.4

7. Buffer G: 20 mM Tris, 1 mM PMSF (phenylmethylsulfonyl fluoride), pH = 7.4

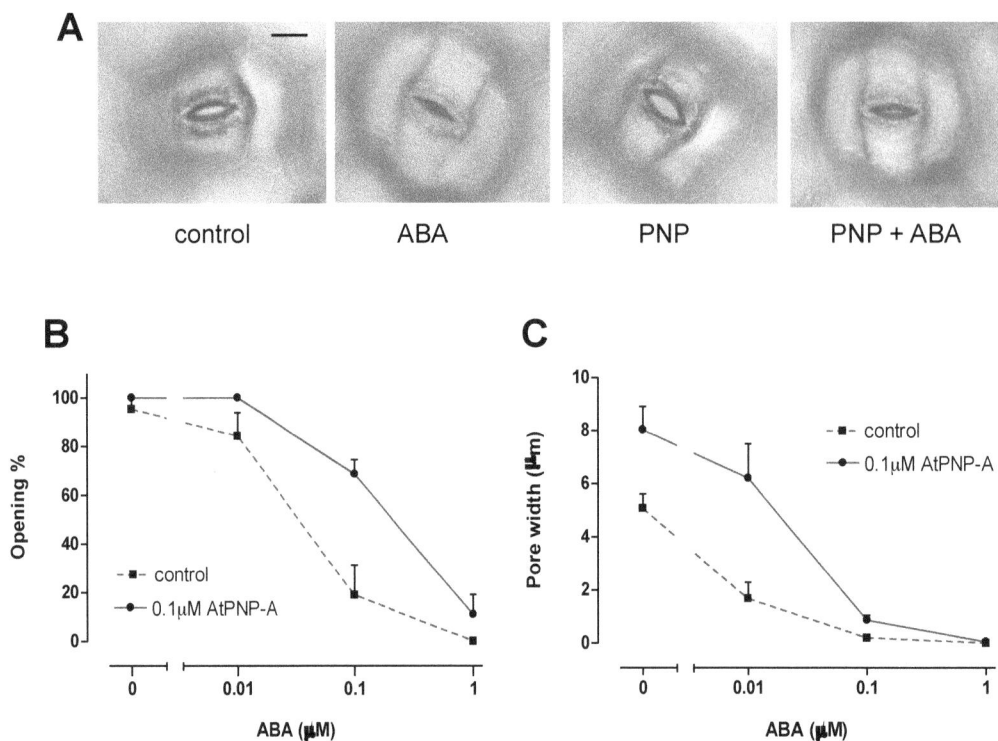

Figure 1: A *Tradescantia* guard cells after 1 h without treatment or with treatments of ABA (100 nM), AtPNP-A (100 nM) or both ABA and AtPNP-A (bar = 20 μm). **B** Addition of AtPNP-A (0.1 μM) in ABA treated leaves increasing stomatal opening rate after 2 h (guard cells with apertures greater than 0.5 μm counted as open). **C** Addition of AtPNP-A (0.1 μM) in ABA treated leaves enhancing guard cell aperture width. Figure reproduced with permission from Wang *et al.* (2007) http://www.publish.csiro.au/nid/102/paper/FP06316.htm)

Solutions for protein SDS-PAGE analysis

1. 5 × Loading buffer: 0.313 M Tris (pH 6.8), 10 % SDS, 0.05 % bromophenol blue, 50 % glycerol, stored at -20 °C.

2. Stacking gel components: 6.4 ml distilled H_2O, 2.5 ml 0.5 M Tris-HCl (pH 6.8), 100 μl 10 % (w/v) SDS, 1 ml 40 % Acrylamide/Bis, 50 μl 10 % ammonium persulfate, and 10 μl TEMED (N, N, N', N',-tetramethyl-ethylenediamine).

3. Resolving gel components: 4.5 ml distilled H_2O, 2.5 ml 1.5 M Tris-HCl (pH 8.8), 100 μl 10 % (w/v) SDS, 3 ml 40 % Acrylamide/Bis, 50 μl 10 % ammonium persulfate, and 5 μl TEMED.

4. Destained solution I: 50 % (v/v) methanol, 10 % (v/v) acetic acid, 40 % (v/v) distilled H_2O.

5. Destained solution II: 5 % (v/v) methanol, 7 % (v/v) acetic acid, 88 % (v/v) distilled H_2O.

6. 10 × SDS running buffer: 15 g Tris, 72 g Glycine, 5 g SDS in 500 ml, pH ≈ 8.3.

7.   Coomassie blue solution: 0.05 % (w/v) Coomassie blue, 50 % (v/v) methanol, 10 % (v/v) acetic acid, 40 % (v/v) distilled H_2O.

Solutions for protein western blot analysis

1.   Transfer buffer: 3.03 g Tris, 14.4 g Glycine, and 200 ml Methanol made to 1000 ml, stored at 4 °C.

2.   PBS solution: 8 g NaCl, 0.2 g KCl, 1.15 g $Na_2HPO_4 \cdot 7H_2O$, 0.2 g KH_2PO_4 dissolved in 1 liter of distilled water, pH 7.3.

3.   PBST solution: 0.1 % Tween-20 in PBS solution.

Plant material

Tradescantia multiflora Sw. plants were grown in pots exposed to normal daylight. The youngest fully expanded leaves were used for stomatal assay.

Stomatal assay solution

10 mM PIPES [Piperazine-N,N'-bis(2-ethanesulphonic acid)], 50 mM KCl, 1 mM $MgCl_2$, 100 µM $CaCl_2$, pH = 6.3.

Instruments

Econo System (Bio-Rad), Vivaspin 20 (3000 MWCO PES) ultrafiltration spins column (Sartorius), centrifuge, Qubit fluorometer (Invitrogen), Quant-iT™ protein assay kit (Invitrogen), electrophoresis chamber, membrane transfer cassette and chamber, calibrated ocular micrometer, and microscope.

2.1.3   Methods

Rapid screening of AtPNP-A expression

1.   The expression vector pCR T7/NT-TOPO containing *AtPNP-A* gene (Morse et al., 2004) was transformed into BL21 Star (DE3) pLysS One Shot competent cells (Invitrogen) according to the manufacturer's guideline. Transformed cells were cultured on LB agar plate added with 100 µg/ml ampicillin and 34 µg/ml chloramphenicol at 37 °C.

2.   After 16 h incubation, several colonies from the plates were selected to separately inoculate 3 ml LB liquid culture containing ampicillin (100 µg/ml) and chloramphenicol (34 µg/ml) at 37 °C with shaking (220 rpm) overnight.

3.   These overnight cultures were used to make bacterial stocks stored at -80 °C. Also 10 ml fresh LB medium (containing 100 µg/ml ampicillin and 34 µg/ml) with the addition of 0.5 ml overnight culture was grown at 37 °C with shaking (220 rpm) for rapid screening of protein expression. When the cell density reached about 0.4, 1 mM IPTG (isopropyl-β-D-thiogalactopyranoside) was added into the medium. Samples (0.5 ml) were taken at 0 h, 1 h and 3 h time points for the assessment of protein expression. All bacterial cells were harvested after a 3 h incubation.

4.   Bacterial cells were resuspended in 0.4 ml buffer A with gentle vortexing and centrifuged at 10000 - 15000 × g for 20 - 30 min. The supernatant was mixed with 0.1 ml 50 % Ni-NTA agarose on a stir wheel for 1 h. Thereafter the mixture was loaded to a filter column and allowed to flow through. The

column was washed three times with 0.6 ml buffer B and then recombinant AtPNP-A was eluted twice with 0.2 ml buffer F for expression assessment.

5. Eluted samples were initially mixed with 5 × loading buffer in 4:1 ratio and denatured by heating at 95 °C for 5 min. Denatured samples were separated in a stacking gel first and then in a resolving gel. Electrophoresis was run in 1 × SDS running buffer at 200 V for 35 min. Then the polyacrylamide gel was stained by Coomassie blue solution for 2 h. Thereafter the gel was destained in solution I for 1 h and continuously in solution II for 16 h. The destained gel was kept in distilled H_2O for checking (Figure 2A). The bacteria with the best levels of protein expression were kept as a stock.

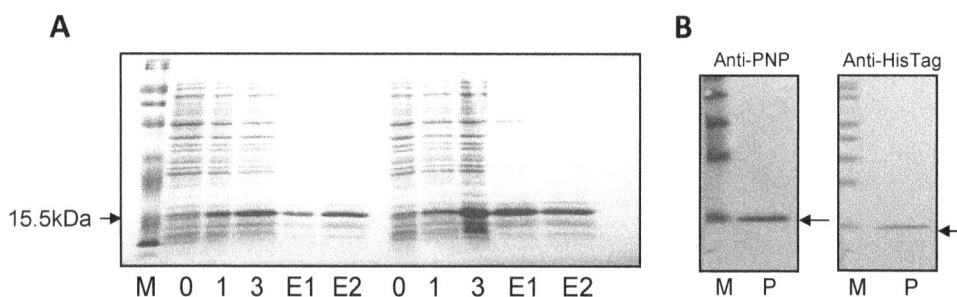

Figure 2: A SDS-PAGE analysis of two bacterial colonies in rapid screening of AtPNP-A expression. Lanes 0, 1, 3 represent lysates in 0 h, 1 h and 3 h time points; lanes E1 and E2 are the first and second eluted proteins. **B** Western blotting analysis of recombinant AtPNP-A using PNP and HisTag antibodies.

Batch purification of recombinant AtPNP-A

1. The stock with the best protein expression was streaked on a LB plate containing ampicillin (100 µg/ml) and chloramphenicol (34 µg/ml) and incubated at 37 °C overnight. Then one single colony was resuspended in 10 ml LB medium containing ampicillin (100 µg/ml) and chloramphenicol (34 µg/ml) at 37 °C with shaking (220 rpm) overnight. This overnight culture was used to inoculate 200 ml broth culture at 37 °C with shaking (220 rpm). At a cell density reaching about 0.4 (OD ≈ 0.4), 1 mM IPTG was added to induce protein expression. After 3 h shaking incubation, total bacterial cells were collected by centrifugation (5000 × g for 30 min at 4 °C) and pelleted cells were stored at 20 °C.

2. Pellets were thawed for 15 min on ice and resuspended in buffer A at 5 ml per gram wet weight. The continuing steps were completed at room temperature. Cells were stirred for 60 min on a rotary shaker and then centrifuged at 10000 × g for 30 min. Lysate was mixed with 50 % Ni-NTA agarose (4:1 ratio) on a stir wheel for 60 min.

3. The lysate-resin mixture was carefully loaded into an empty column with a cap still attached. The cap was removed, and the flow-through was allowed through. The column was washed with buffer B twice (2 × 4 ml) and then buffer C twice (2 × 4 ml). Finally the column was equilibrated with buffer D (4 ml).

4. Protein refolding was completed by gradual dilution of buffer D with buffer E. This procedure was performed using the Econo System (Bio-Rad). The gradient was set as follows: Buffer E was added to the running buffer (mixture of buffer D and E) for 0 % in 0 min, 20 % in 18 min, 50 % in 45 min, 80 % in 72 min, 100 % in 90 min, 100 % in 105 min. The flow rate was adjusted to approximately 2 ml/min.

5. After refolding, recombinant AtPNP-A was eluted using buffer F at least seven times (7×1 ml). Eluted protein was concentrated using Vivaspin 20 (3000 MWCO PES) ultrafiltration spin columns by centrifugation at $3000 \times g$ for 2 h at 4 °C. A desalting step was followed by centrifugation with buffer G at $3000 \times g$ for $60 \sim 90$ min at 4 °C. Protein concentration was determined by Quant-iT^{TM} protein assay kit. Concentrated protein was stored at -20 °C in aliquots and also used for western blotting to confirm identity.

6. The concentrated proteins were run in polyacrylamide gels and then transferred to nitrocellulose membranes (code: RPN303D, Amersham Biosciences). The transfer was completed in an ice-cooled chamber (Bio-Rad) with pre-cooled transfer buffer. The running conditions were set at 100 V for 1 h.

7. Transferred membranes were first saturated in a saturation solution containing PBST solution and 1 % bovine serum albumin for 1 h and then probed with primary antibodies for 2 h at room temperature. AtPNP-A antibody (Wang et al., 2010) was prepared in the saturation solution with 1:50 ratio, while HisTag antibody (Novagen) was prepared in the saturation solution at 0.5 µg/ml. After being washed with PBST solution for three times at 5 min intervals, the AtPNP-A antibody probed membrane was incubated with secondary anti-rabbit IgG (from Sigma, 5 µl in 15 ml saturation solution), while the HisTag probed membrane was incubated with secondary anti-mouse IgG (from Sigma, 5 µl in 15 ml saturation solution). Both membranes were incubated for 1 h, and then washed first with PBST solution (3×5 min) and followed by PBS solution (1×5 min). Washed membranes were detected by incubating with TM/B peroxidase substrate solution (Chemicon / Millipore) for about 5 min (~ 10 ml per membrane). Both detected bands were of the expected size (Figure 2B).

Stomatal assay

1. Leaves from *T. multiflora* were cut into 2×10 mm^2 pieces. Three leaf sections (the sections for all treatments coming from the same leaves) were immersed into stomatal assay solution for each treatment and placed under white light at 23 °C.

2. The opening rate and pore width of about 20 stomata from each leaf section were checked under the microscope with a calibrated ocular micrometer (lower epidermis facing the microscope lens) after 1 or 2 h incubation.

3. Finally, all measured data was analyzed and compared.

2.1.4 Notes

1. Certain eukaryotic proteins are toxic to bacteria, causing premature termination of translation. This can be prevented by reducing rare coding sequence from recombinant protein while not affecting the protein function or replacing the original signal peptide (Sahdev *et al.*, 2008). In the above experiment, the signaling peptide of AtPNP-A was removed as it inhibited bacterial cell growth.

2. To determine the growth rate of bacterial culture, cell density (OD_{600}) can be measured every hour after 90 min shaking incubation. Induction of expression by adding IPTG mostly occurs at OD_{600} of 0.6. However, if bacterial growth is too slow, induction would be started at OD_{600} of 0.4. It is reccommended to take a bacterial sample as 0 time control before the addition of IPTG. The optimal expression times have to be examined individually for different proteins. Induction times vary for different types of proteins.

3. In some cases, expression of recombinant proteins may lead to the formation of inclusion bodies which are insoluble cytoplasmic granules in bacteria. Extraction of insoluble proteins usually requires the use of denaturing agents such as urea. To test the solubility of a recombinant protein, native protein purification (see section 2.2.3 below) can be employed first where all fractions are analyzed by SDS-PAGE. If the protein of interest is in soluble fractions, then native purification should be adopted, otherwise denaturing purification is reccommended.

4. Protein folding pattern and inclusion body formation are strongly linked to the hydrophobic interactions that are temperature dependent. Generally protein expression at low temperature yields more soluble and properly folded products (Sahdev *et al.*, 2008). Thus bacterial induction growth may be completed at a range of 15 ~ 25 °C to enhance protein solubility.

5. The generation of recombinant protein fragments is often due to proteolytic degradation. It may be helpful to add the protease inhibitor PMSF or a protease inhibitor cocktail to decrease proteolysis especially during cell lysis and protein purification. To reduce the background proteins, 1 mM imidazole (or more if necessary) can be included in washing buffers. The viscosity may also be eliminated by either adding Dnase I or alternatively passing the solution three times through a needle attached to a syringe.

2.2. Experiment: Role of Phosphorylation on Protein Function

2.2.1 Introduction

Protein phosphorylation often plays a significant role in signal transduction processes of the cell through its regulation of protein function (Ciesla *et al.*, 2011; Olsen *et al.*, 2006). This phenomenon is known as phosphoregulation and it acts as an 'on' and 'off' switch in the regulation of many proteins thereby altering their biological function and activity. Most proteins under the influence of phosphoregulation exhibit different activities at different phosphorylation states. For instance, a protein may need to be in a phosphorylated state for it to perform its biological function at optimal activity with dephosphorylation of the protein representing a turned off state of the protein where biological activity is minimal.

Through the use of phosphomimetics, recombinant protein technology can be used to investigate the role of phosphorylation in regulating protein function or activity. Phosphomimetics is the mutagenic substitution of a protein's phosphorylation sites with neutral or charged amino acid residues in order to mimic a desired phosphorylation state of a protein. Mutagenic substitutions of phosphorylation sites with a negatively charged amino acid residue, for example aspartate, would yield a mutant that mimics a phosphorylated form of the protein. By the same token, mutagenic substitutions with a neutral amino acid residue, for example alanine, would yield a dephosphorylated form of the protein. In order to carry out a phosphomimetic experiment, the phosphorylation sites of a target protein have to be defined and this is usually done by mass spectrometry. In this experiment, phosphorylation sites of an archetypical receptor kinase from *Arabidopsis thaliana*, were mutated to generate 'on' and 'off' phosphorylated states of the protein (phosphomutants). The effect of phosphorylation on the regulation of this receptor kinase was investigated by measuring the kinase activity of the phosphomutants. The phosphomutants were recombinantly expressed in bacterial cells as His-tag fusions before affinity-purification on a Ni-NTA column (Figure 3A). A comparative analysis of the kinase activities of the two phosphomutants showed that the 'on' state phosphomutant had higher kinase activity relative to that of the 'off' state phosphomutant (Figure 3B).

2.2.2   Materials

Components for recombinant protein expression and purification

1. Media: SOC media, 50 mg/ml carbenicillin, Luria Broth (LB) media fortified with 10 mM $MgCl_2$ and 0.1 % glucose before use, 20 % filter-sterilized L-arabinose.

2. Protein expression vector (pDEST17) containing cDNA of the phosphomutants

3. BL21-AI *E. coli* competent cells for protein expression (obtained from Invitrogen)

4. Cell lysis/wash buffer: 100 mM NaH_2PO_4, 300 mM NaCl, 45 mM imidazole, pH 8.0

5. EDTA-free cocktail of protease inhibitor tablets (Roche), 100 mM PMSF stock solution

6. 10 mg/ml lysozyme stock solution.

7. Ni-NTA agarose beads for purification of His-tagged proteins.

8. Protein elution buffer: 100 mM NaH_2PO_4, 300 mM NaCl, 250 mM imidazole, pH 8.0.

9. Equipment: Sonicator, Rotary shaker, Spectrophotometer, Centrifugal concentrators

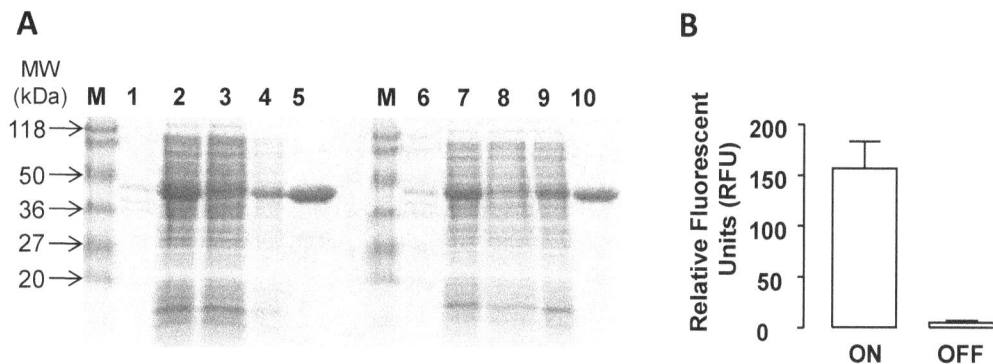

Figure 3: A SDS-PAGE analysis of protein fractions of the affinity purification of 'on' (lanes 1 - 5) and 'off' (lanes 6 - 10) phosphomutants of the receptor kinase. Lanes 1 and 6 shows the pellet fractions lanes 2 and 7 correspond to the crude lysate fractions, lanes 3 and 8 show the flow through fractions, lanes 4 and 9 show the column wash fractions and lanes 5 and 10 correspond to the fractions eluted from the Ni-NTA agarose column. The M lanes show the protein molecular weight marker. **B** Comparative analysis of the kinase activity of 'on' and 'off' state phosphomutants. Kinase activity was measured as relative fluorescence units (RFU) of the phosphorylated SOX peptide. Experiments were done in triplicate and the error bars represent standard error.

Kinase Assay components

1.   Quantified recombinantly expressed protein sample.

2.   Fluorescent Omnia® Ser/Thr Peptide 1 kit (Life Technologies).

3.   FluoroNunc™ Maxisorp™ white 96 well microtiter plate

4.   A fluorescence microplate reader capable of measuring fluorescence at excitation and emission wavelengths of 360 and 485 nm, respectively.

2.2.3   Methods

Recombinant protein expression

1.   A 10 ml LB culture containing 50 µg/ml carbenicillin and 0.1 % glucose in 50 ml flask was inoculated with 500 µl of frozen glycerol stock containing a pDEST17 expression plasmid inserted with cDNA of the kinase. (see Note 1)

2.   The culture was then incubated at 37 °C overnight in a shaking incubator. The 10 ml of the overnight starter culture was added to 500 ml of fresh LB in a 2 L flask with 50 µg/ml carbenicillin and the OD was monitored at 600 nm (OD_{600}).

3.   When the OD_{600} reached a value between 0.4 and 0.5, protein expression was induced with 0.2 % L-arabinose and then the culture was allowed to grow at 25 °C for 4 hours.

4.   Cells were harvested by centrifugation at 8000 g for 10 minutes and the supernatant was discarded.

5.   The pellet was kept at -20 °C until needed for protein extraction.

6.   1 tablet of EDTA-free protease inhibitor cocktail and 1 ml of lysozyme solution from a 10 mg/ml stock solution were added per pellet from a 500 ml culture.

7.   The mixture was incubated on ice with gentle shaking for 30 minutes.

8.   After 30 minutes, the mixture was sonicated on ice for 10 sets of 10 second bursts at 300 W with a 10 second cooling period between each burst.

9.   The sonicated lysate was then centrifuged at 10 000 g for 30 minutes at 4 °C in order to pellet cell debris. The supernatant contains the crude lysate of your bacterial extract and this fraction was retained for protein purification. (see Note 2)

Purification of recombinant protein

1.   4 ml of the crude lysate was added to 2 ml of 50 % equilibrated Ni-NTA slurry. (see Note 3).

2.   The resultant mixture was then incubated on a rotary shaker at 4 °C for at least 1 hour.

3.   The crude lysate and Ni-NTA mixture was loaded into a plastic column with a bottom cap and the bottom outlet was removed before collecting the flow through fraction. A 5 µl aliquot of the flow through fraction was saved for SDS-PAGE analysis.

4.   The column was then washed twice with 5 ml of wash buffer and the wash fractions were collected. 20 µl of these fractions were saved for SDS-PAGE analysis.

5. The protein was eluted with 4 ml of elution buffer and 20 µl of the eluted fraction was kept for SDS-PAGE analysis.

6. The purification factions were analyzed by SDS-PAGE including the crude lysate fraction from the extraction procedure, so as to assess the expression profile of the recombinant protein (Figure 3A).

Determination of kinase activity of phosphomutants

1. Stock solutions for the kinase assay were set up using reagents provided in the Omnia® Ser/Thr Peptide 1 kit (Invitrogen).

2. 2 sets of triplicate experimental reactions were set up, with one set for each phosphomutant. A separate set of 3 control reactions was prepared using all the components of the kinase assay except the protein. For each set, a 4X master mix was prepared so as to minimize inconsistencies due to pipetting error. The total volume of each reaction was made up to 75 µl. (see Note 4)

3. The amount of protein that should be used for each reaction in a single well was determined. Each reaction should contain 1 µg of protein (i.e. 1 µg of protein per 75 µl reaction).

4. The master mix was then added to each well and made up to a total volume of 75 µl with the desired amount of protein.

5. Before measuring fluorescence, the excitation and emission wavelengths on the microplate reader were set at 360 and 485 nm, respectively.

6. The reaction was undertaken for 10 minutes with fluorescence readings being recorded for the entire duration of the reaction. For end point kinetics, the initial and the final values of the measured fluorescence units were used to calculate relative fluorescence units (RFU) for each reaction. The data was then analyzed using GraphPad Prism® software (GraphPad Software, Inc., La Jolla, CA, USA). (see Note 5)

2.2.4   Notes

1. If starting up with colonies from a freshly streaked plate prepare 3 - 5 separate inoculations from isolated colonies. However a verified high protein yielding seed stock is preferable. Expression bacterial stocks kept at -80 °C in BL21-AI do lose their expression capability and it is sometimes worthwhile re-transfecting cells. It is imperative to test for expression if the seed stocks have been kept for more than 3 months. To propagate plasmid, keep in DH5α (bacterial stock at -80 °C) and also keep plasmid stocks for transfection (at -20 °C)

2. You can top up the sonicated mixture with water in order to meet centrifuge volume requirements. Keep 5 µl of the supernatant for SDS-PAGE analysis.

3. The Ni-NTA slurry should be equilibrated with buffer as it is often stored in a 20 % ethanol solution. To equilibrate the Ni-NTA beads wash with deionized sterile water using 5 column volumes (i.e. wash 2 ml resin with 10 ml water). Centrifuge this mixture at 2500 g for 5 minutes so as to pellet the beads. Remove water by discarding the supernatant and repeat this wash step to a total of 2 times using deionized water each time. Equilibrate the beads by the addition of 5 column volumes of lysis buffer before pelleting the beads by centrifugation. Discard the supernatant and add fresh lysis buffer to the beads.

4. When preparing the master mix for the experimental reactions leave room for the amount of protein to be added for each reaction. The protein is to be added immediately before beginning to record fluorescence units.

5. RFU was calculated as the difference between the initial and final fluorescence units for each reaction.

3   Enzymatic Reporter Used in the Assay of Gene Expression

3.1   Experiment: Plant Natriuretic Peptide Controls its Expression via Feedback Regulation

3.1.1   Introduction

Plants are a highly complicated and organized living organism. The role of each plant regulator often resides in the network and feedback systems (Wang & Irving, 2011). Specific activity of each plant regulator stimulates plant actions. Simultaneously, the activity of the regulator itself may be also modulated by diverse cellular compounds or molecular changes during the signaling process. As a plant regulator, PNP release may respond to numerous stimuli and then over time generate different responses. Besides other components, PNP is an element of its own signal transduction chain as well where it may have effects on PNP production. It is essential to elucidate the regulation at the molecular level to give an insight into the entire story of PNP expression and signaling.

Usually it is difficult to detect the transcriptional activity of a particular gene in the tissue where it functions. This problem can be circumvented by merging the upstream promoter sequences of any gene to the coding region of a reporter gene whose product is easily detectable for assessing gene expression. Currently one of the most widely applied reporter gene is luciferase. Luciferase is an oxidative enzyme originally isolated from fireflies. When luciferase acts on the appropriate luciferin substrate in the presence of ATP, light is emitted. The light can be detected by light sensitive apparatus such as a luminometer (Baldwin, 1996; Promega, 2009).

An example testing induction of *AtPNP-A* is given here. In the test, *luciferase (LUC)* gene is constructed under the control of *AtPNP-A* promoter. After the "*AtPNP-A* promoter::*LUC*" DNA is delivered into protoplasts, luciferase gene serves as a tool to document the transcriptional change of *AtPNP-A* gene in response to different amounts of recombinant AtPNP-A. From the outcome of LUC assay, *AtPNP-A* promoter showed concentration-dependent responses to recombinant AtPNP-A (Figure 4). Recombinant AtPNP-A at higher concentration (10 µg/ml) upregulated the *AtPNP-A* expression; but the highest concentration (20 µg/ml) of recombinant AtPNP-A was not different to the control. Apparently AtPNP-A controlled its own expression via a feedback loop. In the initial stage AtPNP-A induces itself via positive feedback; thus AtPNP-A can be amplified in a very short time. However, when AtPNP-A production reaches the threshold level, the self-regulation turns to negative feedback to suppress the continued expression of AtPNP-A avoiding any harmful effects of overexpression (Wang, Donaldson, *et al.*, 2011; Wang, Gehring, *et al.*, 2011).

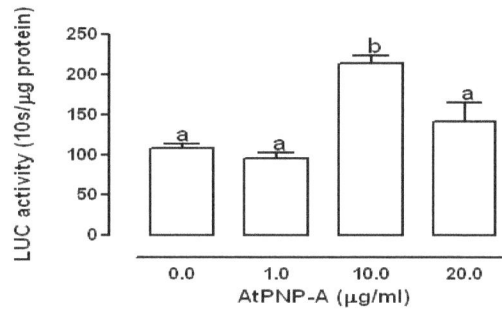

Figure 4: LUC activity was measured in protoplasts transfected with "*AtPNP-A* promoter::*LUC*" construct after 18 h incubation with different concentrations of recombinant AtPNP-A. Columns with different letters were significantly different (P < 0.05 one way ANOVA using Tukey-Kramer post-test). Figure reproduced with permission from Wang, Donaldson, *et al.* (2011).

3.1.2   Materials

Plant material

1. Seeds of *Arabidopsis thaliana* (Col-0) were washed on a sterile filter paper (inserted in a funnel) with 70 ~ 80 % ethanol and then 2 ml of sterilization solution [0.6 % (w/v) sodium hypochlorite, 0.1 % (v/v) Triton X-100]. The seeds were subsequently rinsed with sterile distilled water 3 ~ 5 times.

2. Sterilized seeds were placed on Murashige and Skoog (MS) basal medium (Sigma) supplemented with 3 % (w/v) sucrose and 0.4 % (w/v) agar. The medium was adjusted to pH 5.7. After stratification at 4 °C in the dark for 2 ~ 3 days, the seeds were cultured in 16 h light-period for 14 days at 23 °C. Thereafter the plantlets were transferred into soil with a 12 h light-period at 23 °C.

3. Leaves of 5 ~ 6 week-old plants were used for protoplast experiments.

Cloning kits

1. Taq enzyme (Qiagen)

2. dNTP (Astral Scientific Pty Ltd)

3. ultra-clean PCR clean-up DNA purification kit (MO BIO Laboratories Inc)

4. Gateway® BP Clonase™ II Enzyme Mix (Invitrogen)

5. Gateway® LR Clonase™ II Enzyme Mix (Invitrogen)

Solutions for protoplast transfection

1. Osmotic solution: 0.4 M mannitol, 3 mM MES, 7 mM $CaCl_2$, pH 5.7

2. Enzyme solution: 1 % (w/v) cellulase R-10 (Yakult, Japan), 0.3 % (w/v) Macerozyme R-10 (Yakult, Japan), 0.4 M mannitol, 3 mM MES, 7 mM $CaCl_2$, pH 5.7

3. Washing solution: 154 mM NaCl, 125 mM $CaCl_2$, 5 mM KCl, 2 mM MES, pH 5.7

4. Transfection solution: 0.4 M mannitol, 15 mM $MgCl_2$, 4 mM MES, pH 5.7

5. PEG solution: 4 g PEG 4000 (Fluka, #81240) mixed with 3 ml distilled H_2O, 2.5 ml 0.8 M mannitol and 1 ml 1 M $CaCl_2$, prepared freshly in use

6. Incubation solution: 0.4 M mannitol, 4 mM MES, 20 mM KCl, pH 5.7

Preparation for LUC assay

1. Luciferase Plant Cell Lysis Buffer (Promega)

2. Luciferase Assay Reagent (Promega)

3. NOVO Star microplate reader (BMG Labtechnologies)

4. Qubit® fluorometer (Invitrogen) and Quant-iT™ protein assay kit (Invitrogen).

3.1.3   Methods

Amplification of attB-PCR product

1. The Gateway cloning technology was utilized to construct the "*AtPNP-A* promoter::LUC" plasmid. According to the guidelines [Gateway® Technology (Version E), Invitrogen], two attB-PCR primers were designed to amplify 1547 bp full promoter region upstream to *AtPNP-A* gene (gene code: At2g18660).

2. Forward primer was:

    5′ - GGGGACAAGTTTGTACAAAAAAGCAGGCTTTTTTATTTTACTTTTTGGGCT - 3′

3. Reverse primer was:

    5′ - GGGGACCACTTTGTACAAGAAAGCTGGGTCCATTTTCTTTAACTTGTTTGT - 3′

4. PCR was completed using the standard protocol described in the Qiagen Taq PCR handbook (Qiagen). A plasmid containing 2.5 kb *AtPNP-A* upstream region was used as DNA template (Wang, Gehring, et al., 2011). Approximately 2 ng to 20 ng plasmid DNA was added to 50 μl PCR reaction mixture containing 1× PCR buffer, 1.5 mM $MgCl_2$, 200 μM of each dNTP (Astral Scientific Pty Ltd), 0.4 μM of each primer, and 1.25 units Taq enzyme. The PCR was run in a MyCycler thermal cycler (Bio-Rad) with initial denaturation at 94 °C for 5 min; and then 30 cycles of DNA amplification (denaturation at 94 °C for 30 s, annealing at 50 °C for 1 min, extension at 72 °C for 1.5 min); and final extension at 72 °C for 10 min; and maintenance at 4 °C for 5 min. PCR samples were checked by DNA electrophoresis in a 2 % agarose gel. Accurately sized PCR product was cleaned by the ultra-clean PCR clean-up DNA purification kit (MO BIO Laboratories Inc.).

Creating the entry vector by BP reaction

1. BP reaction was performed according to the guidelines (Gateway® BP Clonase™ II Enzyme Mix, Invitrogen). Plasmid pDONR 207 (Invitrogen) was used as a donor vector. BP mixtures were incubated overnight at 25 °C.

2. The BP reaction was stopped by incubation with proteinase K. Then 1 μl of each BP mixture was added to 50 μl of Std13 competent cells (Invitrogen) and gently mixed by tube-tapping. The mixed cells were incubated on ice for 15 min, then heated in a 42 °C water bath for 2 min, and followed by

15 min on ice again. Thereafter 1 ml of SOC medium (20 g bacto-tryptone, 5 g bacto-yeast extract, 0.5 g NaCl, made to 1 liter, pH 7.0; 2.5 ml of 1 M KCl and 10 ml of 1 M MgSO$_4$ added before use) was added to the transformed cells.

3. The transformed cells were incubated at 37 °C for 1 h with shaking (220 rpm) and then spun at 3000 × g for 2 min. About 800 μl of supernatant was discarded. Resuspended cells were plated respectively as 20 μl and 100 μl aliquots on B medium plates containing 10 μg / ml gentamycin, and were incubated at 37 °C for 16 h.

4. Three bacterial colonies were selected to separately inoculate 5 ml LB liquid culture containing 10 μg / ml gentamycin. After 16 h shaking (220 rpm) at 37 °C, plasmids were extracted from these cultures using the Miniprep kit (Qiagen).

5. Extracted plasmids were amplified by PCR using pDONR 201/207 primers (Invitrogen) to determine the sizes of inserts. PCR running conditions were set as the above attB-PCR running conditions except that the annealing temperature was tested at 50 °C, 52 °C, 54 °C and 56 °C respectively.

6. Plasmids with correct PCR sizes were sent for sequencing using:

   • pDONR 201/207 forward primer: 5′ – TCGCGTTAACGCTAGCATGGATCTC – 3′

   • pDONR 201/207 reverse primer: 5′ – GTAACATCAGAGATTTTGAGACAC – 3′.

7. Sequencing results were analysed using the following tools:

   • The *Arabidopsis* Information Resource (TAIR) (http://www.arabidopsis.org),

   • ApE Plasmid Editor (http://www.biology.utah.edu/jorgensen/wayned/ape)

Creating the expression vector by LR reaction

1. LR reaction was completed according to the guidelines (Gateway® LR Clonase™ II Enzyme Mix, Invitrogen). The *LUC* Trap-3 (GW) plasmid (GenBank accession No AY968054) (Calderon-Villalobos et al., 2006) was used as a destination vector. LR mixture was incubated at 25 °C overnight and then inactivated by proteinase K. The mixture was then transformed into DH5α competent cells (Invitrogen). The transformation procedure was the same as creating entry plasmids. Transformed cells were plated on LB medium containing 50 μg/ml kanamycin.

2. After 16 h incubation at 37 °C, two bacterial colonies were chosen to separately inoculate 5 ml LB liquid culture containing 50 μg / ml kanamycin. These cultures were incubated with 16 h shaking (220 rpm) at 37 °C.

3. Plasmids were extracted from the cultures using Miniprep kit (Qiagen). Extracted plasmids (~ 1 μg each) were digested with EcoR I enzyme (one cutting site in the *AtPNP-A* promoter region while another in the plasmid backbone) and then checked in a 2 % agarose gel. Plasmids with the correctly sized DNA bands were chosen for sequencing, and then analyzed. The sequencing primers were as followed:

   • Primer 1: (attB-PCR forward primer, located in the *AtPNP-A* promoter region)
     5′ – GGGGACAAGTTTGTACAAAAAAGCAGGCTTTTTTATTTTACTTTTTGGGCT – 3′

   • Primer 2: (located in the *LUC* region), 5′ – AGTACTCAGCGTAAGTGATG – 3′

Protoplast transfection

1. Protoplasts were isolated from 5 ~ 6 week-old leaves using a protocol adapted from (Yoo et al., 2007). Leaves were cut into 1 mm-wide strips and plasmolyzed in osmotic solution for 30 min. Then about 600 mg leaf material was incubated in 10 ml enzyme solution for 2 ~ 3 h in the dark and slowly rotated (~50 rpm). After incubation, the enzyme solution was passed through a nylon filter (60 μm diameter) and spun at $100 \times g$ for 5 min. Protoplast pellets were washed with washing solution and then spun at $100 \times g$ for 5 min. Washed protoplasts were suspended in washing solution at 4 °C for 30 min and spun down at $100 \times g$ for 5 min. Pelleted protoplasts were resuspended in transfection solution before protoplast transfection.

2. For protoplast transfection, all samples were pooled together to complete the transfection process first. Accordingly in each sample, 5×10^4 protoplasts were combined with 20 μg plasmid DNA. Then an equal volume of polyethyleneglycol (PEG) solution (PEG volume = DNA volume + Protoplast volume) was added and gently mixed with the protoplasts. After the protoplast mixture was incubated for 20 min, washing solution (washing solution volume = $4 \times$ PEG solution volume) was separated into three aliquots and each was added to the mixture at 5 min intervals. Each addition of washing solution was followed with gentle mixing. Thereafter the mixture was spun at $100 \times g$ for 5 min. Protoplast pellets were suspended in incubation solution. Finally transfected protoplasts were separated into aliquots in 1 ml solution each for different treatments. The samples were incubated in a 24-well plate (1 ml solution / well) at 23 °C in the dark for 18 h.

3. After 18 h of incubation, different samples were collected separately and spun at $100 \times g$ for 5 min. Protoplast pellets of each sample were homogenized in 100 μl of Luciferase Plant Cell Lysis Buffer (Promega) by vigorous vortex for 10 s. Cell lysate was centrifuged at $13000 \times g$ for 30 s and the supernatant was stored at -80 °C for LUC reporter gene assay.

Luciferase (LUC) assay

1. Cell lysate (from -80 °C) was defrosted at 4 °C and then added to a 96-well Geriner plate (Geriner Bio-One) with 20 μl per well.

2. A NOVO Star microplate reader (BMG Labtechnologies) was used to detect LUC activity. The auto-injection system was programmed for measurement. The injector of the NOVO Star microplate reader automatically injected 100 μl of Luciferase Assay Reagent (Promega) into every sample well, and then the measurement head detected luminescence intensity from the injected well immediately.

3. LUC activity was normalized by 10 second of time period and 1 μg of protein amount. Protein concentrations of samples were determined by a Qubit® fluorometer (Invitrogen) using a Quant-iT™ protein assay kit (Invitrogen).

3.1.4 Notes

1. To reduce variance, it is better to prepare buffers once which are enough for all protoplast transfection experiments.

2. Depending on the response of promoter to stimulus, plasmid DNA can be increased up to 40 μg for 5×10^4 protoplasts transfection.

3. In the beginning of new signal stimulation, it is recommended to test a broad range of incubation times and dose gradients to find the optimal expression conditions.

4. The LUC activity is sensitive to temperature and other factors, so it is helpful to store all samples at -80 °C first and then test their LUC activities at the same time.

4   Fluorescent Tag Fused to Detect Protein Cellular Localization

4.1   Experiment: Plant Natriuretic Peptides Are Mobile Molecules

4.1.1   Introduction

Fluorescent proteins are popular molecular probes used for protein visualization. Through recombinant DNA technology, a fluorescent protein tag can be fused to a target protein. Fluorescent fusion protein possesses unique advantages in objective imaging such as the use of green fluorescent protein (GFP) in live organisms. Generally GFP is composed of 238 amino acids (~ 27 kDa) and was first isolated from the jelly fish *Aequorea victoria* (Chalfie *et al.*, 1994). It fluoresces green when exposed to blue light. A hexapeptide containing a cyclic-tripeptide (serine, dehydro-tyrosine and glycine) portion, which is covalently linked through the protein's peptide backbone, is necessary for fluorescence. This unique structure is supposed to be formed via post-translational modification (Cody *et al.*, 1993; Heim *et al.*, 1994). Besides the original jellyfish GFP (wtGFP), currently a wide variety of engineered GFPs are available for imaging experiments. Modified forms of GFP show various excitation and emission ranges, and are more sensitive in application. The most commonly used variants are red-shifted GFPs such as enhanced green fluorescent protein (EGFP) and enhanced yellow fluorescent protein (EYFP). EGFP has a maximum excitation at 484 nm (wavelength) and a maximum emission at 507 nm; while EYFP has a maximum excitation at 514 nm and a maximum emission at 527 nm (Cormack *et al.*, 1996; Delagrave *et al.*, 1995; Heim *et al.*, 1994). Fluorescent protein usually can be fused to either the N-terminus or the C-terminus of a broad range of target proteins without affecting their native functions. Also its fluorescence is not species-specific and is relatively resistant to photo-bleaching (Stearns, 1995).

Although the function and structure of AtPNP-A had been studied actively, little was known about the cellular processing of AtPNP-A. To broaden and deepen the understanding of AtPNP-A processing, it is vital to clarify the cellular localization of AtPNP-A. In the following experiment, GFP was employed as a detectable tag for AtPNP-A visualization (Wang, Gehring, *et al.*, 2011). Using the Gateway cloning technology, AtPNP-A containing signaling peptide was engineered to be C-terminus fused with GFP (signalPNP::GFP). After direct onion epidermal transformation, it was found that AtPNP-A was secreted outside the cells under the direction of its signaling peptide (Figure 5).

4.1.2   Materials and Methods

1. Similarly, Gateway cloning technology was employed to construct the "signalPNP::GFP" expression vector. In accord with the Gateway guidelines (basic procedures detailed in section 3.1.3), full length *AtPNP-A* DNA was cloned into the vector p2GWF7.0 (Karimi *et al.*, 2005; Karimi *et al.*, 2002) as the "signalPNP::GFP" expression vector for subsequent experiment.

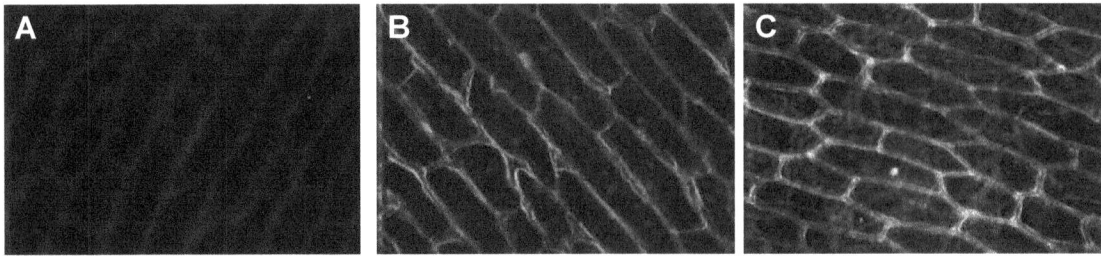

Figure 5: **A** Control onion lower epidermal explants (mock transfection without the construct) show little fluorescence. **B & C** Fluorescent protein (signalPNP::GFP) was detected in extracellular area after 24 h and 48 h transfection respectively. Figure reproduced with permission from Wang, Gehring, et al. (2011).

2. Lower onion epidermis was peeled into thin sections (about 5×20 mm^2). These sections were sterilized by 70 % ethanol and 0.6 % sodium hypochlorite for 10 s each, followed by washing three times with sterile water and once with MS medium containing 0.3 % sucrose.

3. The sterile sections were cultured on the MS medium with 0.3 % sucrose and 0.4 % agar in the dark at 25 °C for 24 h.

4. Thereafter the sections were dipped into osmotic solution (MS medium containing 0.4 M mannitol and 0.3 % sucrose) for 10 min, and then transferred into transformation solution (MS medium with 0.3 % sucrose and 2 μg/mL "signalPNP::GFP" plasmid while control without the plasmid). The transformation was carried out in the dark for 8 h with gentle shaking (50 rpm).

5. After incubation, onion sections were washed by MS medium containing 0.3 % sucrose briefly and cultured onto fresh solid MS medium as above in the dark at 25 °C.

6. Transformation results were checked using fluorescent microscopy (excitation wavelength = 488 nm) at 24 h and 48 h respectively.

4.1.3   Notes

1. To adopt the above transformation method, plasmid DNA size should be smaller than 10 kb or PCR product may be directly tried.

2. Onion epidermal layers need to be peeled as thin as possible (single layer is the best).

4.2   Experiment: Mammalian Cells Enabled to Express Plant Natriuretic Peptides

4.2.1   Introduction

In the human body, natriuretic peptides are involved in regulating blood volume, blood pressure, ventricular hypertrophy, pulmonary hypertension, fat metabolism and long bone growth (Potter *et al.*, 2006). Obviously, natriuretic peptides serve as important regulators for human health. The plant regulator AtPNP-A shares a homologous part of its molecular structure with hANP (Wang *et al.*, 2010) and is predicted to probably play similar roles as ANP (Meier *et al.*, 2008).Therefore it was of interest to see whether AtPNP-A could be expressed not only in plant cells but also in mammalian cells. This is also a crucial first step to test the possibility of utilizing AtPNP-A to mimic ANP in future health applications. Herein mammalian cells are adopted as a research platform to track the AtPNP-A cellular processing (Wang *et al.*, 2010). Using Gateway cloning technology, AtPNP-A without its signaling peptide (26-126 amino acids) was constructed to be C-terminus fused with GFP (PNP::GFP). The construct was transfected into mammalian cells. The results showed that AtPNP-A could be expressed in mammalian cells and did not affect the continuing growth of the transfected mammalian cells (Figure 6).

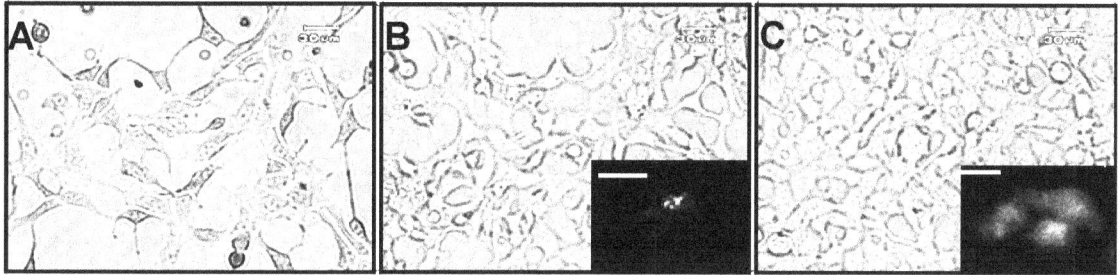

Figure 6: Fusion protein (PNP::GFP) expressed in HEK-293T cells. **A** 24 h cultured cells before transfection. **B** Growing cells after 24 h transfection (inset: confocal image showing PNP::GFP protein mainly located with vesicular regions such as endoplasmic reticulum and Golgi apparatus, bar = 20 μm). **C** Confluent cells after 48 h transfection (inset: confocal image showing PNP::GFP protein distributed throughout the cells, bar = 20 μm). Figure reproduced with permission from Wang *et al.* (2010).

4.2.2   Materials and Methods

Culture of mammalian cells

1. The mammalian cell line 293T/17 [HEK 293T/17], which originates from human kidney embryonic cells, was obtained from the American Type Culture Collection (ATCC), the Global Bioresource Center (ATCC® No: CRL-11268™). HEK 293T/17 cells were cultured in Dulbecco's Modified Eagle's Medium (GIBCO®, Invitrogen) supplemented with 10 % fetal bovine serum (GIBCO®, Invitrogen) at 37 °C in a 5 % CO_2 incubator.

2. For cell subculture, the old culture medium was discarded and cells were washed briefly with sterile 1 × PBS solution (composition as section 2.1.2). Following the removal of PBS solution, a small amount (2 ~ 3 ml) of Trypsin-EDTA (0.25 % Trypsin, 0.5 mM EDTA in 1 × PBS) was added to the flask / plate to disperse the cell layer at 37 °C in a 5 % incubator for 5 min, and then 6 ~ 8 ml culture medium was added to inhibit trypsin activity. The cells were gently aspirated into a 15 ml tube and spun down at 200 × g for 5 min. Cell pellets were suspended in new culture medium in a dilution ratio of 1:4 to 1:8. The medium was renewed every 2 ~ 3 days.

3. The cell viability and density were checked by staining with 0.4 % Trypan Blue.

Mammalian cell transfection

1. Applying Gateway cloning technology (basic procedures detailed in section 3.1.3), *AtPNP-A* gene without its signaling fragment was constructed into plasmid pcDNA™6.2/C-EmGFP (Invitrogen) as the "PNP::GFP" expression vector for mammalian cell transfection.

2. HEK 293T/17 cells were set to a density of 2×10^5 / ml and cultured in a Costar 6-well plate (Corning Inc.) with 2 ml medium per well.

3. Transfection was undertaken the following day. The "PNP::GFP" plasmid DNA (2.5 µg) was added to 500 µl Opti-MEM® I reduced serum medium (Invitrogen) with thorough mixing; and then 6.25 µl Lipofectamine™ LTX reagent (Invitrogen) was added to the diluted DNA with thorough mixing again. This mixture (for one well) was incubated at room temperature for 30 min, and then added to the well containing cells with back and forth gentle rocking for a while. The cells were incubated at 37 °C in a 5 % CO_2 incubator.

4. Medium was changed after 4 h; and expression status was checked by confocal microscopy after 24 h.

4.2.3   Notes

1. Cells should be 50 ~ 80 % confluent at the time of transfection. So the cell growth needs to be monitored by preceding tests. Accordingly the cell density is adjusted when cells are subcultured the day prior to transfection.

2. If microscope is of the upright style, a sterile cover slip can be put inside each well for cell culture. When required, the cover slip is simply taken out, placed on a slide and covered with some culture medium and another cover slip for checking expression status.

5   Concluding Remarks

Currently there is no single technology likely to solve complete problems in protein science. Recombinant technology contributes some important advances in protein science research such as enabling the design of simplified experiments with easier and more thoroughly controlled procedures. Utilization of recombinant technology with the support of other state of the art research platforms will accelerate the pace of protein science. The experimental protocols described here provide a basic guide on the application of recombinant technology and/or some hints for researchers to design and scale their experiments according to their situations.

Acknowledgements

This work was supported by the Australian Research Council's Discovery project scheme. Victor Muleya is supported by a scholarship from the Monash Institute of Pharmaceutical Sciences, Monash University.

References

Alberts, B., Johnson, A., Lewis, J., Raff, M., Roberts, K., & Walter, P. (2008). Molecular Biology of the Cell (5th ed.). New York: Garland Science.

Alterovitz, G., Xiang, M., Liu, J., Chang, A., & Ramoni, M.F. (2008). System-wide peripheral biomarker discovery using information theory. Pacific Symposium on Biocomputing, 13, 231-242.

Anderson, N.L., & Anderson, N.G. (1998). Proteome and proteomics: new technologies, new concepts, and new words. Electrophoresis, 19, 1853-1861.

Baldwin, T.O. (1996). Firefly luciferase: the structure is known, but the mystery remains. Structure, 4, 223-228.

Blackstock, W.P., & Weir, M.P. (1999). Proteomics: quantitative and physical mapping of cellular proteins. Trends of Biotechnology, 17, 121-127.

Brown, T. (2006). Gene Cloning and DNA Analysis: An Introduction. Cambridge, MA: Blackwell Publisher.

Calderon-Villalobos, L.I.A., Kuhnle, C., Li, H., Rosso, M., Weisshaar, B., & Schwechheimer, C. (2006). LucTrap vectors are tools to generate luciferase fusions for the quantification of transcript and protein abundance in vivo. Plant Physiology, 141, 3-14.

Chalfie, M., Tu, Y., Euskirchen, G., Ward, W.W., & Prasher, D.C. (1994). Green fluorescent protein as a marker for gene expression. Science, 263, 802-805.

Ciesla, J., Fraczyk, T., & Rode, W. (2011). Phosphorylation of basic amino acid residues in proteins: important but easily missed. Acta Biochimica Polonica, 58, 137-148.

Cody, C.W., Prasher, D.C., Westler, W.M., Prendergast, F.G., & Ward, W.W. (1993). Chemical structure of the hexapeptide chromophore of the Aequorea green-fluorescent protein. Biochemistry, 32, 1212-1218.

Cormack, B.P., Valdivia, R.H., & Falkow, S. (1996). FACS-optimized mutants of the green fluorescent protein (GFP). Gene, 173, 33-38.

Delagrave, S., Hawtin, R.E., Silva, C.M., Yang, M.M., & Youvan, D.C. (1995). Red-shifted excitation mutants of the green fluorescent protein. Nature Biotechnology, 13, 151-154.

Gehring, C.A., & Irving, H.R. (2003). Natriuretic peptides - a class of heterologous molecules in plants. The International Journal of Biochemistry & Cell Biology, 35, 1318-1322.

Heim, R., Prasher, D.C., & Tsien, R.Y. (1994). Wavelength mutation and posttranslational autoxidation of green fluorescent protein. Proceedings of the National Academy of Sciences USA, 91, 12501-12504.

Karimi, M., De Meyer, B., & Hilson, P. (2005). Modular cloning in plant cells. Trends in Plant Sciences, 10, 103-105.

Karimi, M., Inze, D., & Depicker, A. (2002). GATEWAY^{TM} vectors for Agrobacterium-mediated plant transformation. Trends in Plant Sciences, 7, 193-195.

Kwezi, L., Meier, S., Mungur, L., Ruzvidzo, O., Irving, H., & Gehring, C. (2007). The Arabidopsis thaliana brassinosteroid receptor (AtBRI1) contains a domain that functions as a guanylyl cyclase in vitro. PLoS one, 2, e449.

Kwezi, L., Ruzvidzo, O., Wheeler, J.I., Govender, K., Iacuone, S., Thompson, P.E., Gehring, C., & Irving, H.R. (2011). The phytosulokine receptor is a guanylate cyclase enabling cyclic GMP-dependent signalling in plants. Journal of Biological Chemistry, 286, 22580-22588.

Lian, L.-Y., & Roberts, G. (2012). Protein NMR Spectroscopy: Principal Techniques and Applications: Wiley-VCH.

Maron, J.L., Alterovitz, G., Ramoni, M., Johnson, K.L., & Bianchi, D.W. (2009). High-throughput discovery and characterization of fetal protein trafficking in the blood of pregnant women. Proteomics Clinical Applications, 3, 1389-1396.

Maurya, B.D., Pawar, S.V., Chate, P.B., Kayarkar, N.A., Durgude, S.G., Boraste, A., Kadam, P., & Gomase, V.S. (2009). Proteomics: emerging analytical techniques. International Journal of Genetics, 1, 17-24.

Meier, S., Irving, H., & Gehring, C. (2008). Plant natriuretic peptides - emerging roles in fluid and salt balance. In D.L. Vesely (Ed.), Cardiac Hormones. Kerala, India: Transworld Research Network.

Morse, M., Pironcheva, G., & Gehring, C. (2004). AtPNP-A is a systemically mobile natriuretic peptide immunoanalogue with a role in Arabidopsis thaliana cell volume regulation. FEBS Letters, 556, 99-103.

Ole, N.J. (2004). Modification-specific proteomics: characterization of post-translational modifications by mass spectrometry. Current Opinion in Chemical Biology, 8, 33-41.

Olsen, J.V., Blagoev, B., Gnad, F., Macek, B., Kumar, C., Mortensen, P., & Mann, M. (2006). Global, in vivo, and site-specific phosphorylation dynamics in signaling networks. Cell, 127, 635-648.

Potter, L.R., Abbey-Hosch, S., & Dickey, D.M. (2006). Natriuretic peptides, their receptors, and cyclic guanosine monophosphate-dependent signaling functions. Endocrine Review, 27, 47-72.

Promega (Producer). (2009). Introduction to Bioluminescence Assays.

Sahdev, S., Khattar, S.K., & Saini, K.S. (2008). Production of active eukaryotic proteins through bacterial expression systems: a review of the existing biotechnology strategies. Molecular & Cellular Biochemistry, 307, 249-264.

Stearns, T. (1995). Green fluorescent protein: the green revolution. Current Biology, 5, 262-264.

Wang, Y.H., Ahmar, H., & Irving, H.R. (2010). Induction of apoptosis by plant natriuretic peptides in rat cardiomyoblasts. Peptides, 31, 1213-1218.

Wang, Y.H., Donaldson, L., Gehring, C., & Irving, H.R. (2011). Plant natriuretic peptides: control of synthesis and systemic effects. Plant Signaling & Behavior, 6, 1606-1608.

Wang, Y.H., Gehring, C., Cahill, D.M., & Irving, H.R. (2007). Plant natriuretic peptide active site determination and effects on cGMP and cell volume regulation. Functional Plant Biology, 34, 645-653.

Wang, Y.H., Gehring, C., & Irving, H.R. (2011). Plant natriuretic peptides are apoplastic and paracrine stress response molecules. Plant & Cell Physiology, 52, 837-850.

Wang, Y.H., & Irving, H.R. (2011). Developing a model of plant hormone interactions. Plant Signaling & Behavior, 6, 494-500.

Wilkins, M.R., Pasquali, C., Appel, R.D., Ou, K., Golaz, O., Sanchez, J.-C., Yan, J.X., Gooley, A.A., Hughes, G., Humphery-Smith, I., Williams, K.L., & Hochstrasser, D.F. (1996). From protein to proteomes: large scale protein identification by two-dimensional electroporesis and amino acid analysis. Nature Biotechnology, 14, 61-65.

Yoo, S.-D., Cho, Y.-H., & Sheen, J. (2007). Arabidopsis mesophyll protoplasts: a versatile cell system for transient gene expression analysis. Nature Protocols, 2, 1565-1572.

Staphylococcal Exfoliative Toxins: Purification and Determination of Activity of Epidermolytic Proteases

Joanna Pogwizd

Faculty of Biochemistry, Biophysics and Biotechnology
Jagiellonian University, Krakow, Poland

Grzegorz Dubin

Faculty of Biochemistry, Biophysics and Biotechnology
Jagiellonian University, Krakow, Poland
Malopolska Centre of Biotechnology, Krakow Poland

1   Introduction

Staphylococcus aureus is an opportunistic pathogen responsible for a range of human diseases. This gram positive bacterium produces an entire spectrum of extracellular proteins, most of which play role in virulence of Staphylococcus (Iandolo, 1989). Although, as a group, the extracellular enzymes are essential for staphylococcal virulence, most of them do not have the characteristics of typical toxins. As multiple studies have demonstrated most of staphylococcal extracellular enzymes do not produce any specific symptoms when purified and administered in the absence of the bacterium. Moreover, the bacterial virulence is not markedly reduced when only a single of the extracellular factors is knocked out. Yet, staphylococci produce several typical toxins, directly responsible for deleterious symptoms observed in some infections. These toxins include toxic shock syndrome toxin-1 (TSST-1), staphylococcal enterotoxins (SEA, SEB, SEC, SED, SEE, SEG, SEH, and SEI) and the exfoliative toxins (ETA and ETB) (Dinges *et al.*,2000; Proft, 2009). Of the above, exfoliative toxins are especially interesting due to their extraordinary mechanism of action, unlike that found in any other bacterial toxins.

   Exfoliative toxins (also known as epidermolytic toxins) are glutamic acid-specific serine proteases which cause blistering of the superficial epidermis by hydrolyzing a single peptide bond between extracellular domains 3 and 4 of desmoglein-1. Desmoglein-1 is a desmosomal cadherin. Desmosomal cadherins are responsible for the integrity of desmosomes – structures providing attachment between epithelial cells. Degradation of desmoglein-1 leads to disturbance of desmosomes and skin blistering, the major manifestation of Staphylococcal Scalded Skin Syndrome (SSSS), also known as Ritter's disease. SSSS predominantly affects infants. The most threatening secondary effects include dehydration and secondary infections.

   This chapter will allow the reader to become acquainted with methods of recombinant expression, purification and determination of the level of activity of staphylococcal epidermolytic toxins. Biological activity, structure and function of those exotoxins are also briefly discussed to allow understanding of the unique properties of the described toxins.

1.1   Staphylococcal Scalded Skin Syndrome

Staphylococcal Scalded Skin Syndrome, also known as Ritter's disease is an exfoliative dermatitis (Ladhani *et al.*, 1999). The disease, directly caused by the exfoliative toxins of *Staphylococcus aureus*, is characterized by superficial blistering of skin and almost exclusively affects infants. At an early stage the symptoms include fever, malaise, lethargy, and poor feeding. These are followed by an erythematous rash and the formation of large, fragile, fluid-filled blisters. The blisters are ruptured easily by mechanical factors leaving affected areas of the body without the protection of epidermis (Lyell, 1973). Blisters are usually sterile. Toxin (but not bacteria) spreads from the primary site of infection throughout the body causing the described symptoms. With the large areas of skin uncovered the affected subject is prone to dehydration and secondary infections.

   High similarity of symptoms of SSSS to other skin diseases like toxic epidermal necrolysis, epidermolysis bullosa, bullous erythema multiforme, or listeriosis, and thermal or chemical burns causes problems with diagnosis (Ladhani *et al.*, 1999). The most appropriate method to distinguish SSSS form other exfoliative dermatitis is the PCR reaction for toxin-encoding genes or random amplified polymorphic DNA analysis (Johnson *et al.*, 1991).

Treatment of SSSS includes the use of antibiotics to eliminate the strain of *S. aureus* which produces the toxins. Antibiotic resistance is not yet a major problem but selected problematic cases have been reported and resistance may become an issue in the future (Yamaguchi *et al,* 2002; Noguchi *et al,* 2006). Recent reports demonstrated that 2–3% of MSSA strains carry the *eta* or *etb* gene (Megevand, *et al,* 2009; Sila *et al,* 2009), whereas around 10% of MRSA are *eta* positive (Sila *et al,* 2009). Even though the prevalence of ETs in MRSA is higher than among MSSA there is no clear evidence of correlation between methicillin resistance and ability to produce epidermolytic toxins.

Apart from antibiotic treatment, prevention against dehydration and secondary infections is of great importance (Cribier *et al.*, 1994; Melish & Glasgow, 1971). With proper treatment mortality among children is less than 5% (Gemmell, 1995). The disease is very rare in adults, but because of frequent complications some reports claim nearly 60% mortality in this age group (Cribier *et al.*, 1994). However, the data in the adult age group are incomplete because of the low incidence of the disease.

1.2   Exfoliative Toxins in SSSS

Clinical features of SSSS were first described over 100 years ago by a German doctor, Baron Gottfried Ritter von Rittershain (Von Rittershain, G.R., 1878). However, the relationship between staphylococcal infection, and blistering was characterized only in 1967 by Lyell (Lyell, 1967). The existence of toxin was later confirmed by Melish and Glasgow who demonstrated that sterile fluid obtained from intact bullae and sterile culture medium from *S. aureus* of phage group II were able to produce a positive Nikolsky sign (skin blistering) in neonatal mice (Melish & Glasgow, 1970). Soon after, the exfoliative toxin was purified and characterized (Kapral & Miller, 1971). The initial report was soon confirmed by other researchers (Arbuthnott *et al.*, 1971; Melish *et al.*, 1972).

Initial studies identified two major serotypes of exfoliative toxins which were termed ETA and ETB (Wiley & Rogolshy, 1977). Both serotypes were shown to be proteins of approximately 27 kDa. Mature form of ETA and ETB toxins are 242 and 246 residues long, respectively, after their signal sequence is cleaved off during secretion (Lee *et al.*, 1987). ETA and ETB share 55% sequence identity; the toxins are chromosome- and plasmid-encoded, respectively (Bailey *et al.*, 1980; O'Toole & Foster, 1987). A survey of GenBank resources and recent literature demonstrates ~12% prevalence of toxin encoding genes among *S. aureus* strains (Megevand, *et al,* 2009). In Europe, USA, and Africa, ETA is more prevalent, and is expressed by more than 80% of toxin-producing strains (de Azavedo & Arbuthnott, 1981; Adesiyun *et al.*, 1991). Only in Japan, are ETB-producing strains more prevalent than those expressing ETA (Kondo *et al.*, 1975).

Determination of the amino acid sequences of the purified toxins has allowed the corresponding genes to be cloned (O'Toole & Foster, 1986; Johnson *et al.*, 1979) and the toxins to be expressed in heterologous hosts. Recombinant toxins produced in *Escherichia coli* retained their toxic activity in a mouse model, providing final confirmation that exfoliative toxins are the sole factors responsible for blister formation in SSSS (Lee *et al.*, 1987).

1.3   Activity of Exfoliative Toxins

Although ETA and ETB toxins were isolated and their toxic nature thoroughly characterized, for many years the molecular mechanism of epidermolysis remained a mystery. The close resemblance between the sequence of the toxins and the staphylococcal V8 protease (Lee *et al.*, 1987; O'Toole & Foster, 1987) and the fact that the catalytic triad of V8 protease is present in both ETA and ETB (Dancer *et al.*; 1990) became evident as soon as the primary structure of the toxins was determined. Since the similarity of ETs to the serine proteases has been demonstrated many investigators struggled to experimentally demonstrate the anticipated proteolytic activity, although for a long time unsuccessful. Nonetheless multiple indirect lines of supporting evidence were collected. For example, the functional role of Ser195 (presumed catalytic triad serine residue) was confirmed by site-directed mutagenesis (Prevost *et al.*, 1991; Bailey & Smith, 1990). Substitutions of Ser195 by glycine or cysteine resulted in biologically inactive toxins when tested on the newborn mouse skin model. It was also demonstrated that both ETA and ETB have low but significant *N-t*-butoxycarbonyl L-glutamic acid α-phenyl (boc-L-Glu-*O* phenyl) esterase activity (Bailey & Redpath, 1992). Esterase activity is characteristic for serine proteases. The activity was not present in a mutant form of ETA where the Ser195 was replaced by glycine. The esterase activity of ETB was abolished by diisopropylphosphorofluoridate, a broad-range serine protease inhibitor (Bailey & Redpath, 1992). But still no protein substrate could have been identified and the overall picture remained ambiguous especially that reports claiming superantigen function of epidermolytic toxins appeared at that time (Vath *et al.*, 1997; Vath *et al.*,1999)

Further increasing the ambiguity as to the proteolytic nature of ETs, multiple serine protease inhibitors tested did not inhibit the activity of ETs (Dancer *et al.*; 1990). Although crystal structures of both serotypes of exfoliative toxins were determined [Figure 1] and were almost identical to those of the serine proteases of the chymotrypsin family and specifically to that of the glutamic-acid-specific proteases (Cavarelli *et al.*, 1997; Vath *et al.*; 1999; Papageorgiou *et al.*, 2000) the conformation of the oxyanion hole, one of the important features of the catalytic machinery of serine proteases, was not pre-formed in the structures of epidermolytic toxins.

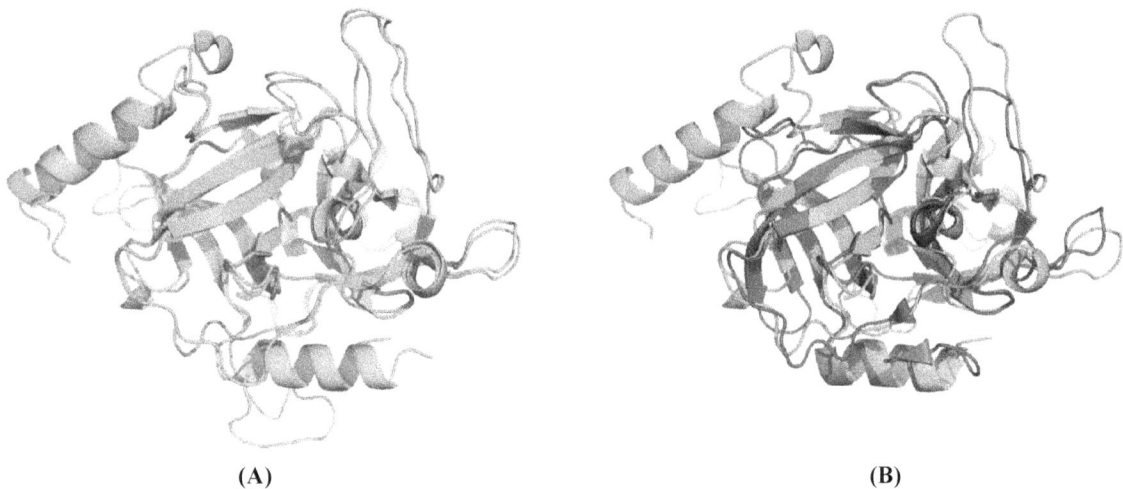

(A)   (B)

Figure 1: Exfoliative toxins belong to the chymotrypsin family of serine proteases and are structurally similar to staphylococcal glutamylendopeptidase (V8 protease). *Panel A*: ribbon representation of overlaid crystal structures of ETA (green) and ETB (blue). *Panel B*: overlay of crystal structures of ETA (green) and V8 protease (red).

1.4   Desmoglein-1 - A target of Exfoliative Toxins in Skin

As described in the previous section, despite multiple indirect suggestions the proteolytic nature of epidermolytic toxins as well as their molecular target remained obscure for a long time. It took almost 30 years since the discovery of the toxic nature of SSSS and characterization of responsible toxins to demonstrate their physiological target. The finding of a specific substrate recognized by the toxins (which in fact remains the only known target of epidermolytic toxins) was facilitated by research on an autoimmune disease *Pemphigus foliaceus*. The clinical features of *Pemphigus foliaceus* include loss of upper parts of epidermis (acantholysis) due to disruption of intercellular adhesion of keratinocytes. In the late 80s it was demonstrated that the symptoms in *Pemphigus foliaceus* are directly associated with autoantibodies that are specific for the extracellular region of the desmosomal glycoprotein, desmoglein-1 (Dsg1) (Feldman, 1993; Eyre *et al.*, 1987). The superficial blisters observed in *Pemphigus foliaceus* are reminiscent of those observed in SSSS and therefore it has been hypothesized that Dsg1 is the likely target of exfoliative toxins. This presumption was confirmed both *in vivo* and *in vitro*. It was demonstrated that ETs target and hydrolyze Dsg1. This finding provided a full molecular explanation of the mechanism of action of epidermolytic toxins (Amagai *et al.*; 2000; Amagai *et al.*, 2002; Hanakawa *et al.*, 2002). Preliminary results were confirmed by the detailed characterization of the mechanism of recognition and hydrolysis of desmoglein-1 (Hanakawa *et al.*, 2004; Aalfs *et al.*, 2010). Cleavage sites were characterized using recombinant extracellular domain of Dsg1 (Amagai *et al.*, 2000; Amagai *et al.*, 2002). It has been shown *ex vivo* and on isolated proteins, that the toxins are extremely specific in their activity, hydrolyzing only a single peptide bond located between the extracellular domain 3 (EC3) and 4 (EC4) of desmoglein-1 (Simpson *et al.*, 2010; Funakoshi & Payne, 2010). Other closely related desmogleins are not affected. Even some desmoglein-1 homologs form closely related species are not affected which constitutes the basis of species specificity of epidermolytic toxins. The extraordinary specificity of ETs clearly explains the reason of the problems to demonstrate their proteolytic activity in the previous studies. Fragmentation of desmoglein-1 leads to disintegration of desmosomes, resulting in a loss of cell connections and blistering of the skin (Hanakawa *et al.*, 2002). Cleavage depends on the conformation of Dsg1 - unfolded protein is not hydrolyzed (Hanakawa *et al.*, 2003). The folding of Dsg1 domains dependents on calcium ions. Their removal causes denaturation of the protein which results in inability of ETs to recognize and hydrolyze Dsg1.

The question remains why the blistering occurs only in superficial layer of skin (*stratum granulosum*) and not other layers of skin or mucosa where the integrity of cell-cell adhesion also depends on desmosomes. This question is easily explained when the distribution of different desmogleins is taken into account. Dsg1 is expressed in all strata of the skin, whereas other desmogleins are expressed only in deeper strata (Arnemann *et al.*, 1993). Therefore, in the deep layers of the skin, the disruption of Dsg1 by ETs is compensated by other desmogleins and exfoliation only occurs in the *stratum granulosum* [Figure 2], where only desmoglein-1, but not other desmogleins, is responsible for the integrity of desmosomes. The distribution of desmogleins differs in the mucosa where desmoglein-1 occurs in low quantities. Dominant form of desmoglein in mucosa is desmoglein-3 which is not recognized by exfoliative toxins. Therefore disruption of desmoglein-1 is compensated by the presence of desmoglein-3 and no blistering occurs. The molecular determinants of the extreme substrate specificity of ETs (the fact that of 4 closely related human desmogleins [Figure 3] only desmoglein-1 is hydrolyzed) are still not fully explained at structural level and constitute one of the most interesting research topics in this field.

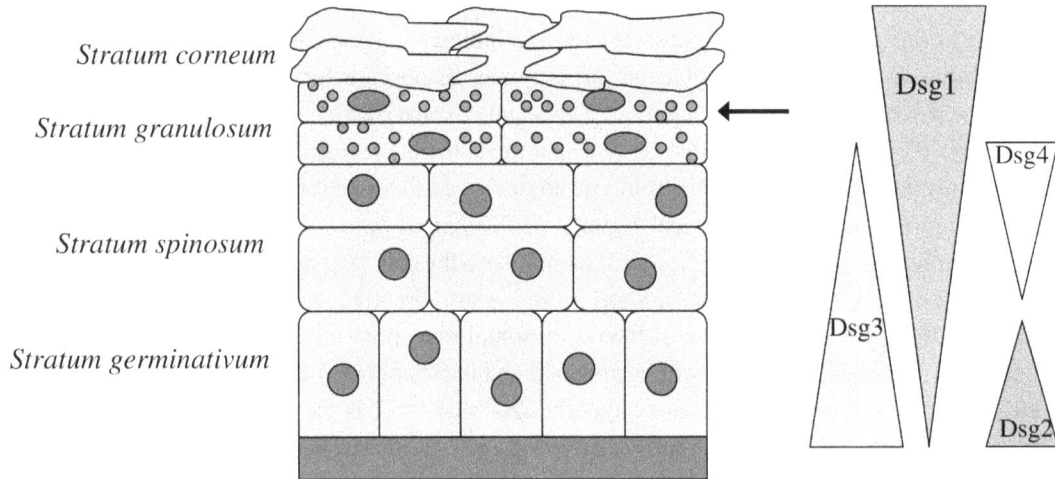

Figure 2: Desmosomal cadherin expression pattern in epidermis. The figure shows the location and relative levels of expression of different desmogleins in respective layers of epidermis. The site of ET induced epidermal splitting is marked with an arrow.

```
HUMAN_DSG1 : QSSYTIEIQENTLNSNLLETRVIDLDEEFSANWMAVIFFISGNEGNWFEIEMNERTNV : 58
HUMAN_DSG2 : NKVLEGMVEENQVNVEVTRIKVFDADEIGSDNWLANFTFASGNEGGYFHIETDAQTNE : 58
HUMAN_DSG3 : DSQYSARIEENILSSELLRFQVTDLDEEYTDNWLAVYFFTSGNEGNWFEIQTDPRTNE : 58
HUMAN_DSG4 : KTSYSASIEENCLSSELIRLQAIDLDEEGTDNWLAQYLILSGNDGNWFDIQTDPQTNE : 58
```

```
HUMAN_DSG1 : GILKVVKPLDYEAMQSLQLSIGVRNKAEFHHSIMSQYKLKASAISVTVLNVIEGPVF : 115
HUMAN_DSG2 : GIVTLIKEVDYEEMKNLDFSVIVANKAAFHKSIRSKYKPTPIPIKVKVKNVKEGIHF : 115
HUMAN_DSG3 : GILKVVKALDYEQLQSVKLSIAVKNKAEFHQSVISRYRVQSTPVTIQVINVREGIAF : 115
HUMAN_DSG4 : GILKVVKMLDYEQAPNIQLSIGVKNQADFHYSVASQFQMHPTPVRIQVVDVREGPAF : 115
                                                          *
```

Figure 3: Amino-acid sequence alignment of EC3 domains of four human desmogleins. Significant homology of desmogleins is clearly visible. Asterisks indicates the glutamic acid residue after which DSG-1 is hydrolyzed by ETs. Although the glutamic acid is conserved in all desmogleins only desmoglein 1 is hydrolyzed.

2   Methodology

A fundamental step in studying individual proteins is to obtain the protein of interest as a homogenous preparation. A variety of strategies have been developed for purifying proteins. These strategies address different requirements of downstream applications including scale and throughput. There are however several basic steps indifferent the scale and required for almost any protein purification including: 1) cell lysis; 2) specific binding to a matrix; 3) washing; and 4) elution. These basic and some additional, protein specific stages are going to be outlined in more details based on the example of epidermolytic toxin purification from a heterogenous host.

2.1   Protein Expression

A prerequisite of any purification is to obtain a reliable and abundant source of the protein of interest. This can either be achieved on the basis of an extended search of natural producers (for example multiple different strains of the microorganism of interest may be tested) or, as often done in these days, through artificial modification of a well known microorganism such as for example *Escherichia coli*, a bacterium widely used in today's science. Only the latter process is going to be further considered. First the expression construct must be prepared. These constitute fragments of DNA (usually plasmids) which encode the protein of interest and appropriate signals recognized by the target microorganism which will ensure stable maintenance of the DNA, its transcription into mRNA and finally translation into protein. A choice of such DNA fragments is available commercially and usually the only manipulation done by particular researcher is to introduce the fragment encoding the gene of interest into a common template. However, previous to this relatively straightforward manipulation, appropriate plasmid must be chosen including all necessary elements especially the affinity tag. Affinity purification tags can be fused to the protein of interest which increases its solubility, but most of all allow fast and easy purification following a procedure that is based of the properties of the tag and does not have to be adjusted every time a different protein of interest is purified. Affinity tags can by added to the N- or C-terminus of protein of interest (Lichty *et al.*, 2005) or, very rarely, inside the protein of interest. The biochemical features of different tags influence the purification scheme of the protein of interest here exemplified by epidermolytic toxin. Due to its numerous benefits, in our laboratory we use pGEX-4T-1 vector to express and purify the exfoliative toxin. pGEX-4T-1 is a commercially-available plasmid that encodes GST fusion tag and includes a multiple cloning site permitting convenient insertion of a gene encoding any protein of interest. The GST fusion protein is easily purified by affinity chromatography using a Glutathione-Sepharose matrix utilizing mild conditions. Removal of the GST moiety from the protein of interest is accomplished through hydrolysis using a specific protease. The site of hydrolysis is located between the GST moiety and the recombinant polypeptide. The digestion can be carried out either in solution or on the column. The cleaved-off GST is easily removed from the final preparation by a second round of chromatography on the Glutathione-Sepharose or by ion exchange chromatography. Some benefits of GST affinity tag and the pGEX family of expression vectors are summarized in Table 1.

After selecting the appropriate affinity tag the protein expression vectors are prepared using standard methods of genetic manipulation as described in multiple elaborations and laboratory manuals. (ex. Biochemistry, Level II: Practical Manual; Peter Kill). Briefly, in a most common case, polymerase chain reaction (PCR) is used to amplify the encoding gene. The target vector and the insert are digested with restriction enzymes, mixed and ligated to create an expression plasmid. These are than transferred into appropriate expression host and the expression optimization is initiated.

Protein expression is a complex process. It is influenced by multiple factors like temperature, time, concentration of the inducer, host strain and many other which have to be experimentally optimized to ensure best possible efficiency and quality of the final product. To obtain recombinant ETA we used *E. coli* BL21 strain mainly because of relatively good expression and protease-deficiency. Protease deficiency ensures that the recombinant protein is not unspecifically degraded and that the final preparation is not contaminated with foreign proteolytic activity. The strain also usually provides a high level of expression of GST fusion proteins and therefore is one of the strains of choice for initial expression trials.

Properties of pGEX family of expression vectors and GST purification tag
GST tag can be used in any expression system
Single step purification procedure yields pure product
Easily scalable purification
pGEX vectors enable tag cleavage and protein purification in a single step
Site-specific proteases enable cleavage of the tag whenever required
GST tag is easily detected using an enzymatic assay or an immunoassay
Simple purification. Mild elution conditions minimize risk of damage to functionality and antigenicity of target protein
GST tag can help stabilize folding of recombinant proteins
pGEX vectors contain inducible promoter

Table 1: Basic properties and benefits of pGEX family of expression vectors and GST purification tag.

In our case the main optimization of expression process involved selecting the appropriate timing and temperature of the experiment. Short protocol for optimization of time and temperature of ETA expression is given below and may be easily adjusted to optimization of other parameters as well.

1. Prepare starting cultures of appropriate expression strain by inoculating one bacterial colony from an agar plate into a 5 ml sample of LB medium with selection antibiotic. Incubate cultures overnight with shaking at 37 ° C.

2. Next morning, add 500 microliters of the overnight culture to a new flask containing 50 ml of LB with selection antibiotic and incubate with shaking at 37 °C.

3. Allow cultures to grow until the absorbance at 600 nm reaches 0.6 (exponential growth phase). Measure the absorbance using a spectrophotometer blanked with LB media. Induce protein expression by addition of IPTG and allow cultures to grow until different time points. Suggested time points are 3, 8, 16 and 24 hours.

4. Check the absorbance at each chosen time point and save aliquots diluted with LB to cell density equal to that obtained at the first time point. Note that the cultures usually reach OD of more than 1 which is usually impossible to measure on common spectrophotometers and dilution before measurement is necessary. Centrifuge the samples and separate the supernatant and bacterial pellet. Freeze the samples at -20 ° C for further analysis.

5. Repeat the above steps, but try different temperatures by placing 50 ml cultures in conditioned shakers. Suggested temperatures are 37° C, 30° C, 21° C, 16°, and 4° C. Allow to grow until different time points as described in point 3 and collect aliquots as described in point 4. You may also try to induce the cells at different density (ex. 0.3; 1.2 instead of 0.6).

6. Run an SDS-PAGE gel to analyze all collected samples. Determine expression levels of the protein of interest in each sample. One may also wish to use different detection methods such as

immunoblotting or enzymatic detection. For future expression use conditions with the highest expression of the protein of interest.

The above described experiments allowed to determine the optimal expression conditions for GST-ETA fusion: IPTG concentration of 0.5 mM, time of expression 16 h and temperature of 21° Celsius. Expression at other temperatures and times gave lower level of ETA overexpression.

Once the optimal expression conditions are established the expression is scaled up typically to several liters (convenient in laboratory scale) but scaling up to much larger quantities is often carried out in the industry. Once the culture is finished the cells are pelleted and disrupted to release the protein to be purified. Sonication was used as a method of choice during purification of exfoliative toxin. During sonication ultrasounds are applied to the sample. The probe is placed in the sample and the high-frequency oscillation causes the bacterial cells to break open. The most important issue during sonication is to keep the temperature of the sample low. Sonication tends to overheat the sample which is deleterious to most proteins. The entire process is therefore performed in a water-ice bath and appropriate cycling of impulse and off times must be adjusted for each type of sample and container.

2.2   Affinity Chromatography and Tag Cleavage

Soluble fraction of bacterial lysate obtained by sonication is recovered by high speed centrifugation and is used for the next step of toxin purification, which is affinity chromatography. At this step hundreds of proteins are contained in the preparation. It is most challenging to obtain the protein of interest with any unspecific methodology. However, the affinity chromatography uses specific binding interactions, in our case between GST fusion tag and glutathione coupled to a solid support (GST Gene Fusion System Handbook, GE Healthcare). The lysate (protein mixture) is passed over the column containing immobilized glutathione, molecules of GST-ETA fusion protein are retained on the solid support by virtue of GST affinity towards glutathione. The vast majority of remaining proteins pass through the column unaffected. In the next step all remaining contaminating proteins are washed away. The bound fusion protein is finally eluted from the support by addition of excess soluble glutathione. The specificity of interaction between GST and glutathione ensures that high purity preparation is obtained in a single step. Elution is performed under mild conditions (using reduced glutathione) so that the function of the protein of interest is almost always retained.

Each specific affinity system requires its own set of conditions and presents its own particular challenges for a given research purpose. Despite unquestionable advantages of the GST fusion, due to its large size (26 kDa) it is necessary to remove it from the protein of interest. This can be accomplished with protease treatment that hydrolyzes the linker between GST tag and the protein of interest. The construct used to obtain ETA in the current study contains thrombin recognition site. In the discussed case only specific hydrolysis is observed [Figure 4], but it is often the case that several tag removing enzymes have to be evaluated to select the one which does not affect the protein of interest (none of the commonly used proteases is exclusively specific and most will affect the protein of interest when the protease is used in high concentration and the incubation time is long). Fortunately, at least several different enzymes are commonly used and commercially available (including PreScission, TEV, thrombin and factor X) while the literature contains description of several other enzymes which can be used in difficult cases. The amount of enzyme and the cleavage time have to be usually optimized experimentally.

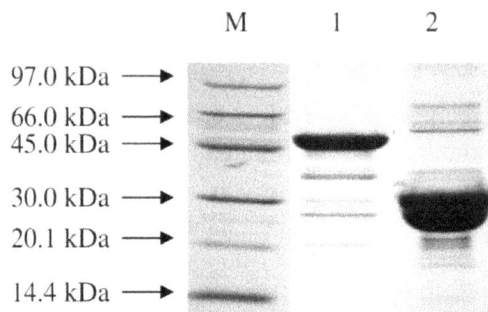

Figure 4: SDS-PAGE analysis of the preparation obtained after Glutathione Sepharose chromatography. Lanes: M - low molecular weight marker, 1 - purified fusion protein, 2 - preparation after incubation with thrombin. Sodium dodecyl sulfate polyacrylamide gel electrophoresis (SDS-PAGE) was carried out in 12% acrylamide gel. Prior electrophoresis, the samples were heated to 100°C for 5 min in SDS-PAGE loading buffer containing, 2% SDS and 5% 2-mercaptoethanol, and centrifuged at 12,000 g for 5 min. Protein size marker contains phosphorylase b (97.0 kDa), albumin (66.0 kDa), ovalbumin (45.0 kDa), carbonic anhydrase (30.0 kDa), trypsin inhibitor (20.1 kDa) and α-lactalbumin (14.4 kDa). SDS-PAGE was carried out at 120 V for 2 h at room temperature. The gel was stained with Coomassie Brilliant Blue G-250.

2.3   Final Polishing (Removal of Contaminating Affinity Tag)

After GST-tag removal ETA was separated from GST tag which, although cleaved off, still remained in the sample. The common way to remove GST is to first remove excess of reduced glutathione by dialysis and second to remove the GST by another step of affinity chromatography on Glutathione Sepharose. In our case a more convenient way was to make use of significant difference in charge between ETA and GST and separate the proteins by ion-exchange chromatography. Such procedure did not necessitate the dialysis and was therefore shorter. Ion-exchange chromatography separates proteins based on their molecular charge. The protein preparation was loaded on the Mono Q column directly after cleavage. ETA does not bind in the utilized conditions and pure preparation is recovered in column flow through. GST is latter removed using salt (NaCl) gradient. The proteins were detected with online UV spectrophotometer [Figure 5A]. The quality and purity of fractions was assessed by SDS-PAGE-electrophoresis [Figure 5B].

The protein concentration was determined in the fraction containing ETA. The preparation was aliquoted, appropriately labeled and frozen at -20°C for further use. It is most important to appropriately label all preparations at least with the name of the protein, its concentration and lot number. The lot number should correspond to a certificate of analysis to be carefully preserved in the laboratory notebook including the chromatogram from the last chromatography step, the buffer the preparation was frozen in, the protein concentration and the method of determination thereof (as the results will significantly differ with different methods), SDS-PAGE analysis and activity analysis (see below). The value of appropriate analysis of protein preparations and keeping track of every lot number cannot be overestimated. Some preparations are used months or even years after purification and results of multiple studies depend on the initial quality. Do always keep the quality of protein preparations high and traceable!

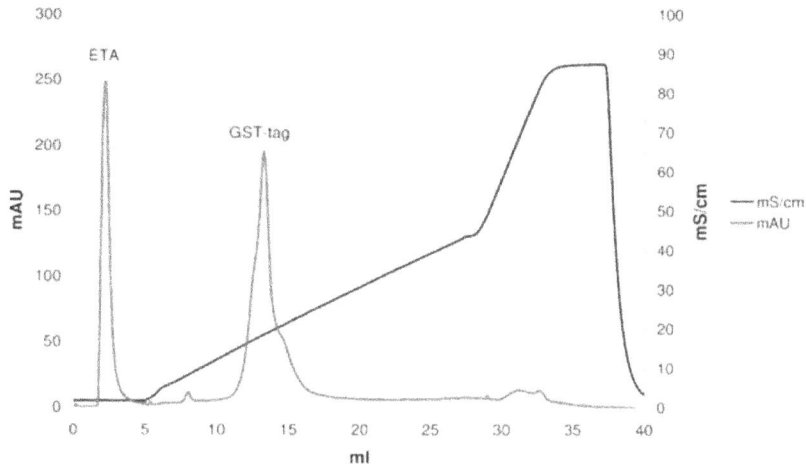

(A)

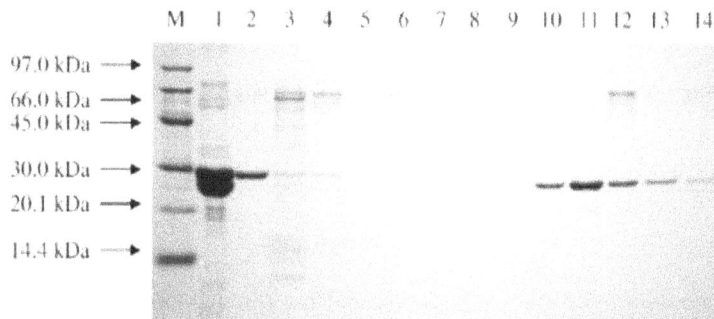

(B)

Figure 5: Ion exchange separation of GST and ETA after fusion protein processing with thrombin. *Panel A*: Ion-exchange chromatogram of ETA purification on MonoQ in Tris-HCl pH 8.0 (elution using NaCl gradient). The peaks containing unbound ETA and NaCl gradient eluted GST are marked. *Panel B*: SDS-PAGE analysis of fractions obtained from anion-exchange chromatography depicted in panel A. Lanes: M - low molecular weight marker, 1 - GST and ETA mixture directly after cleavage with thrombin as loaded on the column, 2- unbound ETA, 3-8 intermediate fractions, 9 – 14 eluted GST-tag.

2.4   ETA Activity Assay

As we already know both ETA and ETB exhibit low but nonetheless easily detectable *N-t*-butoxycarbonyl L-glutamic acid α-phenyl (boc-L-Glu-*O*-phenyl) esterase activity. It has been demonstrated that the esterase activity correlates with exfoliation capability in a mouse model (Dancer *et al.*, 1991). Therefore esterase activity has been used by many researchers to determine the quality of toxin preparations – an assay much less time consuming than animal experiment and moreover providing not only qualitative or semi quantitative, but truly quantitative measure of activity. Procedure of the esterase assay is provided below:

1. Prepare 500mM *N-t*-butoxycarbonyl L-glutamic acid α-phenyl ester (Fluka, 15115) in 1,4-dioxane

2. Add five microliters of 500 mM substrate to 1ml samples containing different concentrations of ETA (0, 5, 10 and 15µg/ml) in 20 mM Tris/phosphate buffer (pH 7.8).

3. Record the absorbance of the samples at 270nm after 5 minutes. [Figure 6].

Esterase avtivity of ETA

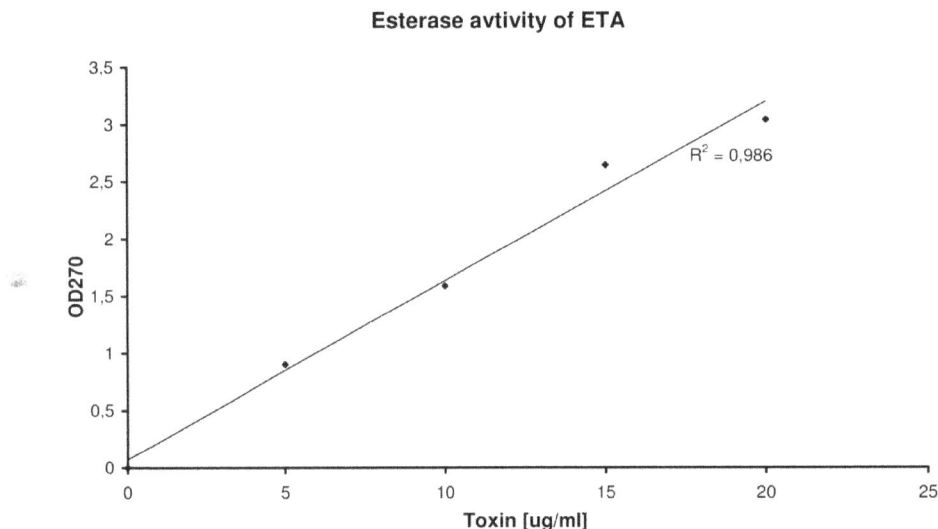

Figure 6: Esterase activity of ETA. ETA preparation was tested for esterolytic activity with the use of *N*-t-Boc-L-Glutamic acid α-phenyl ester as a substrate. Esterase activity was measured spectrophotometrically as changes of absorbance at 270 nm.

3   Conclusions

In this chapter were described the basic properties of epidermolytic toxins, proteases responsible for the symptoms of Staphylococcal Scalded Skin Syndrome a condition characterized by intraepidermal separation of outer layers of the skin. The toxins are serine proteases with extremely high substrate specificity. The exfoliation of the epidermis occurs due to hydrolysis of desmoglein-1 which is a calcium-binding transmembrane glycoprotein.

We present step-by-step methodology for obtaining proteolytically active toxin in a heterologous expression system and methods for quantitative determination of toxin activity. The presented procedures facilitate further research on exfoliative toxins which will not only allow us to better understand the pathogenesis of SSSS, but also provide useful information on normal skin physiology and other toxin-mediated diseases.

Acknowledgements

This work was supported in part by grant IP2011 010871 form the Polish Ministry of Science and Higher Education (to GD). We acknowledge the financial support from the European Union structural funds (grants POIG.02.01.00-12-064/08 and POIG.02.01.00-12-167/08).

References

Aalfs, A. S., D. A. Oktarina, et al. (2010). "Staphylococcal scalded skin syndrome: loss of desmoglein 1 in patient skin." Eur J Dermatol 20(4): 451-456.

Adesiyun, A. A., W. Lenz, et al. (1991). "Exfoliative toxin production by Staphylococcus aureus strains isolated from animals and human beings in Nigeria." Microbiologica 14(4): 357-362.

Amagai, M., N. Matsuyoshi, et al. (2000). "Toxin in bullous impetigo and staphylococcal scalded-skin syndrome targets desmoglein 1." Nat Med 6(11): 1275-1277.

Amagai, M., T. Yamaguchi, et al. (2002). "Staphylococcal exfoliative toxin B specifically cleaves desmoglein 1." J Invest Dermatol 118(5): 845-850.

Arbuthnott, J. P., J. Kent, et al. (1971). "Toxic epidermal necrolysis produced by an extracellular product of Staphylococcus aureus." Br J Dermatol 85(2): 145-149.

Arnemann, J., K. H. Sullivan, et al. (1993). "Stratification-related expression of isoforms of the desmosomal cadherins in human epidermis." J Cell Sci 104 (Pt 3): 741-750.

Bailey, C. J., J. de Azavedo, et al. (1980). "A comparative study of two serotypes of epidermolytic toxin from Staphylococcus aureus." Biochim Biophys Acta 624(1): 111-120.

Bailey, C. J. and M. B. Redpath (1992). "The esterolytic activity of epidermolytic toxins." Biochem J 284 (Pt 1): 177-180.

Bailey, C. J. and T. P. Smith (1990). "The reactive serine residue of epidermolytic toxin A." Biochem J 269(2): 535-537.

Cribier, B., Y. Piemont, et al. (1994). "Staphylococcal scalded skin syndrome in adults. A clinical review illustrated with a new case." J Am Acad Dermatol 30(2 Pt 2): 319-324.

Dancer, S. J., R. Garratt, et al. (1990). "The epidermolytic toxins are serine proteases." FEBS Lett 268(1): 129-132.

Dancer, S. J. and W. C. Noble (1991). "Nasal, axillary, and perineal carriage of Staphylococcus aureus among women: identification of strains producing epidermolytic toxin." J Clin Pathol 44(8): 681-684.

Dinges, M. M., P. M. Orwin, et al. (2000). "Exotoxins of Staphylococcus aureus." Clin Microbiol Rev 13(1): 16-34.

de Azavedo, J. and J. P. Arbuthnott (1981). "Prevalence of epidermolytic toxin in clinical isolates of Staphylococcus aureus." J Med Microbiol 14(3): 341-344.

Eyre, R. W. and J. R. Stanley (1987). "Human autoantibodies against a desmosomal protein complex with a calcium-sensitive epitope are characteristic of pemphigus foliaceus patients." J Exp Med 165(6): 1719-1724.

Feldman, S. R. (1993). "Bullous dermatoses associated with systemic disease." Dermatol Clin 11(3): 597-609.

Funakoshi, T. and A. S. Payne (2010). "Cleavage isn't everything: potential novel mechanisms of exfoliative toxin-mediated blistering." Am J Pathol 177(6): 2682-2684.

Gemmell, C. G. (1995). "Staphylococcal scalded skin syndrome." J Med Microbiol 43(5): 318-327.

Hanakawa, Y., N. M. Schechter, et al. (2002). "Molecular mechanisms of blister formation in bullous impetigo and staphylococcal scalded skin syndrome." J Clin Invest 110(1): 53-60.

Hanakawa, Y., N. M. Schechter, et al. (2004). "Enzymatic and molecular characteristics of the efficiency and specificity of exfoliative toxin cleavage of desmoglein 1." J Biol Chem 279(7): 5268-5277.

Hanakawa, Y., T. Selwood, et al. (2003). "Calcium-dependent conformation of desmoglein 1 is required for its cleavage by exfoliative toxin." J Invest Dermatol 121(2): 383-389.

Iandolo, J. J. (1989). "Genetic analysis of extracellular toxins of Staphylococcus aureus." Annu Rev Microbiol 43: 375-402.

Johnson, A. D., L. Spero, et al. (1979). "Purification and characterization of different types of exfoliative toxin from Staphylococcus aureus." Infect Immun 24(3): 679-684.

Johnson, W. M., S. D. Tyler, et al. (1991). "Detection of genes for enterotoxins, exfoliative toxins, and toxic shock syndrome toxin 1 in Staphylococcus aureus by the polymerase chain reaction." J Clin Microbiol 29(3): 426-430.

Kapral, F. A. and M. M. Miller (1971). "Product of Staphylococcus aureus responsible for the scalded-skin syndrome." Infect Immun 4(5): 541-545.

Kondo, I., S. Sakurai, et al. (1975). "Two serotypes of exfoliatin and their distribution in staphylococcal strains isolated from patients with scalded skin syndrome." J Clin Microbiol 1(5): 397-400.

Ladhani, S., C. L. Joannou, et al. (1999). "Clinical, microbial, and biochemical aspects of the exfoliative toxins causing staphylococcal scalded-skin syndrome." Clin Microbiol Rev 12(2): 224-242.

Lee, C. Y., J. J. Schmidt, et al. (1987). "Sequence determination and comparison of the exfoliative toxin A and toxin B genes from Staphylococcus aureus." J Bacteriol 169(9): 3904-3909.

Lichty, J. J., J. L. Malecki, et al. (2005). "Comparison of affinity tags for protein purification." Protein Expr Purif 41(1): 98-105.

Lyell, A. (1967). "A review of toxic epidermal necrolysis in Britain." Br J Dermatol 79(12): 662-671.

Lyell, A. (1973). "Toxic epidermal necrolysis." Nurs Mirror Midwives J 136(2): 42-45.

Melish, M. E. and L. A. Glasgow (1970). "The staphylococcal scalded-skin syndrome." N Engl J Med 282(20): 1114-1119.

Megevand, C., A. Gervaix, et al. (2009). "Molecular epidemiology of the nasal colonization by methicillin-susceptible Staphylococcus aureus in Swiss children." Clin Microbiol Infect 16(9): 1414-1420.

Melish, M. E. and L. A. Glasgow (1971). "Staphylococcal scalded skin syndrome: the expanded clinical syndrome." J Pediatr 78(6): 958-967.

Melish, M. E., L. A. Glasgow, et al. (1972). "The staphylococcal scalded-skin syndrome: isolation and partial characterization of the exfoliative toxin." J Infect Dis 125(2): 129-140.

Noguchi, N., H. Nakaminami, et al. (2006). "Antimicrobial agent of susceptibilities and antiseptic resistance gene distribution among methicillin-resistant Staphylococcus aureus isolates from patients with impetigo and staphylococcal scalded skin syndrome." J Clin Microbiol 44(6): 2119-2125.

O'Toole, P. W. and T. J. Foster (1986). "Molecular cloning and expression of the epidermolytic toxin A gene of Staphylococcus aureus." Microb Pathog 1(6): 583-594.

O'Toole, P. W. and T. J. Foster (1987). "Nucleotide sequence of the epidermolytic toxin A gene of Staphylococcus aureus." J Bacteriol 169(9): 3910-3915.

Papageorgiou, A. C., L. R. Plano, et al. (2000). "Structural similarities and differences in Staphylococcus aureus exfoliative toxins A and B as revealed by their crystal structures." Protein Sci 9(3): 610-618.

Prevost, G., S. Rifai, et al. (1991). "Functional evidence that the Ser-195 residue of staphylococcal exfoliative toxin A is essential for biological activity." Infect Immun 59(9): 3337-3339.

Proft, T. (2009). "Microbial Toxins: Current Research and Future Trends." Caister Academic Press: Norfolk, UK. (pp. 147–166).

Sila, J., P. Sauer, et al. (2009). "Comparison of the prevalence of genes coding for enterotoxins, exfoliatins, panton-valentine leukocidin and tsst-1 between methicillin-resistant and methicillin-susceptible isolates of Staphylococcus aureus at the university hospital in Olomouc." Biomed Pap Med Fac Univ Palacky Olomouc Czech Repub 153(3): 215-218.

Simpson, C. L., S. Kojima, et al. (2010). "Plakoglobin rescues adhesive defects induced by ectodomain truncation of the desmosomal cadherin desmoglein 1: implications for exfoliative toxin-mediated skin blistering." Am J Pathol 177(6): 2921-2937.

Vath, G. M., C. A. Earhart, et al. (1997). "The structure of the superantigen exfoliative toxin A suggests a novel regulation as a serine protease." Biochemistry 36(7): 1559-1566.

Vath, G. M., C. A. Earhart, et al. (1999). "The crystal structure of exfoliative toxin B: a superantigen with enzymatic activity." Biochemistry 38(32): 10239-10246.

Von Rittershain, G.R. (1878). "Die exfoliative dermatitis jungener senglinge" Z. Kinderheilks. 2, 3-23.

Wiley, B. B. and M. Rogolsky (1977). "Molecular and serological differentiation of staphylococcal exfoliative toxin synthesized under chromosomal and plasmid control." Infect Immun 18(2): 487-494.

Yamaguchi, T., Y. Yokota, et al. (2002). "Clonal association of Staphylococcus aureus causing bullous impetigo and the emergence of new methicillin-resistant clonal groups in Kansai district in Japan." J Infect Dis 185(10): 1511-1516.

Production of Extremophilic Proteins using *Escherichia coli*-based Expression Systems

Rushyannah R. Killens-Cade, Rebecca L. Kitchener, Stephanie L. Mathews,
Steven Schreck, Mikyoung L. Ji, Rachel Turner, Christine MacInnes,
Amy M. Grunden

Department of Microbiology
North Carolina State University, USA

1   Introduction

Many industrial and biotechnological applications utilize biocatalysts or enzymes. Due to the harsh nature of some of these processes, there is an increasing demand for enzymes that can not only withstand but thrive in extreme environmental conditions such as high or low temperatures, pH, salinity, pressure, high metal concentrations, high radiation, oxygen deprivation, or lack of water and nutrients (Gomes and Steiner, 2004). Extremophilic microorganisms, or extremophiles, are capable of surviving in these extreme environments. To date, most known extremophiles are archaea; however, in recent years, extremophilic bacteria and eukaryotic species have been identified and characterized (van den Burg, 2003).

Biocatalysts isolated from these organisms are termed extremozymes and have significant potential for use in agricultural, chemical, biomedical and biotechnological processes as they are stable and active under extreme conditions. By studying these extremozymes, several common factors that lead to their enhanced stability have been identified. Changes in amino acid residues in key locations, ionic interactions, oligomerization, surface charges, and catalytic mechanisms have been identified in extremophilic enzymes (Demirjian *et al.*, 2001). While there is a growing commercial demand for extremozymes, the fact that the organisms that produce them cannot grow under so-called "normal" laboratory fermentation conditions presents a challenge. Specialized bioreactors do exist for this purpose and have been utilized; however, production of these enzymes can be further optimized by cloning and over-expression of the extremophilic genes that code for them in suitable mesophilic hosts (van den Burg, 2003). In most cases, cloning and over-expression of enzymes in mesophilic systems does not affect conformation or activity of the enzyme (de Miguel Bouzas *et al.*, 2006). A majority of recombinant extremozymes currently in use have been produced in *Escherichia coli* although *Bacillus*, *Pseudomonas*, *Lactobacillus*, and *Lactococcus* have also proved to be acceptable expression systems (van den Burg, 2003). Eukaryotic host systems such as the yeast *Pichia* have been successfully employed as well.

Psychrophilic or psychrotolerant organisms are found living in environments where temperatures never exceed 5°C, such as polar regions, oceans, and the upper atmosphere (Gomes and Steiner, 2004). There is industrial interest in reducing energy consumption by using low temperature operation and cold active enzymes that have the commercial potential to optimize detergents (enabling cold washing), milk processing, textile finishing, brewing, cheese-making and animal feeds (Demirjian *et al.*, 2001). Additionally, their use in bioremediation strategies of solids and water polluted with hydrocarbons and oils has been proposed (Gomes and Steiner, 2004, van den Burg, 2003). Molecular adaptations in psychrophilic enzymes such as decreased ionic interactions, decreased core hydrophobicity, decreased hydrogen bonds, reduced disulfide bridges, reduced oligomerization and increased surface hydrophobicity allow them to function at lower temperatures when compared to their mesophilic counterparts (Cavicchioli *et al.*, 2011). At lower temperatures these enzymes are more flexible overall which enhances their catalytic ability (Gomes and Steiner, 2004).

In this chapter, we provide over-expression, purification and biochemical characterization methods for an antioxidant enzyme, glutathione reductase, from *Colwellia psychrerythraea*, which is a strictly psychrophilic gamma proteobacteria found in cold marine environments such as Arctic and Antarctic sea ice (Demming *et al.*, 1998; Junge *et al*, 2002). *C. psychrerythraea* potentially has to contend with high levels of reactive oxygen species (ROS) as a result of exposure to high UV-light in its native environment (Mock and Thomas, 2005). In order to cope with the oxygen toxicity, several antioxidant enzyme-encoding genes are found in the *C. psychrerythraea* genome (Methe et al., 2005). One of these genes codes for the antioxidant enzyme glutathione reductase which reduces oxidized glutathione (GSSG) to form reduced glutathione (GSH) (Scrutton *et al.*, 1987). Reduced forms of glutathione provide protection from oxygen induced cellular damage, generation of DNA precursors as well as maintenance of reduced thiol groups (Holmgren, 1976; Kehrer and Lund, 1994).

As with psychrophiles, thermophilic organisms are classified based on their optimal growth temperatures. Thermophiles are organisms that grow above 55°C while hyperthermophiles require temperatures above 80°C for optimal growth (de Miguel Bouzas *et al.*, 2006). Thermoactive or thermostable enzymes are used in the detergent, food, feed, starch, textile, leather, pulp and paper and pharmaceutical industries (Gomes and Steiner, 2004). Thermoactive enzymes have several advantages over their mesophilic counterparts such as improved solubility of reaction components due to elevated temperatures, increased resistance to contamination during reactions, and higher reaction rates, but perhaps the most notable advantage is the relative ease of the purification process during production. When the enzyme is expressed in a mesophilic host, a heat treatment step used before column purification can denature most host cell proteins and allow for their subsequent removal by centrifugation. On a molecular level, thermoactive proteins exhibit increased ionic interaction and hydrogen bonds, increased hydrophobicity, and decreased flexibility at elevated temperatures which contribute to increased stability with respect to mesophilic enzymes (Gomes and Steiner, 2004).

One of the types of thermophilic enzymes which are of particular industrial interest are proteases, with proteases constituting more than 65% of the enzymes utilized in industrial applications (Rao *et al.*, 1998). Proteases are classified into two groups: endopeptidases, which cleave peptide bonds within a protein and exopeptidases, which cleave amino acids located at the termini. Proteolytic enzymes from thermophilic bacteria and archaea have been shown to retain their catalytic properties in the presence of detergents, denaturants such as urea and dithiothreitol and high temperatures making them sturdy biocatalysts in industrial reactions (de Miguel Bouzas *et al.*, 2006).

One particular type of thermostable protease with a variety of industrial and medical applications are the proline dipeptidases, or prolidases, from *Pyrococcus horikoshii* that function *in vivo* at 98–100°C to hydrolyze dipeptides with a prolyl residue in the C-terminus and a non-polar amino acid residue in the N-terminus (Theriot *et al.*, 2011). Prolidases can also hydrolyze organophosphorus (OP) compounds found in many pesticides and chemical warfare agents (CWAs). Organophosphorus acid anhydrolase (OPAA) isolated from *Alteromonas* sp. JD6.5 is a prolidase with optimal activity at 50°C that has been utilized successfully in nerve agent detoxification strategies; however, the enzyme is limited by decreased stability at increased temperatures as well as in the presence of solvents and denaturants (Cheng *et al.*, 1993). The prolidases from *P. horikoshii* are highly thermostable at 90°C for extended periods of time and have shown activity against the nerve agents soman and DFP at a broad range of temperatures and pH making them appealing candidates for incorporation into field applications such as enzyme cocktails used for OP decontamination (Theriot *et al.*, 2011). In this chapter, methods for the cloning, over-expression, purification and biochemical characterization of two *P. horikoshii* prolidases (PH1149 and PH0974) are presented.

Another industrial application area that benefits from thermoactive and thermostable enzymes is that of plant biomass deconstruction to produce sugar streams for biofuel generation. Plant biomass is predominantly composed of cellulose, hemicellulose, lignin, and pectin. Cellulose is the most abundant component of plant cell walls and is composed of D-glucose linked by β-1,4-glucosidic bonds. (Jorgensen *et al.*, 2007) Efficient cellulose degradation is a complex process that involves the combined action of at least three enzymes: exo-1,4-β-D-glucanases (cellobiohydrolase), endo-1,4-β-D-glucanases (endoglucanase), and 1,4-β-D-glucosidases. Cellulase enzymes are used commercially in the fermentation of cellulosic biomass to biofuels, in the processing of coffee, in the textile industry, as an additive in laundry detergents, as well as in the pulp and paper industry. However, cellulase enzyme efficiency is often an obstacle for application in these areas. One such example is found in cellulosic biofuel production; pre-treatment strategies aim to increase enzymatic convertibility and most methods heat the biomass to 100-200°C, making it one of the most energy intensive steps in the process (Jorgenesen *et al.*, 2007). Often high temperatures used in this step inhibit enzyme efficiency during the subsequent steps in biofuel production. Thermostable cellulase enzymes are in high demand in the cellulosic biofuel production, paper, and laundry manufacturing industries.

Sulfolobus solfataricus is an acidophilic thermophile. This archaeon has optimal growth at pH 2-4 and temperature of 80°C (She *et al.*, 2001). The gene *sso1354* is homologous to other endoglucanase genes in the glycosyl hydrolase family 12. Family 12 enzymes catalyze the hydrolysis of β-1,4, glucosidic linkages in cellulose and arabinoxylans. Endoglucanases cleave bonds within the cellulose chain producing smaller cellulose units that are more accessible to enzymatic degradation. An endoglucanase that has high activity at 80°C and low pH would lend itself well to industrial applications, and the cloning, over-expression, purification, and biochemical characterization methods for *S. sulfolobus* sso1354 (CelA) endoglucanase are included in this chapter.

Recently extremophilic lipases, including thermostable lipases, have also been intensively studied, especially for use in biofuel production applications. The biological function of lipases is to catalyze the hydrolysis of the ester bonds of triglycerides, resulting in free fatty acids, monoglycerides, diglycerides, and glycerol (Gupta *et al.*, 2004). In addition to their natural function as carboxylesterases, lipases also catalyze ester synthesis, inter-esterification, alcoholysis, and acidolysis (Kademi *et al.*, 2005). Besides being lipolytic, lipases are attractive versatile biocatalysts because they are (1) highly stable in organic solvents, (2) do not require cofactors, (3) possess a very diverse substrate range, (4) act under mild conditions, and (5) exhibit a high chemoselectivity, regionselectivity, and enanioselectivity (Jaeger and Reetz, 1998).

Although lipases are ubiquitous in nature, microbial lipases (yeast, fungal and bacterial) are commercially significant due to the versatility of their applied properties and ease of mass production (Hasan and Shah, 2009). They play vital roles in manufacturing of detergent, food, leather, textiles, cosmetics, and paper. Lipases are important components in many industrial laundry and house-hold detergent formulations based on their ability to hydrolyze fatty stains on surfaces, leaving no harmful residue. In addition to using the hydrolytic application of lipases for flavor development, the food industry also relies on the biolipolysis process for the production of leaner meat. In the paper industry, lipases are used to remove the pitch, or hydrophobic components of wood, from the pulp produced for paper manufacturing.

In addition to the novel biotechnological applications of using lipases in detergent formulations, food processing, and paper production, one prospective use of lipases is the conversion of microalgal lipids into free fatty acids, a vital step in the production of microalgae-derived biofuel. With the dwindling supply of fossil fuels, there has been a push towards creating renewable biofuels, and algae have emerged as a promising alternative. However, for algae to be a truly viable alternative, the process of creating biofuels must be more efficient. One way to increase efficiency is to transform algae with thermostable lipases, which will be expressed during the high temperature conversion of lipids to fuel. At high temperatures, the lipases will become active and release the fatty acids previously sequestered during cell growth as part of algal phospholipid membranes. Specifically, we have recombinantly expressed and characterized a lipase from the thermophilic archeaon *Metallosphaera sedula* DSM5348, which is a thermoacidophilic archaeon originally isolated from an acidic drain of a hot water pond at Pisciarelli Solfatara (near

Naples, Italy) that grows optimally at a temperature of 75°C and within a pH range of 1.0 and 4.5 (Huber *et al.*, 1989).

Since some of the most promising algae biofuel production systems feature marine (halophilic) algae, algae-derived biofuel systems could also benefit from the development of suitable lipases meant to function in high salt environments. Halophilic organisms are found in hypersaline environments such as the Dead Sea and the Great Salt Lake. Enzymes from these organisms are exposed to salt concentrations as high as 4 and 5 M, and exhibit several biochemical adaptations such as increased acidic amino acid residues on their surfaces and reduced surface hydrophobicity to decrease aggregation tendencies (Gomes and Steiner, 2004). Currently, halophilic microorganisms are used in the production of solar salt (production of salt from evaporation of shallow ponds), fermented foods, β-carotene, osmotic solutes such as ectoine, and in saline wastewater treatment (Oren, 2010). Herein the methods for the cloning, over-expression, purification and biochemical characterization of lipases from the halophilic bacterium *Chromohalobacter salexigens* are described.

2   Cold-active Antioxidant Enzyme (Glutathione Reductase)

2.1   Bacterial Strains, Plasmids, Enzymes, and Reagents

The *Colwellia psychrerythraea* (Cps) 34H strain was obtained from American Type Culture collection (ATCC), and grown in marine broth 2216 (Difco laboratories, Detroit, MI) at 4°C for 85-96 h with shaking at 180 rpm in order to isolate the genomic DNA. *C. psychrerythraea* cells were harvested by centrifugation, washed with 50 mM potassium phosphate buffer, pH 7.8 and stored at -20°C until used for genomic DNA (gDNA) isolation. *C. psychrerythraea* 34H gDNA was isolated using the Ultra Clean Microbial DNA Isolation Kit from MOBIO Laboratories (Carlsbad, CA). For cloning and maintaining the recombinant protein, *Escherichia coli* XL1-Blue was used. *E. coli gor* mutant strain, MLJ600 [BL21 (λDE3) ΔGOR] produced in A. Grunden's lab, was used for over-expression of recombinant protein. pET21b from Novagen, EMD Biosciences (Madison, WI) served as the expression vector for *C. psychrerythraea* glutathione reductase production. Restriction endonucleases and T4 ligase were purchased from New England Biolabs, Inc. (Ipswitch, MA). DNA Pfu polymerase was purchased from Stratagene (Santa Clara, CA). QIAquick PCR Purification Kit, QIAquick Gel Extraction Kit, and QIAGEN Plasmid Mini Prep Kit were purchased from Qiagen (Valencia, CA) for cloning the gene. The YP-30 Centricon centrifugal filter from Millipore (Billerica, MA) was used for concentrating the recombinant protein. The following chromatography columns were used for purification: 20-ml HiPrep 16/10 DEAE FF, 5-ml HiTrap Phenyl FF and 5-ml Blue Sepharose™ from GE Healthcare Life Sciences (Piscataway, NJ). ß-nicotinamide adenine dinucleotide phosphate, NADPH, the oxidized form of glutathione (GSSG), and glutathione reductase from baker's yeast were purchased from Sigma-Aldrich.

2.2   Cloning of a Cold-active Glutathione Reductase from *C. psychrerythraea*

The *C. psychrerythraea* glutathione reductase gene was amplified with polymerase chain reaction (PCR) using the following primers targeted to Cps 34H gDNA: forward primer containing an *Nde*I site (shown in bold): 5'-**CTAATG**AGTGAACATATGACACAACAT-3' and reverse primer containing a *Sac*I site (shown in bold): 5'-GCAATCAACATT**GAGCTC**GCTTTA-3. The following PCR amplification program was used: 40 cycles consisting of denaturation at 95°C for 1 min, annealing at 56°C for 2 min, and extension at 72°C for 2 min. The glutathione reductase (GR) gene was amplified using *Pfu* polymerase. The amplified PCR product was digested with *Nde*I and *Sac*I restriction enzymes and purified by gel extraction and finally ligated into the *Nde*I-*Sac*I site of plasmid pET21b downstream of T7 promoter. The resulting plasmid construct was transformed into *E. coli* XL1 Blue chemically competent cells. Plasmid DNA was isolated from the transformants using a plasmid mini-prep kit, and the plasmids were screened for inserts by visualization of DNA agarose gels. The cloned GR gene sequence was verified by MWG Biotech (Huntsville, AL).

2.3 Over-expression of a Recombinant Cold-active Glutathione Reductase from *C. psychrerythraea*

The sequence-verified clones were transformed into *E. coli gor* mutant strain, MLJ600 [BL21 (λDE3) ΔGOR]. The transformants were grown overnight at 37°C for large scale over-expression. The *E. coli* mutant MLJ600 cells harboring the recombinant *C. psychrerythraea* glutathione reductase were inoculated to into a 1-L culture for large scale expression. The cultures were incubated at room temperature for 36 h with shaking at 125 rpm in lactose auto-induction media (Studier, 2005) that was supplemented with ampicillin (100 μg/ml). Over-expressed cultures were harvested, and the cell pellets were stored frozen at -80°C.

2.4 Recombinant Cold-active Glutathione Reductase Purification

All of the enzyme purification steps were performed with buffers chilled to 4°C in an ice bath to minimize thermolability. The cell pellets were resuspended in 50 mM Tris-HCl, pH 8.0 with 1 mM EDTA and 1 mM benzamidine and the cell suspensions were passed through a French pressure cell twice at 20,000 psi. The lysed cell suspension was centrifuged in a Sorval GS-3 rotor at 20,000 x g for 30 min to remove cell debris and was filtered using a 0.45 μm syringe filter. The cell extract was applied to a 20-ml HiPrep 16/10 DEAE Sepharose anion exchange column at a flow rate of 1 ml/min equilibrated with binding buffer [50 mM Tris-HCl, pH 8.0 with 1 mM ethylenediaminetetraacetic acid (EDTA)] for the purification. The loaded column was washed with 3 column volumes (CV) of binding buffer to remove any loosely bound protein. 50 mM Tris-HCl, pH 8.0 with 1 mM EDTA and 1 M ammonium sulfate [$(NH_4)_2SO_4$] was used to elute the recombinant glutathione reductase. Glutathione reductase was eluted at a flow rate of 1 ml/min into 4-ml fractions. Fractions containing glutathione reductase were visualized using sodium dodecylsulfate polyacrylamide gel electrophoresis (SDS-PAGE), and were dialyzed into 50 mM Tris-HCl, pH 8.0 with 1 mM EDTA overnight at 4°C. The sample was reapplied to a 5-ml phenyl-sepharose hydrophobic interaction chromatography (HIC) column equilibrated with 50 mM Tris-HCl, pH 8.0, 1 mM EDTA, 1 M $(NH_4)_2SO_4$ and eluted with 50 mM Tris-HCl, pH 8.0, 1 mM EDTA. The flow-through was collected and concentrated using a YP30 Centricon concentrator. The concentrated sample was reapplied to a 5-ml Blue Sepharose™ affinity column equilibrated with 50 mM potassium phosphate (KH_2PO_4), pH 7.0 with 1 mM EDTA and eluted with 50 mM KH_2PO_4, pH 7.0, 1.5 M KCl, and 1 mM EDTA. A Blue Sepharose column was chosen for the purification of glutathione reductase because the protein contains the cofactor ($NADP^+$) which can bind with high affinity to Blue Sepharose resin. The fractions containing glutathione reductase were collected and concentrated using a YP-30 Centricon concentrator. The *C. psychrerythraea* glutathione reductase over-expression and purification scheme is presented in Figure 1. An image of the SDS-PAGE showing the various steps for the *C. psychrerythraea* glutathione reductase purification is shown in Figure 2.

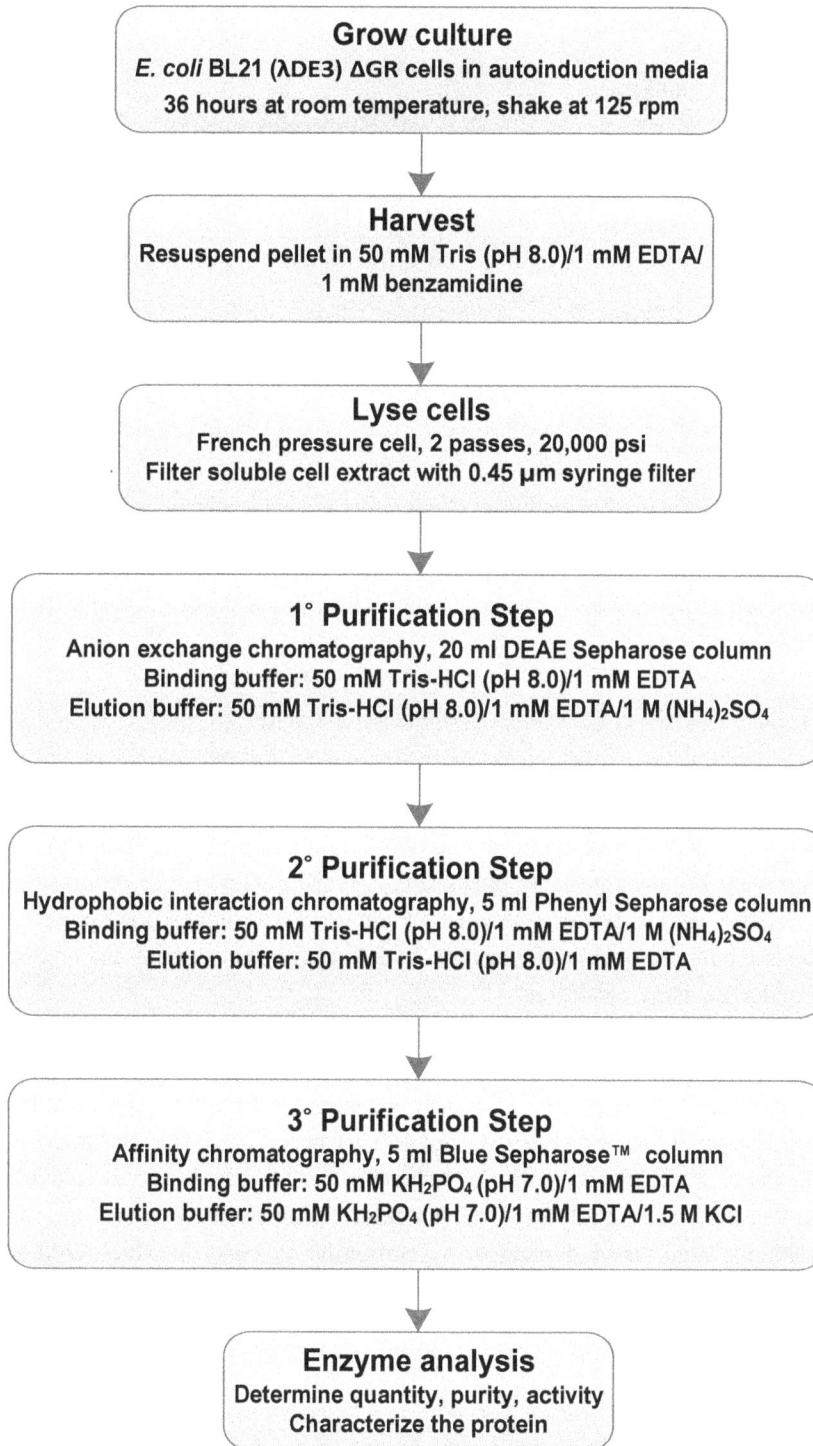

Figure 1: Over-expression and purification steps for recombinant *C. psychrerythraea* glutathione reductase.

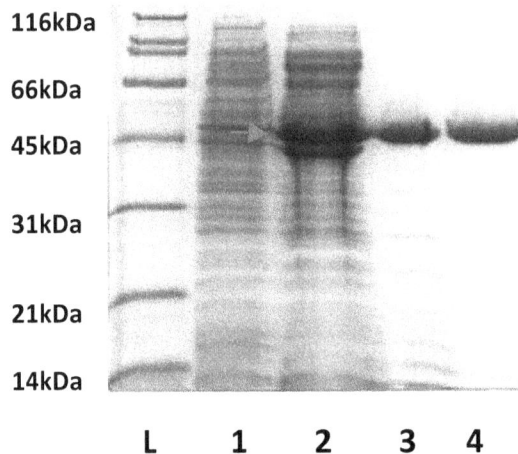

Figure 2: Protein purification of recombinant *C. psychrerythraea* glutathione reductase. L: Molecular Weight Marker, Lane 1: Cell-free extract, Lane 2: Pooled GR from DEAE sepharose column, Lane 3: Flow through of phenyl-sepharose column, Lane 4: Pooled GR from Blue Sepharose™ column. The arrow indicates expected *C. psychrerythraea* glutathione reductase molecular weight of 49 kDa.

2.5 Recombinant Cold-active Glutathione Reductase Characterization

Glutathione reductase activity was measured spectrophotometrically with a Shimadzu Spectrophotometer UV2401-PC at various temperatures. Mesophilic homologs from baker's yeast along with that of purified *C. psychrerythraea* were used to investigate the activity temperature ranges. In a 3 ml reaction mix, the final concentrations were 75 mM potassium phosphate, 2.6 mM EDTA, 1 mM oxidized glutathione, 0.09 mM NADPH, 0.13% (w/v) bovine serum albumin (www.sigmaaldrich.com/etc/medialib/docs/ .../glutathionereductase.pdf). One unit of enzyme is defined as the amount that oxidizes 1 µmol of NADPH per min under the assay conditions.

Glutathione reductase activity assays (Figure 3) showed that the apparent maximal activity of *C. psychrerythraea* glutathione reductase had shifted and was seen at approximately 20°C lower compared to the glutathione reductase from mesophilic yeast. It is commonly observed that maximal specific activities of psychrophilic enzymes are between 30°C and 40°C (Chen *et al.*, 2011, D'Amico *et al.*, 2006, Feller *et al.*, 1992; Huston *et al.*, 2008). Glutathione reductase from *C. psychrerythraea* exhibited its highest activity 40°C and then declined rapidly at 45°C. Therefore, temperature response presented for *C. psychrerythraea* glutathione reductase is typical of psychrophilic enzymes in which cold activity and heat lability at moderate temperatures is seen (Feller & Gerday, 2003, Huston *et al.*, 2008).

2.6 Considerations for Optimizing Purification of Active *C. psychrerythraea* Glutathione Reductase

C. psychrerythraea glutathione reductase was originally cloned into the pBAD/His vector (Invitrogen) to express the protein with an N-terminal polyhistidine (6x-His) tag for purification using a nickel affinity column. However, it was determined that multi-column chromatography was required for the purification because it was observed that the recombinant *C. psychrerythraea* glutathione reductase was present in the flow-through after applying the cell extract to the nickel column. Ultimately the His-tagged glutathione reductase was determined to be inactive. It has been previously shown that polyhistidine tags can disrupt enzyme activity by altering protein folding (Ueda *et al.*, 2003). To avoid protein inactivation, the *C. psychrerythraea* glutathione reductase was cloned into pET-21b so that an untagged version of the protein could be expressed and purified using the methods described above.

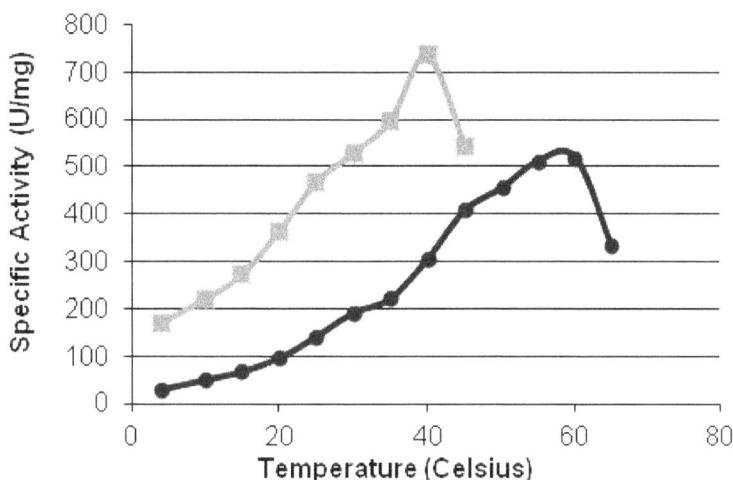

Figure 3: Specific activities for *C. psychrerythraea* glutathione reductase (square) and baker's yeast glutathione reductase (circle) in response to temperature.

3 Thermoactive Peptidase

3.1 Bacterial Strains, Plasmids, Enzymes, and Reagents

Pyrococcus horikoshii gDNA was obtained from ATCC, strain 700860D-5. The T7-polymerase-driven expression vector pET-21b was obtained from Novagen, EMD Biosciences. Primers were designed using MacVector software (Accelrys, San Diego, CA). PCR was carried out using a Bio-Rad thermal cycler (Bio-Rad Laboratories, Inc., Hercules, CA), *P. horikoshii* prolidase-specific primers from Eurofins MWG Operon (Huntsville, AL) and *Pfu* polymerase and dNTPs from Stratagene. The pCR-Script plasmid was obtained from Stratagene and *E. coli* strain XL1-Blue was from Novagen, EMD Biosciences (Madison, WI). Plasmids were sequenced by MWG Biotech. The arginine, leucine, and isoleucine tRNA-encoding plasmid pRIL from Stratagene was used for over-expression of the enzyme in *E. coli* BL21(λDE3) cells from Novagen-EMD Biosciences. The following chromatography columns were utilized for purification: 5-ml Hi-Trap Phenyl HP and 5-ml Hi-Trap Q-FF Column from GE Healthcare Life Sciences. All SDS-PAGE steps utilized 12.5% SDS-polyacrylamide pre-cast gels from Bio-Rad Laboratories, Inc. and were run on the Bio-Rad Mini-PROTEAN® system. Methionyl-proline (Met-Pro) substrate was obtained from Bachem Bioscience, Inc. (King of Prussia, PA).

3.2 Cloning of Thermoactive Peptidases from *Pyrococcus horikoshii*

The genes for *P. horikoshii* prolidase (PH1149) and *P. horikoshii* prolidase homolog 1 (PH0974) were amplified by PCR and cloned into the T7-polymerase-driven expression vector pET-21b (Theriot *et al.*,

2010). For *Ph*prol, the following primers were utilized: forward primer (5'-AAGATCAAGGAGG T**CATATG**GACATAA-3', containing an *Nde*I restriction site shown in bold) and reverse primer (5'-CCTACTA**AAGCTT**GCTAGATGAGTTCTC-3', containing a *Hin*dIII restriction site in bold). *Ph1*prol primers were: forward primer (5'-AAC**CATATG**AGGCTTGAAAAGTTCATTCAC-3', containing an *Nde*I restriction site shown in bold) and reverse primer (5'-TGA**GTCGAC**AGTAGTAGAATAA TAACA-3', containing a *Sal*I restriction site shown in bold). Native *Pyrococcus furiosus* DNA polymerase (0.2 µl) was used for amplification in a 50 µl reaction containing 5.0 µl 10X Taq buffer, 0.4 µl dNTP (25 mM), 0.5 µl forward primer (40 µM), 0.5 µl reverse primer (40 µM), 0.5 µl Taq polymerase and 1.0 µl *P. horikoshii* gDNA (100 ng/µl). The following PCR protocol was used: two initial denaturation cycles for 4 min at 94°C, 1 min at 55°C for annealing, 1 min at 72°C for extension, 39 cycles of 94° for 1 min and a final cycle at 72°C for 7 min. PCR yielded 1.08- and 1.07-kbp products for *Ph*prol and *Ph1*prol, respectively, which were visualized by electrophoresis using a 1% agarose gel.

The *Ph1*prol gene was then cloned into the *Eco*RV site of the expression plasmid yielding the plasmids *Ph*prol-script and *Ph1*prol-script which were transformed into *E. coli* XL1-Blue cells and plated on Luria-Bertani (LB) agar containing ampicillin (100 µg/ml) and X-gal (40 µg/ml). Plates were incubated overnight at 37°C and colonies were selected for plasmid isolation using blue-white screening. Plasmids containing the *Ph* or *Ph1* prolidase inserts were isolated from white colonies and digested with *Nde*I and *Hin*dIII to excise the *Ph*prol gene and *Nde*I and *Sal*I to excise the *Ph1*prol gene. The excised gene was subsequently cloned into the *Nde*I and *Hin*dIII or *Nde*I and *Sal*I sites in the pET-21b expression vector yielding the plasmid pET-*Ph1*prol which was then sent out for sequencing to ensure that the sequence was not altered during the cloning process.

3.3   Over-expression of *P. horikoshii* Prolidase and *P. horikoshii* Prolidase Homolog 1

The *Ph*prol and *Ph1*prol expression plasmids and the pRIL plasmid were transformed into competent *E. coli* BL21(λDE3) cells encoded for isopropyl-β-D-thiogalactopyranoside (IPTG)-inducible expression of T7-RNA polymerase on the chromosome, plated on Luria-Bertani agar (LB) with ampicillin and chloramphenicol, and incubated overnight at 37°C for selection of viable transformants. For large-scale protein expression, a 1-L culture of auto-induction media (Studier, 2005) supplemented with 100 µg/ml of ampicillin and 34 µg/ml of chloramphenicol was inoculated. Cells were grown for 14 h in an incubator-shaker at 37°C and 200 rpm. The cells were harvested by centrifugation and were stored at -80°C. Recombinant protein expression was monitored throughout the over-expression process by SDS-PAGE.

3.4   Recombinant Thermoactive Peptidase Purification

The frozen cell pellet, stored at -80°C, was thawed on ice and resuspended in Tris buffer (50 mM Tris-HCl, pH 8.0) using 3 ml Tris per 1 g of cell paste. 3 µl of both 1 mM benzamidine-HCl and 1 mM DTT were also added per gram of cell paste to prevent degradation by host cell proteases. To recover the protein of interest, diluted cell slurry was passed three times through a French pressure cell at 20,000 psi and kept on ice in between passes to cool the lysate. The lysate was then centrifuged at 38,720 x g for 30 min at 4°C and the supernatant was collected for further recovery. The supernatant was heat-treated at 80°C under anaerobic conditions for 30 min in a water bath to denature most host cell proteins unable to withstand that temperature. Heat-treated supernatant was centrifuged at 38,720 x g for 30 min to remove the denatured protein, and the resulting extract containing the *Ph* or *Ph1* prolidase was collected for purification. Enzyme activity was analyzed in both pre- and post-heat treatment samples.

Prior to the first column purification step, [NH$_4$]$_2$SO$_4$ was added to the extract to a final concentration of 1.5 M. The extract was loaded onto a 5 ml phenyl-sepharose column and purified using 50 mM Tris-HCl pH 8.0 with 1.5 M (NH$_4$)$_2$SO$_4$ as the binding/equilibration buffer and 50 mM Tris-HCl, pH 8.0 as the elution buffer. The protein was eluted using a linear gradient (10-100% elution buffer) and 1-mL fractions were collected throughout the elution process. Wash and flow-through were also collected for testing. All fractions were visualized using SDS-PAGE and were tested to determine enzyme activity. Fractions containing active prolidase were pooled and dialyzed overnight at 4°C into 4 L of 50 mM Tris-HCl, pH 8.0 to remove residual (NH$_4$)$_2$SO$_4$. The prolidase pool was further purified using a 5-ml Q Sepharose™ anion exchange chromatography (AEC) column. The binding/equilibration buffer for AEC was 50 mM Tris-HCl, pH 8.0 and the elution buffer was 50 mM Tris-HCl, pH 8.0, 1 M NaCl. Fractions were again visualized using SDS-PAGE and tested for enzyme activity. Fractions were pooled based on the gel images and the pooled stock was stored at -80°C. Prolidase stock purity was estimated to be greater than 95% by visual inspection of the gel images and electrophoretic microchip analysis.

An image of the SDS-PAGE for the purification of *P. horikoshii* prolidases, *Ph*prol and *Ph1*prol is presented in Figure 4A. The over-expression and purification scheme for the thermophilic protease, endoglucanase, and lipase enzymes is presented in Figure 5.

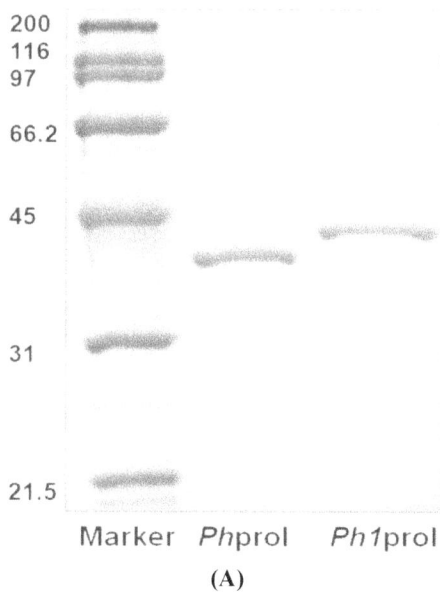

(A)

Sample	*Ph*prol	*Ph1*prol
Cell extract	168 ± 23	219 ± 42
Heat-treated	580 ± 54	395 ± 9
Q-column fractions	1,038 ± 135	1852 ± 256
Recovered protein (mg)	20.2	52.3

(B)

Figure 4: A. 12.5% SDS-PAGE showing purified *P. horikoshii* prolidases, *Ph*prol and *Ph1*prol (1 µg). Molecular marker includes (in kDa): myosin (200), β-galactosidase (116), phosphorylase b (97), serum albumin (66.2), ovalbumin (45), carbonic anhydrase (31), and trypsin inhibitor (21.5). From (Theriot, 2010). **B.** Representative *Ph*prol and *Ph1*prol specific activities throughout the purification process. Prolidase assays were done at 100°C in 50 mM MOPS, pH 7.0 with CoCl$_2$ (1.2 mM) and the substrate Leu-Pro (4 mM). One unit of prolidase activity is defined as the amount of enzyme that liberates one µmole of proline per min. From (Theriot, 2010).

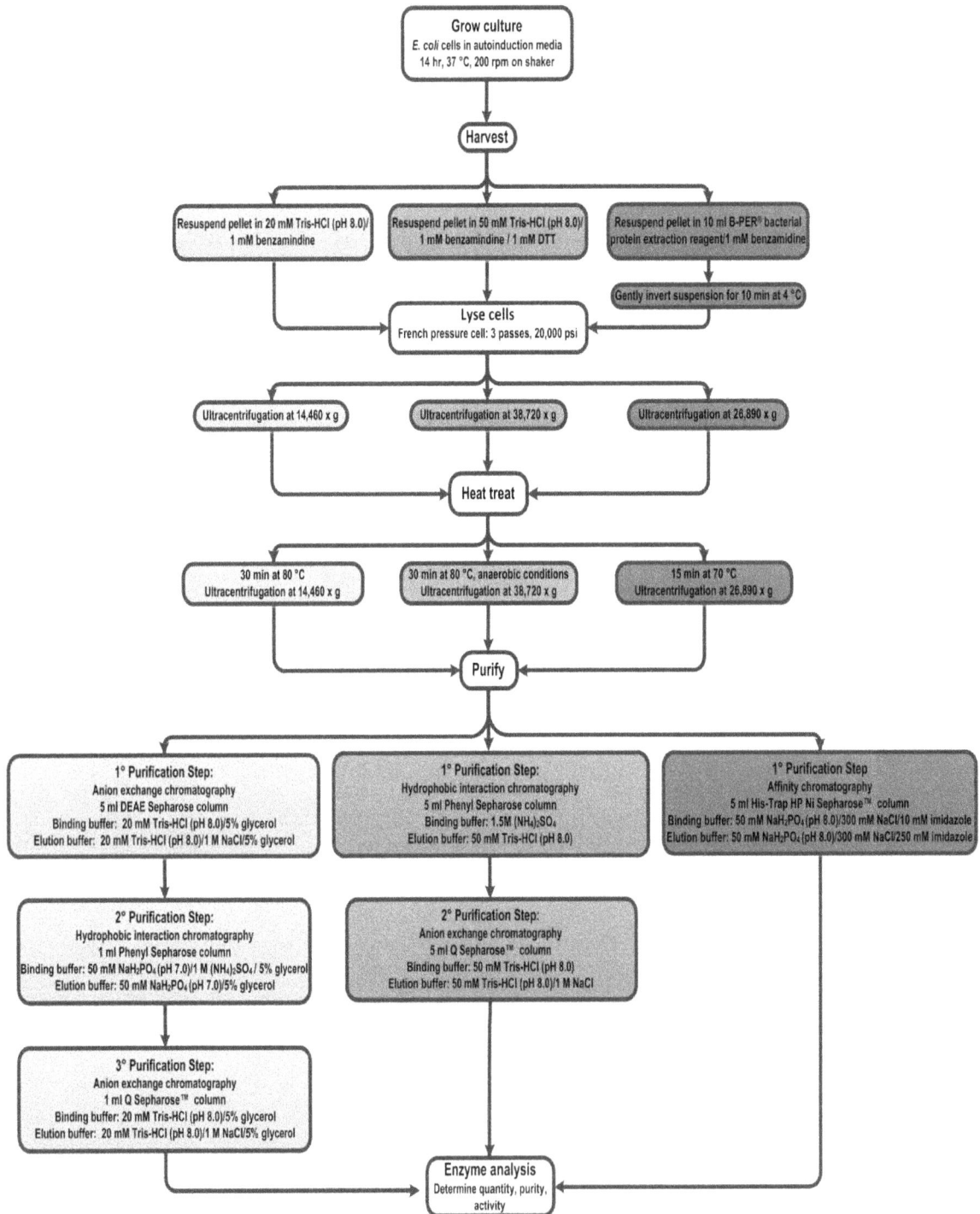

Figure 5: Over-expression and purification steps for recombinant thermophilic prolidase, endoglu-canase and lipase. Steps specific for the thermoactive endoglucanase are shown in light grey, for the thermoactive peptidase in medium grey, and thermoactive lipase in dark grey.

3.5   Recombinant Thermoactive Peptidase Characterization

Prolidase enzyme activity was determined using a modified version of Chinard's original method for photometric determination of free proline (Chinard, 1952, Ghosh et al., 1998). All samples were assayed in triplicate. The assay reaction mixture contained 50 mM 3-[*N*-morpholino] propanesulfonic acid (MOPS) buffer at pH 7.0, 200 mM NaCl, water, 5% (vol/vol) of 50% glycerol, 100 µg/ml bovine serum albumin (BSA), 1.2 mM $CoCl_2$ and enzyme. The reaction mixture was heated at 100°C for 5 min to allow the enzyme and metal to interact. The reaction was initiated by the addition of 4 mM dipeptide substrate Met-Pro and the final reaction volume was 500 µl. The reaction was allowed to proceed at 100°C for 10 min and was stopped by lowering the pH with 500 µl of glacial acetic acid. In order to colorimetrically visualize the free proline left behind by the enzymatic reaction, 500 µl of ninhydrin reagent (3% wt/vol) was added to the reaction mixture and heated for 10 min at 100°C. The reaction was then cooled to room temperature, transferred to plastic cuvettes, and analyzed on a bench-top spectrophotometer measuring absorbance at 515 nm. Data analysis to determine enzyme activity was performed in Microsoft Excel using an extinction coefficient of 4,570 M^{-1} cm^{-1} for the ninhydrin-proline complex. One unit of prolidase activity is defined as the amount of enzyme that hydrolyzes 1 µmol of proline per min and is expressed as U/mg. Full biochemical characterization of *Ph*prol and *Ph1*prol including substrate specificity, temperature and pH profiles, thermostability, metal preference, and kinetics were performed by Theriot et al. (Theriot *et al.*, 2010, Theriot *et al.*, 2011). Figure 4B shows activity assay results (in U/mg) for both the *Ph*prol and *Ph1*prol during various stages of purification.

Figure 6 demonstrates the response of *Ph*prol and *Ph1*prol to temperatures ranging from 40-100°C, clearly showing that efficient enzyme activity requires elevated temperatures.

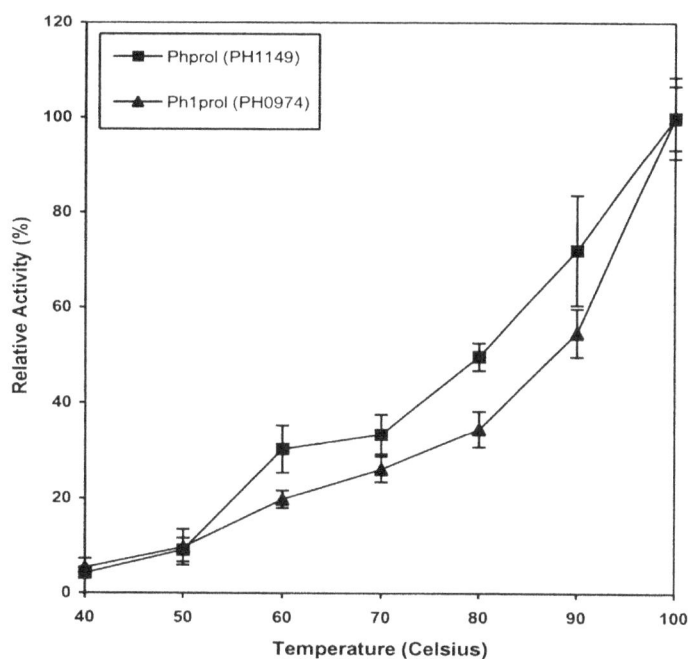

Figure 6: Activity of *P. horikoshii* prolidases resulting from incubating the reaction assays at temperatures ranging from 40 – 100°C. Prolidase assays contained 14.8 ng of *Ph*prol and 6.2 ng of *Ph1*prol, Met-Pro (4 mM) and $CoCl_2$ (1.2 mM). 100% specific activity corresponds to 1938 U/mg for *Ph*prol and 2355 U/mg for *Ph1*prol. From (Theriot, 2010).

4   Thermoactive Endoglucanase

4.1   Bacterial Strains, Plasmids, Enzymes, and Reagents

Sulfolobus solfataricus gDNA was gifted by Dr. Robert Kelly at North Carolina State University (NCSU). The *E. coli* XL1-Blue strain (Novagen, EMD Biosciences) was used for cloning and maintaining the recombinant plasmid. *E. coli* BL21 (λDE3) (Novagen, EMD Biosciences) cells were used for the over-expression of the proteins. The expression plasmid pET28a was obtained from Novagen, EMD Biosciences. Restriction endonucleases, T4 DNA ligase, and DNA polymerase were purchased from New England Biolabs. Synthetic oligonucleotides were synthesized by Eurofins MWG Operon. iProof DNA polymerase was purchased from Bio-Rad Laboratories, Inc. The PCR products were purified using QIAquick PCR purification kit (Qiagen). DEAE Sepharose, phenyl-sepharose, and Q Sepharose™ columns were purchased from GE Healthcare Life Sciences. Slide-A-Lyzer® dialysis cassettes were obtained from Thermo Scientific (Rockford, IL). Carboxymethyl cellulose, cellobiose, xylan from oat spelts, and pectin were purchased from Sigma Aldrich.

4.2   Cloning of a Thermoactive Endoglucanase from *Sulfolobus solfataricus*

PCR was used to amplify the *S. solfataricus* gene 1354 for subsequent cloning into the T7-polymerase-driven expression vector pET28a using the following primers *sso1354FfNhe*I (5'-GGGGG**GCTAGC**ATGGGGGGAATCATTTACTTGCATCAACAGTCTCTCAGCGTTAAACCCG-3'; forward primer containing a *Nhe*I restriction site shown in bold) and *sso1354RSac*I (5'-GGGGGG**GAGCTC**TTAGAGGAGAGTTTCAGAAAAGTTGGATACGGTCCACGAGAAGTATG-3'; reverse primer containing a *Sac*I restriction site shown in bold). Primers were designed using Amplify software version 3.1. PCR amplification was performed using iProof™ DNA polymerase 0.5 µL in a 50 µl reaction solution containing 5.0 µl 5X iProof™ buffer, 1 µl dNTP (25 mM), 0.5 µl forward primer (40 µM), 0.5 µl reverse primer (40 µM), and 1 µl *S. solfataricus* genomic DNA (50 ng/µl). The following protocol was run on a Bio-Rad thermal cycler: one initial cycle for 30 sec at 98°C followed by 30 cycles of 10 sec at 98°C, 30 sec at 65°C, and 45 sec at 72°C, with a 7 min final extension at 72°C. Endoglucanase PCR product size was 970 base pairs. PCR products were electrophoresed through 1% agarose gels for visual inspection. The amplified endoglucanase gene was subsequently cloned into the *Nhe*I and *Sac*I sites of pET28a. Plasmids were transformed into *E. coli* strain XL 1-Blue, and the transformed cells were plated on LB plates supplemented with kanamycin (100µg/ml) and incubated at 37°C overnight. Plasmids were sent to MWG Biotech for sequencing to ensure that no sequence changes occurred in the cloning process.

4.3   Identifying and Removing the Secretion Signal from *S. solfataricus* Thermoactive Endonuclease

Initial expression studies using the full length *Sso1354* gene revealed that the recombinant protein was being made in inclusion bodies or degraded in the membrane. An N-terminal 6x-His tag resulted in a small amount of soluble protein expression; however, a C-terminal 6x-His tag resulted in almost no soluble protein expression. These results suggest that the N-terminal 6x-His tag reduced the efficiency of recognition of the secretion signal allowing some leaky soluble protein expression. The predicted function of this gene should involve secretion from the archaeal cell. Thus, prediction software was used to identify a secretion signal. Simple secretion signals are composed of a stretch of hydrophobic amino acids at the N-terminus of the protein. PRED-Signal (http://bioinformatics.biol.uoa.gr/PRED-SIGNAL/) and

SPOCTOPUS (http://octopus.cbr.su.se/index.php) software utilize hidden Markov models and were used to predict the probability of a secretion signal. Both programs showed high probability of a secretion signal at the N-terminus, thus the primer used for *Sso1354* cloning omits the first 18 amino acids of the protein. Using this construct, soluble expression of the recombinant protein was achieved using the over-expression methods detailed below.

4.4   Over-expression of a Recombinant Thermoactive Endoglucanase from *S. solfataricus*

S. solfataricus Cel7A expression plasmid and the rare arginine, leucine, and isoleucine tRNA- encoding plasmid pRIL (Stratagene) were transformed into *E. coli* BL21 (λDE3) cells with IPTG-inducible expression of T7-RNA polymerase encoded on the chromosome. Transformants were selected on LB-kanamycin-chloramphenicol plates after incubation at 37°C overnight. Large-scale protein expression was done by inoculating 2-L cultures of autoinduction media (Studier, 2005) supplemented with 100 μg/ml kanamycin and 34 μg/ml chloramphenicol for plasmid maintenance. Cells were grown with shaking (200 rpm) at 37°C for 14 h. Cells were harvested by centrifugation at 14,460 x g for 50 min, and stored at -4°C until used for cell lysate preparations. Recombinant protein expression was evaluated throughout this process using SDS-PAGE analysis.

4.5   Recombinant Thermoactive Endoglucanase Purification

Cell pellets containing *S. solfataricus* Cel7A protein were suspended in 20 mM Tris-HCl, pH 8.0 containing 1 mM benzamindine-HCl. The cell suspension was passed through a French pressure cell (20,000 psi) three times. The lysed suspension was centrifuged at 14,460 x g for 30 min to remove cell debris. The supernatant was heated at 80°C for 30 min. *E. coli* cell debris and denatured protein were removed by centrifugation of the heated supernatant at 14,460 x g for 30 min. The clarified extract was applied to a 5-ml DEAE column. For DEAE chromatography, the binding buffer used was 20 mM Tris-HCl, pH 8.0 with 5% glycerol to reduce protein-protein interaction, and the elution buffer was 20 mM Tris-HCl, pH 8.0 with 1 M NaCl and 5% glycerol. The fractions with active enzyme were dialyzed and applied to a 1 ml phenyl-sepharose column after the addition of $(NH_4)_2SO_4$ to a final concentration of 1 M, and glycerol to a final concentration of 5%. Phenyl-sepharose chromatography was performed using a binding buffer of 50 mM NaH_2PO_4, pH 7.0, 1 M $(NH_4)_2SO_4$, 5% glycerol and elution buffer 50 mM NaH_2PO_4, pH 7.0, 5% glycerol,. Active fractions were dialyzed and applied to a 1 ml Q Sepharose™ column equilibrated with binding buffer (20 mM Tris-HCl, pH 8.0 with 5% glycerol). The elution buffer was 20 mM Tris-HCl, pH 8.0 with 1 M NaCl and 5% glycerol. All fractions were visualized on 12.5% SDS-polyacrylamide gels, and western blots were performed to confirm the presence of recombinant protein using antibody to the 6x-His tag. The over-expression and purification scheme used for recombinant *S. solfataricus* Cel7A is shown in Figure 5.

4.6   Recombinant Thermoactive Endoglucanase Characterization

Endoglucanase enzyme assays were done at 70°C in 1.5 ml reaction mixtures containing 50 mM sodium acetate buffer, pH 5.0, and 0.5% (wt/vol) solutions of soluble polysaccharide substrates, unless otherwise indicated. Enzymatic activity was measured by monitoring the release of reducing sugars. Briefly, 2 ml of substrate-enzyme solution were added to a 2-ml solution containing 4 volumes of Somogyi reagent I and 1 volume of Somogyi reagent II (Wood and Bhat, 1988). The solution is mixed and boiled for 15 min. After the solution has cooled to room temperature, 2 ml the of Nelson reagent is added followed by 4 ml of distilled water (Wood and Bhat, 1988). The solution is mixed by carefully inverting and absorbance was read at 520 nm (Wood and Bhat, 1988). Non-enzymatic hydrolysis of the substrate was corrected for using control reactions that did not receive any enzyme. Enzyme activity was defined as the amount of enzyme required to release 1 μmol of glucose-equivalent reducing groups per min. SDS-PAGE of the various steps for the *S. solfataricus* Cel7A purification is shown in Figure 7. The endoglucanase activity for recombinant *S. solfataricus* Cel7A in response to temperature is presented in Figure 8 and shows that the highest activity results from incubation of the reaction assays at 80°C, which is consistent with the optimal growth temperature for *S. solfataricus*.

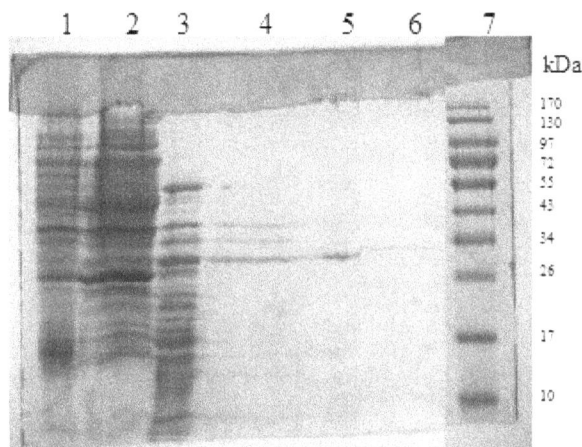

Figure 7: SDS-PAGE visualization of the steps in the recombinant *S. solfataricus* Cel7A protein purification. Lane 1: Whole-cell extract (102.4 μg), Lane 2: Soluble proteins (134.6 μg), Lane 3: Heat-treated soluble proteins (loaded onto DEAE column, 110.8 μg), Lane 4: Protein loaded onto phenyl-sepharose column (19.7 μg), Lane 5: Protein loaded onto Q column (6.5 μg), Lane 6: Active fraction from Q column (4.3 μg), Lane 7: Fisher EZ Run pre-stained protein ladder (6 μL).

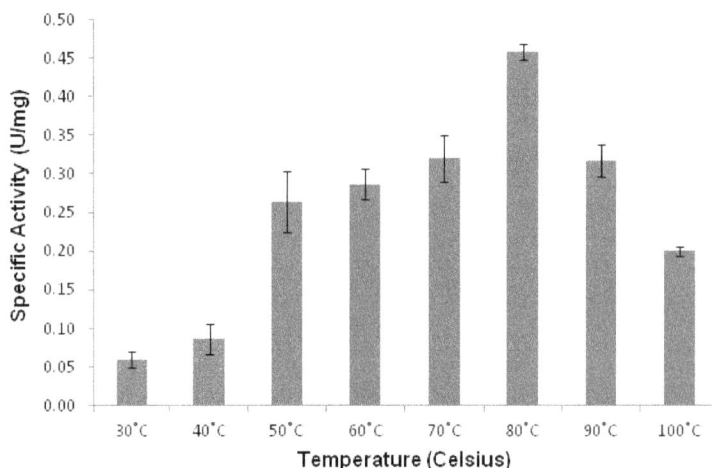

Figure 8: Activity of *S. solfataricus* endoglucanase over a temperature range of 30-100°C. 50 mM sodium acetate pH 5.0 with 0.5% Beechwood xylan was used for each assay.

5 Thermoactive Lipases

5.1 Bacterial Strains, Plasmids, Enzymes, and Reagents

The genomic DNA of *Metallosphaera sedula* DSM5348 was kindly provided by Dr. Robert Kelly of NCSU. The *E. coli* XL1-Blue strain (Novagen, EMD Biosciences) was used for cloning and maintaining the recombinant plasmid. BL21(DE3)LysS (Novagen, EMD Biosciences) cells were used for the over-expression of the proteins. The expression plasmids pET21b and pET28a were obtained from Novagen, EMD Biosciences. Restriction endonucleases, T4 DNA ligase, and DNA polymerase were purchased from New England Biolabs. Synthetic oligonucleotides were synthesized by Eurofins MWG Operon. The PCR products were purified using QIAquick PCR purification kit (Qiagen). The plasmids were purified using the QIAquick gel extraction kit (Qiagen). 4-nitrophenyl-octanoate was purchased from Sigma-Aldrich. The following chromatography column was utilized for the purification step: 5-ml HisTrap Nickel Sepharose™ from GE Healthcare Life Sciences.

5.2 Cloning of a Thermoactive Lipase from *Metallosphaera sedula*

The *Msed_1072Nt* gene was amplified using the forward primer: 5' TTAATACGAC-C**ATATG**CCCCTACATCCAGA GGTAAAGAAATTAC-3', with a *Nde*I site (bold), and the reverse primer: 5'-GATACATT C**GGATCC**GTGGATAGGTTCATCTCGG-3', with a *Bam*HI site (bold). The *Msed_1072Ct* gene was amplified using the forward primer: 5' ATACGAC**CATATG**CCCC TACATCCAGAGGTAAAGAAATTACTTTCCCAGCAGAGG TAAAGAAATTAC-3', with an *Nde*I site (bold), and the reverse primer: 5'-TAC**GGATCC**AGGACAGATCTC AGAACCCCAGCAATGTG 3', with a *Bam*HI site (bold) and Phusion® high fidelity DNA polymerase in a 50 µl PCR reaction solution containing 10 µl 5x Phusion® HF buffer, 1 µl dNTPs (10 mM), 0.5 µl forward primer (40 uM), 0.63 µl reverse primer (40 uM), 0.5 µl Phusion® DNA polymerase, and 2 µl *M. sedula* genomic DNA (50 ng/µl). The PCR reactions were carried out using a thermal cycler (Bio-Rad) under the following conditions: an initial denaturing step at 98°C for 30 sec; 30 cycles at 98°C for 10 sec (denaturing), annealing at 64.4°C [Msed_1072Nt]/67.9C [Msed_1072Ct] for 30 sec, and extension at 72°C for 30 sec; a final extension cycle of 72°C for 7 min, and preservation at 4°C. The amplicons were purified and visualized using a 1% (w/v) agarose gel. The purified DNA products were subjected to a double digestion with *Nde*I and *Bam*HI to render sticky ends needed for cloning. For construction of pET21b-Msed_1072Ct and pET28a-Msed_1072Nt, the plasmids were digested with *Nde*I and *Bam*HI, gel purified, and ligated to the compatible sticky end DNA molecule of Msed_1072Ct and Msed_1072Nt, respectively. CaCl$_2$-competent *E. coli* XL1-Blue cells were transformed with the ligated reaction and plated on solid LB agar media supplemented with ampicillin (100 µg/ml) or kanamycin (50 µg/ml) for selection of pET21b-Msed_1072Ct and pET28a-Msed_1072Nt, respectively. A positive clone of each construct was sequenced by Eurofins MWG Operon (Huntsville, AL) to ensure that no mutations were generated during the amplification process. The sequence information was analyzed by using MacVector (Accelrys) computer software.

5.3 Over-expression of Recombinant Thermoactive Lipase Msed_1072

For the over-expression of *M. sedula* lipase, each construct and the rare arginine, leucine, and isoleucine tRNA encoding plasmid pRIL were transformed into *E.coli* BL21(DE3)pLysS cells. For the control expression samples, the plasmids without the *Msed_1072* gene were also transformed into *E.coli* BL21(DE3)pLysS. The transformants were plated and selected on LB agar plates containing the appropriate antibiotics after incubation overnight at 37°C. The *E. coli* BL21(DE3)pLysS cells harboring the recombinant plasmids were inoculated into a liquid 1-L culture of auto-induction media (Studier, 2005) supplemented with the appropriate antibiotics for large scale expression of the protein. The cells were incubated with shaking at 200 rpm for 16 h at 37°C. Cells were harvested by centrifugation (13,680 x g, 50 min, 4°C) and stored at -20°C prior to preparing cell lysates The expression of the recombinant protein was evaluated by SDS-PAGE using a 12.5% polyacrylamide gel with the Bio-Rad Mini-PROTEAN® apparatus and visualized using Coomassie brilliant blue R250. The molecular mass of the lipase was determined to be approximately 36 kDa by SDS-PAGE. Protein concentrations were determined by the Bradford protein assay from Bio-Rad.

5.4   Recombinant Thermoactive Lipase Purification

The *E.coli* BL21(DE3)pLysS cell pellets containing the Msed_1072Ct and Msed_1072Nt proteins were resuspended and lysed for 10 min with 10 mL B-PER® bacterial protein extraction reagent (Pierce, Rockford, IL) containing 1 mM benezamidine-HCl. The use of the nonionic detergent in the initial lysing step was critical for the solubility of the protein. The cells were further lysed by three passages of the lysate through a French pressure cell (20,000 lb/in^2). Cellular debris was removed by centrifugation (26,890 x g, 45 min, 4°C). The supernatant was collected and heated at 70°C for 15 min. The heat-treated supernatant was centrifuged (26,890 x g, 15 min, 4°C) to remove denatured proteins. The supernatant containing the solubilized His-tagged recombinant proteins was added to a 5 ml HisTrap Ni Sepharose™ column for purification. Prior to the addition of the protein, the Ni^{2+}-charged column was equilibrated with 50 mM sodium phosphate buffer (pH 8.0), 300 mM NaCl, and 10 mM imidazole. After binding the protein to the metal charged column, the column was washed with the equilibration buffer to remove all unbound protein. The thermostable lipase bound to the affinity column was then eluted with a linear 10 mM to 250 mM imidazole gradient. The peak fractions were visualized using 12.5% SDS-PAGE gels. Fractions containing the recombinant proteins were pooled and dialyzed against 50 mM Tris-HCl buffer (pH 7.0) for 16 h at 4°C to remove the imidazole. The over-expression and purification steps used for the isolation of recombinant *M. sedula* lipase are presented in Figure 5. SDS-PAGE of the various steps for the *M. sedula* lipase purification is shown in Figure 9.

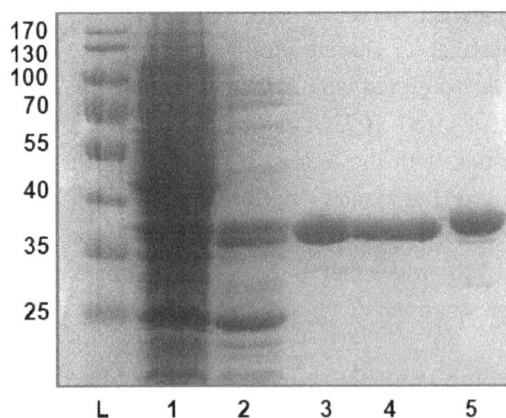

Figure 9: Protein purification of recombinant *M. sedula* lipase, Msed_1072Nt L: Molecular Weight Marker (in kDa), Lane 1: Cell free extract, Lane 2: Heat-treated cell free extract, Lane 3: Pooled Msed_1072Nt from the HisTrap Ni Sepharose, Lane 4: Purified Msed_1072Nt (2.5 μg), Lane 5: Purified Msed_1072Ct (2.5 μg)

5.5   Recombinant Thermoactive Lipase Characterization

Lipolytic activity was determined by a spectrophotometric assay using 4-nitrophenyl-octanoate as substrate, which was dissolved in dimethyl sulfoxide (DMSO) at a concentration of 0.1 M. The 1-ml reaction mixture consisted of 50 mM MOPS buffer, pH 7.0, 0.025% Tween-20, and 1 mM substrate. The amount of liberated *p*-nitrophenol was determined by reading absorbance of the sample at 410 nm. Lipase samples were assayed in 12 technical replicates. One unit (U) of lipase activity was defined as the amount of enzyme required to hydrolyze 1 μmol of substrate per min per mg of protein; thus, activities were expressed in units per milligram of protein.

5.6   Effect of Temperature on Enzyme Activity

The temperature profile for activity of the lipase was determined at 37°C, 60°C, 65°C, 70°C, 75°C, 80°C, 85°C, 90°C, and 95°C. The reaction mixture (as described above) was pre-heated with enzyme at 65°C for 5 min to thermo-activate the enzyme. The reaction was initiated by the addition of substrate and allowed to proceed for 5 min at the various temperatures. The enzyme reaction was stopped by adding 97.5 μl of chilled 0.25 M sodium carbonate. Controls were carried out as above, minus the addition of enzyme, to monitor the background hydrolysis of the substrate. The response of the N-terminal his-tagged and C-terminal His-tagged versions of the recombinant *M. sedula* lipase to temperature is shown in Figure 10 which demonstrates that higher lipase activity is achieved at thermophilic temperatures. The C-terminal His-tagged version of the *M. sedula* lipase (Msed_1072Ct) had greater specific activity than the N-terminal His-tagged version (Msed_1072Nt). The higher observed activity for Msed_1072Ct is believed to be due to the position of the poly-histidine tag. According to the NCBI Conserved Domain database, the substrate binding pocket is located at the N-terminal portion of Msed_1072. Thus, the presence of the tag at the N-terminal end may interfere with the enzyme binding the substrate.

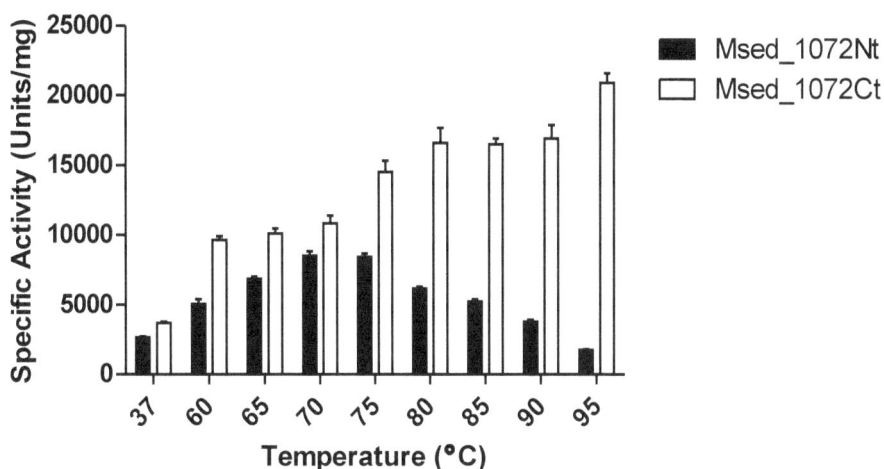

Figure 10: Activity response of Msed_1072Nt and Msed_1072Ct to temperature using 4-nitrophenyl-octanoate as a substrate.

6   Halophilic Lipases

6.1   Bacterial Strains, Plasmids, Enzymes, and Reagents

The gDNA of *Chromohalobacter salexigens* DSM3043 was purchased from ATCC. The *E. coli* XL1-Blue strain (Novagen, EMD Biosciences) was used for cloning and maintaining the recombinant plasmid. BL21(DE3)LysS (Novagen, EMD Biosciences) cells or M15[pRep4] cells (Qiagen) were used for the over-expression of the proteins. The expression plasmids pET21b and pQE-1 were obtained from Novagen, EMD Biosciences and Qiagen respectively. Restriction endonucleases, T4 DNA ligase, and DNA polymerase were purchased from New England Biolabs). Synthetic oligonucleotides were synthesized by Eurofins MWG Operon. The PCR products were purified using QIAquick PCR purification kit (Qiagen). The plasmids were purified using QIAquick gel extraction kit (Qiagen). All 4-nitrophenyl-based substrates were purchased from Sigma-Aldrich. TAGZyme™ DAPase enzyme and Cysteamine-HCl for histidine tag removal were obtained from Qiagen.

6.2   Cloning of Halophilic Lipases from *Chromohalobacter salexigens*

Basic Local Alignment Search Tool (BLAST) analysis was used to identify sequences in the *C. salexigens* genome that are similar to the *E. coli* thioesterases TesA and TesB. The *C. salexigens* open reading frames CSal2620 (YP_574666) and CSal0838 (YP_572894) were identified which have 63.9% homology to TesA and 58.4% homology to TesB, respectively. *C. salexigens* TesA homologue CSal2620 and TesB homologue CSal_0838 genes were amplified by PCR for subsequent cloning of these genes into the T7-polymerase-driven expression vector pET-21b (Novagen) and the T5-polymerase-driven expression vector pQE-1 (Qiagen). The former expression system enables production of C-terminal histidine tag-fused proteins, while the later system allows for production of removable N-terminal histidine tag-fused protein. For PCR amplification of the *C. salexigens* TesA homolog and TesB homolog genes, primers were designed for each gene per expression vector. The primers used to amplify the CSal2620 gene for expression in pET-21b were 5'-**CATATG**GGGCCCGTCGCGAATGTCCATGCCGAT-3'; forward, containing an *Nde*I restriction site shown in bold and 5'-**AAGCTT**TGATTCGTTCCGGTCGGTGTCCCGCGAC AG-3'; reverse, containing a *Hin*dIII restriction site shown in bold. The annealing temp used for amplification with these primers was 55°C. Similarly, the primers used to amplify the CSal0838 gene for expression in pET-21b were 5'-**CATATG**ACGCAACCACTCGACACCCTCGTC GAT-3'; forward, containing an *Nde*I restriction site shown in bold and 5'-**GGATCC**CACTCGACCAGGCGCGT CAGCCCC TCCTGCGCCACCGAGGCCACCAG -3'; reverse, containing a *Bam*HI restriction site shown in bold. The annealing temp used for amplification with these primers was: 65°C. The primers used to amplify the CSal2620 gene for expression in pQE-1 were 5'-**GCATGC**AATGGGGCCCGTCGCGAATGTCCAT GCCGA-3'; forward, containing an *Sph*I restriction site shown in bold and 5'-**AAGCTT**TCATTCGTTC CGGTCGGTGTCCCGCGACAG -3'; reverse, containing a *Hin*dIII restriction site shown in bold. The annealing temp used for amplification with these primers was 67°C. Similarly, the primers used to amplify the CSal0838 gene for expression in pQE-1 were 5'- AGAG**GCATGC**AATGACGCAACCAC-TCGACACCCTCGTCGATCTTCTGGGCCTCGA-3'; forward, containing an *Sph*I restriction site shown in bold and 5'-AGAG**AAGCTT**TCACTCGACCAGGCGCGTCAGCCCCTCCTGCGC CACCG AGGCCAC-3'; reverse, containing a *Hin*dIII restriction site shown in bold. The annealing temp used for amplification with these primers was 67°C. All primers were designed using MacVector (Accelrys, San Diego, CA) computer software. PCR amplification was performed in a 50 µl reaction solution containing

5 µl 10× Taq buffer, 0.4 µl dNTP (25 mM), 0.5 µl forward primer (40 µM), 0.5 µl reverse primer (40 µM), 0.5 µl Taq polymerase, and 1 µl *C. salexigens* genomic DNA (~300 ng/µl). The PCR was performed using a Bio-Rad iCycler thermal cycler programmed with the following parameters: one initial cycle for 5 min at 94 °C for denaturation, followed by 30 cycles of 94 °C for 30 sec, annealing temp listed above depending on primers for 30 sec, 72 °C for elongation for 1 min; and one final cycle at 72 °C for 7 min. The lipase PCR product sizes were 585 bp, and 807 bp for CSal2620 and CSal0838, respectively. PCR products were electrophoresed through a 1% agarose gel for visual inspection.

The amplified lipase genes for CSal2620::pET-21b, CSal2620::pQE-1 and CSal0838::pET-21b were subsequently cloned into the *EcoR*V site of plasmid pCR-Script (Stratagene). Plasmids were transformed into *E. coli* strain XL1-Blue, and the transformed cells were plated on LB plates supplemented with ampicillin (100 µg/ml) and X-gal (40 µg/ml) and incubated at 37°C overnight. Blue-white screening was used to select colonies for plasmid isolation. The amplified lipase genes for CSal0838::pQE-1 were subsequently digested with *Sph*I and *Hin*dIII to generate sticky ends on the amplified products and then cloned into the *Sph*I and *Hin*dIII sites of plasmid pQE-1 (Qiagen). Plasmids were transformed into *E. coli* strain XL1-Blue, and the transformed cells were plated on LB plates supplemented with ampicillin (100 µg/ml) and kanamycin (50 µg/ml) and incubated at 37°C overnight. pCR-Script plasmids containing the insert were isolated and digested with *Nde*I and *Hin*dIII to excise the gene for CSal2620 from the CSal2620::pCR-Script plasmid, *Nde*I and *Bam*HI to excise the gene for CSal0838 from the CSal0838::pCR-Script plasmid, and *Sph*I and *Hin*dIII to excise the gene for CSal2620 from the CSal2620::pCR-Script. The pCR-Script excised lipase genes were subsequently cloned into the *Nde*I and *Hin*dIII or *Nde*I and *Bam*HI (NEB) sites in expression vector pET-21b (Novagen) or the *Sph*I and *Hin*dIII sites in expression vector pQE-1 (Qiagen). All plasmids were sent to MWG Biotech for sequencing to ensure that no sequence changes occurred in the cloning process.

6.3 Over-expression of Recombinant Halophilic Lipases

C. salexigens lipase expression plasmids based on pET-21b were transformed into *E. coli* BL21(λDE3) cells, which have IPTG-inducible expression of T7-RNA polymerase encoded on the chromosome. Transformants were selected on LB–ampicillin (100 µg/ml) plates after incubation at 37°C overnight. Expression plasmids based on pQE-1 were transformed into *E. coli* M15[pRep4] cells (Qiagen). The pQE-1 plasmid contains a T5 phage promoter under the control of two *lac* operator sequences which allows for IPTG induction of cloned gene expression. The M15 strain contains the pRep4 plasmid which provides *lac* repressor in *trans* with pQE-1. Large-scale protein expression was done for all constructs by inoculating 2-L cultures of LB media supplemented with 100 µg/ml of ampicillin for pET-21b based constructs, and 100 µg/ml ampicillin with 50 µg/ml kanamycin was used for pQE-1 systems ensuring plasmid maintenance. Cells were grown with shaking (200 rpm) at 37°C until an OD_{600} of 0.6 to 0.8 was reached. Cells were harvested by centrifugation and stored at −80°C prior to preparing cell lysates. Recombinant protein expression was evaluated throughout this process using SDS-PAGE analysis.

6.4 Recombinant Halophilic Lipase Purification

Cell pellets containing the CSal2620 or CSal0838 proteins were suspended in 50 mM potassium phosphate buffer, pH 8.0 containing 1 mM benzamidine–HCl. The cell suspension was passed through a French pressure cell (20,000 psi) three times. The lysed suspension was centrifuged at 15,000 x g for 60 min at 4°C to remove cell debris. The supernatant was filtered through 0.45 µm syringe filters to further remove debris. The filtered extract was applied to a 5-ml HisTrap HP Nickel Sepharose™ affinity column (GE Healthcare Life Sciences) and washed with five column volumes of wash buffer (50 mM sodium phosphate buffer,pH 8.0, 1.0 M NaCl, 20 mM imidazole). The binding buffer used was 50 mM sodium phosphate buffer, pH 8.0, 1.0 M NaCl, 10 mM imidizole, and the elution buffer was 50 mM sodium phosphate buffer, pH 8.0, 1.0 M NaCl, 250 mM imidizole. The protein of interest was eluted via a linear gradient ranging from 0% to 100% elution buffer. All fractions were visualized on 12.5% SDS-polyacrylamide gels. Following affinity chromatography, the samples containing active protein were pooled and dialyzed using a 10,000 Da molecular weight cutoff (MWCO) dialysis cassette against 50 mM Tris-HCl, pH 8.0, 1.0 M NaCl to remove unwanted imidazole from the fractions. Final protein concentrations were estimated using Bio-Rad's Bradford assay.

6.5   DAPase Removal of Histidine Tags from Recombinant Halophilic Lipases

Purified lipase protein was desalted via dialysis (10,000 MWCO) against TAGZyme™ buffer (20 mM NaH$_2$PO$_4$, pH 7.0, 150 mM NaCl, 0.001% Tween-20). N-terminal fused histidine tags on proteins expressed via the pQE-1 system were removed using the TAGZyme™ DAPase Enzyme kit (Qiagen). Removal of DAPase enzymes from the untagged lipases was accomplished by subtractive immobilized-metal affinity chromatography (IMAC) using Ni-NTA Spin Columns (Qiagen). Final protein concentrations were estimated using the Bradford assay (Bio-Rad). A representative SDS-PAGE for the purification steps for CSal0838 is shown in Figure 11 and the over-expression and purification scheme used for the isolation of recombinant CSal2620 and CSal0838 is provided in Figure 12.

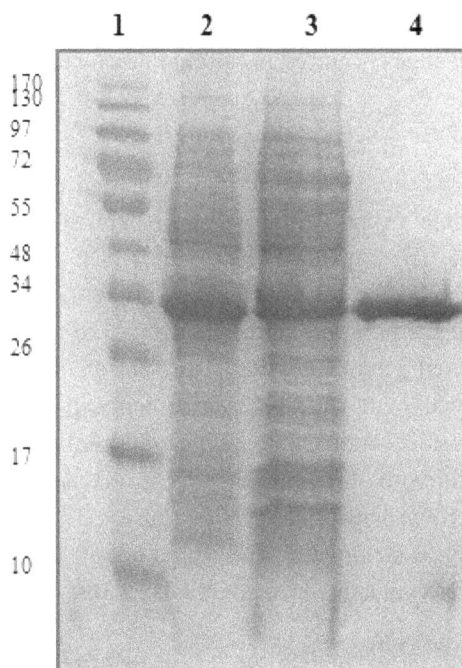

Figure 11: SDS-PAGE showing purification of CSal-0838 halophilic lipase. Lane 1: Protein ladder; Lane 2: Whole cell; Lane 3: Cell-free extract; Lane 4: Purified pooled elution fractions of CSal-0838 (5 µg).

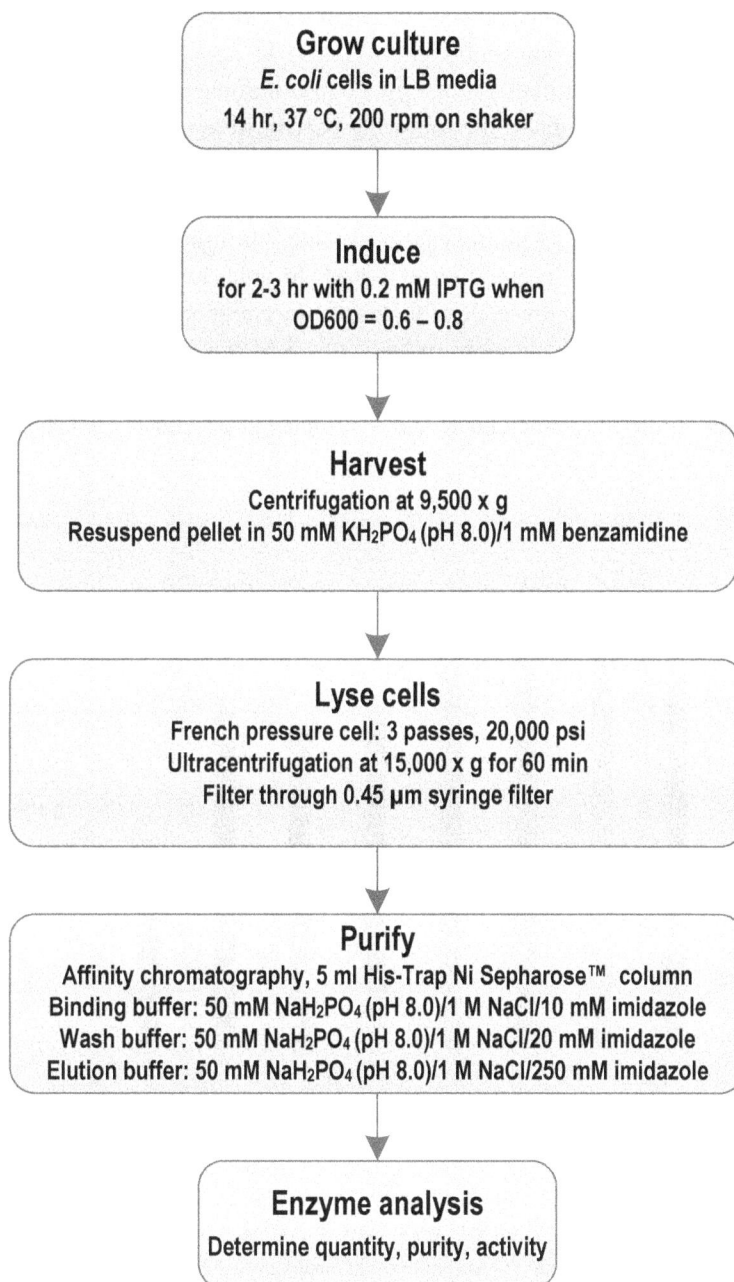

Figure 12: Over-expression and purification steps used for the isolation of recombinant CSal2620 and CSal0838.

6.6 Recombinant Halophilic Lipase Characterization

A typical 1-ml reaction mixture contains 988 μl 50 mM Tris-HCl, pH 8.0, 0.5 M NaCl, 0.001% Tween-20, 10 μl 100 mM o-nitrophenyl linked substrate (ex. 4-nitrophenyl butyrate from Sigma-Aldrich), and 2 μl of enzyme at a dilution sufficient to give an OD_{410} between 0.1 – 0.8. The buffer was heated to 37°C for 5 min, after which the substrate and enzyme were added. The reaction was allowed to continue for 5 min, at which time it was stopped by addition of 250 µl of 0.25 M Na$_2$CO$_3$. The absorbance was immediately read at 410 nm with an extinction coefficient of 13,635 M^{-1} cm^{-1}. One unit of lipase activity is defined as the amount of enzyme that liberates one µmole of o-nitrophenyl per min per mg of enzyme. For assays conducted at different pH values, the following buffers were used: pH 2.0 - 5.5, 50 mM sodium acetate, 50 mM Tris-HCl, 0.001% Tween-20; pH 6.0–9.5, 50 mM Tris-HCl, 0.001% Tween-20. When evaluating substrate specificity the following substrates were used 4-nitrophenyl-acetate, 4-nitrophenyl-butyrate, 4-nitrophenyl-octanoate, 4-nitrophenyl-decanoate, 4-nitrophenyl-dodecanoate, and 4-nitrophenyl-palmitate, each at a final concentration of 1 mM. In order to demonstrate that the recombinant CSal2620 lipase can function in the presence of high salt concentration, a set of activity assays were prepared which contained varying concentrations of NaCl (0 – 5 M NaCl), and the results are shown in Figure 13. It can be seen that the highest activities were observed for NaCl concentrations ranging from 0.25 M – 1.5 M NaCl when 4-nitrophenyl-octonoate and 4-nitrophenyl-decanoate are used as the substrates.

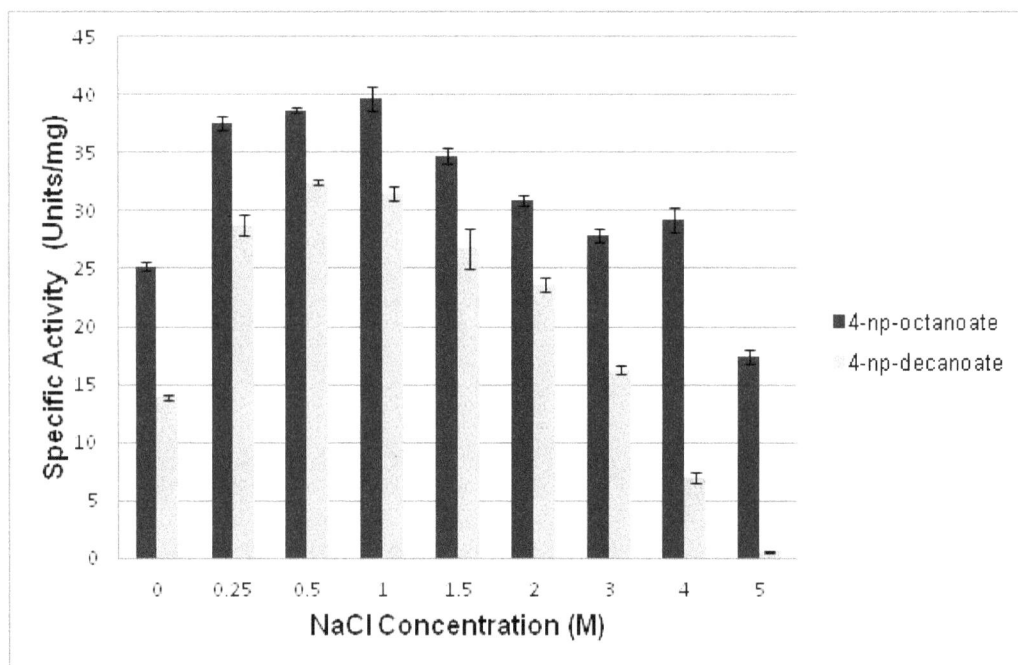

Figure 13: Activity of N-terminal-Tagged CSal2620 in response to varying NaCl concentrations. Purified N-terminal histidine-tagged CSal2620 enzyme was incubated in varying concentrations of NaCl in the presence of either 4-nitrophenyl-octanoate or 4-nitrophenyl-decanoate substrates.

7   General Considerations for Recombinant Protein Expression Construct Design and Over-expression

7.1   Using Synthetic DNA for Expression Vector Construction

Two challenges in successful recombinant expression vector construction have historically been (1) having access to genomic DNA from which to amplify your target gene of interest, which can especially be a problem if the source organisms cannot be cultivated under laboratory conditions and (2) ensuring the target gene has an appropriate codon bias to enable efficient translation in *E. coli*. To help with codon bias in *E. coli*, plasmids such as pRIL (Novagen) that code for *E. coli*'s rare tRNAs (rare argininine, isoleucine and leucine tRNAs) can be transformed along with the recombinant expression plasmid as long as the plasmids are compatible and appropriate anitbiotic selections can be used. However, with the advent of reasonably-priced DNA synthesis services, target genes to be cloned into expression vectors can be synthesized using a sequence optimized specifically for the codon bias of the expression host of choice, which ultimately circumvents the need for both PCR amplification of target genomic DNA and having to provide for the expression of rare tRNAs in the expression host.

7.2   Use of Small-scale Protein Over-expression Protocols to Optimize Recombinant Protein Production

Generally standard expression condition methods recommended by expression vector suppliers are a good starting point for performing successful large-scale (> 1-L cultures) recombinant protein expression. However, often expression of active, soluble, recombinant proteins can be improved by attempting to optimize under small-scale conditions (volumes ranging from 10 to 100 ml of culture media) expression conditions prior to scaling up. Conditions that can be considered for optimization include media type (e.g. LB, autoinduction, minimal media), inducer concentration ranges (e.g. using an IPTG concentration range of 0 to 1 mM in increments of 0.25 mM), induction temperature (e.g. dropping the induction temperature from 37°C to 30°C or room temperature to decrease the rate of protein production in an effort to enhance soluble protein folding or using a brief 42°C heat shock period to induce chaperone production to aid in soluble protein folding), and choice of expression strain (e.g. use of strains that express rare tRNAs or strains that express GroEL chaperones to help with protein folding).

7.3   Use of Affinity Tags to Simplify Recombinant Protein Purification

Generating recombinant proteins fused with affinity tags (e.g. 6x-histidine tags, S-tags, chitin-binding domain tags, etc.) is a very popular approach since the affinity tags generally facilitate easy protein purification and detection by Western blot analysis. It should be noted, however, that the addition of a tag may also effect the activity of the recombinant protein. A tag placed near the active domain may interefere with the binding of substrate or with catalytic activity. Therefore, before choosing a tagging location (i.e. an N-terminal or C-terminal tagging position), sequence analysis of the target protein should be done to determine the location(s) of the binding, catalytic, and cofactor sites that the protein may have in order to decide on a tagging strategy that would potentially be the least disruptive option. If the presence of fused affinity tags does negatively impact protein structure or performance, then vector constructs can be used that have specific peptidase cleavage sites (e.g. thrombin, enterokinase, DAPase, etc.) that can be used to remove the affinity tags as a step of the protein purification.

7.4   General Considerations for Selection of Chromatography Resins for Protein Purification

Although affinity chromatography provides a convenient and efficient method for the purification of most tagged proteins, for some recombinant proteins, the tag is not surface-exposed in the folded protein and consequently the recombinant protein does not bind well to an affinity column, as was the case with our thermoactive endoglucanase (see section 4). In this situation it is important to select alternate chromatography resins. Knowing the general properties of the recombinant protein (such as the protein's pI, degree of hydrophobicity, molecular weight, or whether the protein has special attributes such as flavin cofactors or can bind sugars or nucleic acids) can be a useful guide for the selection of chromatography columns to use for a protein purification strategy. Specifically, the pI and hydrophobicity of the recombinant protein is helpful for choosing chromatography columns and buffers for purification based on cation or anion exchange (e.g. Q, DEAE, and SP columns) or hydrophobic interaction (e.g. butyl or phenyl-sepharose columns).

References

Cavicchioli, R., Charlton, T., Ertan, H., Mohd Omar, S., Siddiqui, K. S. & Williams, T. J. (2011). Biotechnological uses of enzymes from psychrophiles. Microbial Biotechnology, 4, 449-460.

Chen, R. P., Guo, L. Z. & Dang, H. Y. (2011). Gene cloning, expression and characterization of a cold-adapted lipase from a psychrophilic deep-sea bacterium Psychrobacter sp C18. World Journal of Microbiology & Biotechnology, 27, 431-441.

Cheng, T. C., Harvey, S. P. & Stroup, A. N. (1993). Purification and properties of a highly active organophosphorus acid anhydrolase from Alteromonas undina. Applied and Environmental Microbiology, 59, 3138-3140.

Chinard, F. P. (1952). Photometric estimation of proline and ornithine. Journal of Biological Chemistry, 199, 91-95.

D'Amico, S., Collins, T., Marx, J. C., Feller, G. & Gerday, C. (2006). Psychrophilic microorganisms: challenges for life. Embo Reports, 7, 385-389.

De Miguel Bouzas, T., Barros-Velazquez, J. & Villa, T. G. (2006). Industrial applications of hyperthermophilic enzymes: a review. Protein and Peptide Letters, 13, 645-651.

Deming, J. W., Somers, L. K., Straube, W. L., Swartz, D. G. & MacDonell, M. T. (1988). Isolation of an obligately baro-philic bacterium and description of a new genus, Colwellia gen. nov. Systematic and Applied Microbiology, 10, 152-160.

Demirjian, D. C., Morís-Varas, F. & Cassidy, C. S. (2001). Enzymes from extremophiles. Current Opinion in Chemistry and Biology, 5, 144-151.

Feller, G., Lonhienne, T., Deroanne, C., Libioulle, C., VanBeeuman, J. & Gerday, C. (1992). Purification, characterization, and nucleotide-sequence of the thermolabile alpha-amylase from the Antarctic psychrotroph Alteromonas-Haloplanctis A23. Journal of Biological Chemistry, 267, 5217-5221.

Feller, G. & Gerday, C. (2003). Psychrophilic enzymes: Hot topics in cold adaptation. Nature Reviews Microbiology, 1, 200-208.

Ghosh, M., Grunden, A. M., Dunn, D. M., Weiss, R. & Adams, M. W. (1998). Characterization of native and recombinant forms of an unusual cobalt-dependent proline dipeptidase (prolidase) from the hyperthermophilic archaeon Pyro-coccus furiosus. Journal of Bacteriology, 180, 4781-4789.

Gomes, J. & Steiner, W. (2004). The biocatalytic potential of extremophiles and extremozymes. Food Technology and Bio-technology, 42, 223-235.

Gupta, R., Gupta, N., & Rathi P. (2004). Bacterial lipases: An overview of production, purification and biochemical prop-erties. Applied Microbiology and Biotechnology, 64, 763–781.

Hasan, F. & Shah, A. (2009). Methods for detection and characterization of lipases: A comprehensive review. Biotechnol-ogy Advances, 27, 782-798.

Holmgren, A., (1976). Hydrogen donor system for Escherichia coli ribonucleoside-diphosphate reductase dependent upon glutathione. Proceedings of the National Academy of Sciences USA, 73, 2275-2279.

Huber, G., Spinnler, C., Gambacorta, A. & Stetter, K. O. (1989). *Metallosphaera sedula gen. and sp. nov. represents a new genus of aerobic, metal-mobilizing, thermoacidophilic archaebacteria. Systematics and Applied Microbiology, 12, 38-47.*

Huston, A. L., Haeggstrom, J. Z. & Feller, G. (2008). *Cold adaptation of enzymes: Structural, kinetic and microcalorimetric characterizations of an aminopeptidase from the Arctic psychrophile Colwellia psychrerythraea and of human leukotriene A(4) hydrolase. Biochimica Et Biophysica Acta-Proteins and Proteomics, 1784, 1865-1872.*

Jaeger, K. E. & Reetz, M. (1998). *Microbial lipases form versatile tools for biotechnology. Trends Biotechnol, 16: 396-403.*

Jorgensen, H., Kristensen, J. B., Felby, C. (2007). *Enzymatic conversion of lignocellulose into fermentable sugars: challenges and opportunities. Biofuels Bioproducts & Biorefining, 1, 119-134.*

Junge, K. Imhoff, J. F., Staley, J.T. & Deming, J. W. (2002). *Phylogenetic diversity of numerically important arctic sea-ice bacteria cultured at subzero temperature. Microbial Ecolology, 43, 315-328.*

Kademi, A., Danielle, L. & Ajain, H. (2005). *Lipases. In Enzyme Technology (pp. 297–318).*

Kehrer, J.P. & Lund, L. G. (1994). *Cellular reducing equivalents and oxidative stress. Free Radical Biology and Medicine, 17, 65-75.*

Methe, B. A., Nelson, K.E., Deming, J.W., Momen, B., Melamud, E., Zhang, X., et al. (2005). *The psychrophilic lifestyle as revealed by the genome sequence of Colwellia psychrerythraea 34H through genomic and proteomic analyses. Proceedings of the National Academy of Sciences USA, 102, 10913-10918.*

Mock, T. & Thomas, D. N. (2005) *Recent advances in sea-ice microbiology. Environmental Microbiology, 7, 605-619.*

Oren, A. (2010). *Industrial and environmental applications of halophilic microorganisms. Environmental Technology, 31, 825-834.*

Rao, M. B., Tanksale, A. M., Ghatge, M. S. & Deshpande, V. V. (1998). *Molecular and biotechnological aspects of microbial proteases. Microbiology and Molecular Biology Reviews, 62, 597-635.*

Scrutton, N. S., Berry, A. & and Perham, R. N. (1987). *Purification and characterization of glutathione reductase encoded by a cloned and over-expressed gene in Escherichia coli. Biochemistry Journal, 245, 875-880.*

She, Q., Singh, R.K., Confalonieri, F., Zivanovic, Y., Allard, G., Awayex, M.J., Chan-Weiher, C.C, Clausen, I.G., Curtis, B.A., De Moors, A., Erauso, G., Flethcer, C., Gorndon. P.M.K., Jong, I.H., Jeffries, A.C., Kozera, C.J., Media, N., Pend, X., Thi-Ngoc, H.P., Redder, P., Schenk, M.E., Theriault, C., Tolstrup, N., Charlebois, R.L., Doolittle, W.F., Duguet, M., Caasterland, T., Garret, R.A., Ragan, M.A., Sensen, C. W. & Van der Oost, J. (2001). *The complete genome of the crenarchaeon Sulfolobus solfataricus P2. Proceedings of the National Academy of Sciences USA, 98, 7835-7840.*

Studier, F. W. (2005). *Protein production by auto-induction in high density shaking cultures. Protein Expression and Purification, 41, 207-234.*

Theriot, C. M., Semcer, R. L., Shah, S. S. & Grunden, A. M. (2011). *Improving the catalytic activity of hyperthermophilic Pyrococcus horikoshii prolidase for detoxification of organophosphorus nerve agents over a broad range of temperatures. Archaea, 2011, 565127.*

Theriot, C. M., Tove, S. R. & Grunden, A. M. (2010). *Characterization of two proline dipeptidases (prolidases) from the hyperthermophilic archaeon Pyrococcus horikoshii. Applied Microbiology and Biotechnology, 86, 177-188.*

Ueda, E. K. M., Gout, P. W. & Morganti, L. (2003). *Current and prospective applications of metal ion-protein binding. Journal of Chromatography A, 988, 1-23.*

van den Burg, B. (2003). *Extremophiles as a source for novel enzymes. Current Opinion in Microbiology, 213-218.*

Wood, T. M. & Bhat, M. (1988). *Methods for measuring cellulase activities. Methods in Enzymology, 160, 87-112.*

Antioxidant Role of *Escherichia Coli* Glucose-6-Phosphate Dehydrogenase in Metalloid-Mediated Oxidative Stress

Juan M. Sandoval
Departamento de Biología, Facultad de Química y Biología
Universidad de Santiago de Chile, Santiago, Chile

Felipe A. Arenas
Departamento de Biología, Facultad de Química y Biología
Universidad de Santiago de Chile, Santiago, Chile

Claudio C. Vásquez
Departamento de Biología, Facultad de Química y Biología
Universidad de Santiago de Chile, Santiago, Chile

1   Cellular Response to Tellurite-mediated Oxidative Stress

Tellurium is one of the rarest elements in nature, and one of its derivatives, tellurite, is highly toxic for most living organisms. Despite years of research, the mechanism by which this oxyanion exerts its toxicity is still an enigma (Taylor, 1999; Pérez *et al.*, 2007; Zannoni *et al.*, 2008; Chasteen *et al.*, 2009). Characterizing this mechanism is of great interest due to the sustained use of tellurium derivatives in different applications in the electronic, optical and metallurgical industries. In addition to its occurrence in sulfide-rich natural reserves, it is possible to find high local metalloid concentrations in places of waste discharge of mining plants, which can cause potential adverse impacts to the environment and public health (Silver and Phung, 1996; Silver, 1998).

Currently, it is accepted that tellurite exerts its toxic effects mainly through two partially characterized pathways (a) cellular thiol oxidation and (b) superoxide generation, both triggering a toxic metabolic state known as oxidative stress (Turner *et al.*, 1999, 2001; Borghese *et al.*, 2004; Borsetti *et al.*, 2005; Calderón *et al.*, 2006, 2009; Pérez *et al.*, 2007; Tremaroli *et al.*, 2007; Sandoval *et al.*, 2010). In addition, our group has identified different antioxidant cell responses that allow *E. coli* facing the adverse effects caused by the tellurium oxyanion. For instance, induction of *sodA* and *sodB* genes is observed during toxicant exposure; the resulting increase of superoxide dismutase activity helps in dismutating the intracellular superoxide that is concomitantly generated during tellurite reduction (Calderón *et al.*, 2006; Pérez *et al.*, 2007; Chasteen *et al.*, 2009). In addition, induction of *yqhD* (encoding aldehyde oxidoreductase, Pérez *et al.*, 2008) and *btuE* (encoding glutathione peroxidase, Arenas *et al.*, 2010) genes occurs in tellurite-exposed *E. coli*, which in turn results in decreased content of reactive aldehydes and organic hydroperoxides thus alleviating tellurite-mediated oxidative damage.

In this communication, we show that in response to tellurite stress *E. coli* increases the intracellular level of the antioxidant molecule reduced nicotinamide adenine dinucleotide phosphate (NADPH) via glucose-6-phosphate dehydrogenase (G6PDH). The nucleotide seems to be used for reducing tellurite by means of a secondary activity of 6-phosphogluconate dehydrogenase (Gnd). By overproducing G6PDH *E. coli* can better cope with tellurite-mediated oxidative stress through increasing the level of antioxidant molecules and reducing the intracellular level of oxidized macromolecules, including oxidation-sensitive enzymes (Sandoval *et al.*, 2011).

2   Involvement of G6PDH in the Response to Tellurite

Increased ROS concentration -by activation of the *soxRS* regulatory system- seems to be the first signal for the cell to counteract the harmful effects caused by tellurite (Pérez *et al.*, 2007). Activation of the *soxRS* regulon in turn induces the expression of a set of genes involved in eliminating ROS, repair mechanisms and recycling of different cellular components. Among these, the *zwf* gene controls the intracellular levels of NADPH in response to oxidative stress (Pomposiello *et al.*, 2001; Blanchard *et al.*, 2007).

Exposing *E. coli* to tellurite results in induced G6PDH activity in a concentration- and time-dependent manner, transcript and protein levels behaved similarly. After 30 min of treatment with sublethal toxicant concentrations (2 μM), the maximum specific enzymatic activity was ~70-90% regarding the controls (Sandoval *et al.*, 2011). In general, G6PDH activity is altered in response to significant metabolic changes that depend on growth conditions (Rowley *et al.*, 1992). Basal levels of G6PDH expression result from regulating NADPH intracellular levels (Rowley and Wolf, 1991; Rowley *et al.*, 1992). In general, the activation of the *soxRS* regulon by tellurite-mediated stress quickly induces the expression of *zwf* and in tellurite-exposed Δ*soxRS* cells no induction of G6PDH was observed (Sandoval *et al.*, 2011 and our unpublished data).

By synthesizing NADPH, a component used in various antioxidant response systems and a co-factor for the biosynthesis of many cell precursors (Ying, 2008), G6PDH plays a pivotal role in maintaining the cell's redox status. Nearly 60% of the cell's NADPH requirement, via G6PDH, is met by the pentose phosphate pathway (Nicolas *et al.*, 2007). Under tellurite stress, *E. coli* increases NADPH synthesis by ~30% (Sandoval *et al.*, 2011), a result that is in agreement with recent publications indicating that in response to oxidative stress a metabolic cell adaptation occurs favoring NADPH over NADH synthesis (Singh *et al.*, 2007, 2008). In fact, after tellurite exposure the intracellular NADH concentration decreased by ~50% (Sandoval *et al.*, 2011). Although a decrease in NADH synthesis could be counterproductive for energy generation (Singh *et al.*, 2007), it can be still a significant response to reduce the cell's oxidative status. In fact, several NAD^+-dependent enzymes from prokaryotic or eukaryotic origin are selectively inhibited upon tellurite exposure (Siliprandi *et al.*, 1971, 1973; Castro *et al.*, 2008; Reinoso *et al.*, 2012). In this context, cell exposure to oxidizing compounds that trigger the activation of the *zwf* gene results in the alteration of the NADH/NADPH ratio. Along the same lines, it has been determined that due to oxidative stress a shifting of glucose catabolic flux from glycolysis to pentose phosphate pathway occurs and probably represents an antioxidant mechanism of cell response (Ralser *et al.*, 2007; Rungrassamee *et al.*, 2008; Rui *et al.*, 2010). In the presence of tellurite, G6P accumulation was directly correlated with PtsG (glucose-specific transporter of the phosphotransferase system) and Pgi (phosphoglucose isomerase) activities (Sandoval *et al.*, 2011).

3   Effect of G6PDH on Tellurite-induced Oxidative Damage Parameters

The induction of G6PDH in response to tellurite-mediated oxidative stress seems to be an important source of reducing equivalents to cope with the oxidative damage generated by the toxicant. Consistent with this, the absence of the *zwf* gene induces increased cell sensitivity to several oxidative stress elicitors (Giró *et al.*, 2006; Sandoval *et al.*, 2011). However, *zwf* over-expression did not result in a resistance phenotype. This result suggests that the protective effect triggered by G6PDH during the *soxRS*-mediated response occurs in cells in which the stress condition is regulated by the NADPH/$NADP^+$ ratio rather than by the severity of the tested toxicants (Krapp *et al.*, 2011).

NADPH plays an important role in the maintenance of the cell's redox status. Actually, the coenzyme can act *per se* as a scavenger for different radical species (Kirsch and de Groot, 2001). In basal conditions, cells lacking the *zwf* gene showed higher (~15-fold) ROS levels than the wild type strain, a number that was increased to ~80% in the presence of tellurite. Approximately, a 2-fold increase in tellurite-induced oxidative markers as protein carbonylation and membrane lipid peroxidation was observed in *E. coli* Δ*zwf*, a phenotype that could reflect a weaker cell antioxidant environment (NADPH levels) or an increased basal ROS content (Sandoval *et al.*, 2011). In particular, macromolecule damage results most likely from the physiological formation of OH• (hydroxyl radical) and/or, increased, tellurite-mediated reactive aldehyde and organic lipid peroxide content (Pérez *et al.*, 2008; Arenas *et al.*, 2010). G6PDH over-production clearly decreased basal ROS levels in genetically complemented Δ*zwf* cells (~10-fold regarding the mutant strain) and slightly in the presence of the toxicant. Similarly, oxidative markers values were partially/fully restored as compared to those observed in control conditions. Dehydratase activities resulted protected even under conditions of oxidative stress (Sandoval *et al.*, 2011). This particular phenotype was demonstrated using *in vitro* cell-free reconstituted systems, where redox equivalents synthesized by G6PDH are transferred via flavodoxin-NADPH reductase to oxidized dehydratase [Fe-S] centers (Giró *et al.*, 2006).

4   G6PDH as Source of Reducing Equivalents During Tellurite Reduction

Either direct toxicant elimination or metabolism represent new antioxidant mechanisms that have been described for different metals or their derivatives (Chasteen *et al.*, 2009). Once inside the cell, tellurite's oxidizing ability affects different cellular macromolecules. For instance, the glutathione (GSH) pool is depleted upon tellurite exposure (Turner *et al.*, 1999, 2001). In addition, enzymes such as nitrate reductase and various oxidoreductases and terminal oxidases from the electron transport chain contribute to tellurite reduction (Avazeri *et al.*, 1997, Trutko *et al.*, 2000). Our group has reported that tellurite can also be reduced by secondary activities of some NAD(P)H-dependent proteins that have been referred to generically as tellurite reductases (TRs). Also, important metabolic enzymes such as catalase and dihydrolipoyl dehydrogenase are able to reduce tellurite to elemental tellurium in the presence of NADH. Assays carried out *in vitro* showed that tellurite reduction is paralleled by superoxide generation, the molecular signal that induces the activation of *soxRS* regulon response described previously (Calderón *et al.*, 2006; Castro *et al.*, 2008).

NADPH is used normally by enzymes involved in electron transfer reactions. In particular, the difference in coenzyme usage (NADPH vs. NADH) depends on protein function (catabolism vs. anabolism), kinetic rates associated, cofactor availability, growth conditions, etc. (Brumaghim *et al.*, 2003; Singh *et al.*, 2007). Product of the metabolic change resulting from tellurite-mediated oxidative stress, probably the effective concentration of both reduced cofactors can be limiting for the oxyanion-reducing activities (Sandoval *et al.*, 2011). According to our results, NADPH seems to be the preferred coenzyme for tellurite reduction. Crude extracts from *E. coli* revealed that TR activity functions with both cofactors. However, the use of exogenous NADPH increases this activity ~3-4 fold as compared with NADH (same concentration, 1 mM). In *zwf*-expressing strains, therefore exhibiting increased NADPH content, the NADPH-dependent TR activity was further induced (~2-fold, Sandoval *et al.*, ms in preparation). This increased activity may result from a direct effect of NADPH (for example, inducing enzymes involved in tellurite reduction) or by an indirect regulatory effect at the transcription level of genes related to TR activity. Such a NADPH regulatory function has been observed in a number of cellular and/or metabolic eukaryotic processes (Ying, 2008).

The molecular characterization of the *E. coli* TR activity resulted in the identification of 6-phosphogluconate dehydrogenase (Gnd) as the enzyme responsible for tellurite reduction. As with G6PDH, this protein is part of the oxidative branch of the pentose phosphate pathway (Nasoff *et al.*, 1984). Not much information is available about its molecular regulation. Finally, it was interesting to observe that increased NADPH results in the induction of Gnd-associated TR activity (Sandoval *et al.*, unpublished results). Tellurite-mediated deviation of the glucose catabolic flux from glycolysis to the pentose phosphate shunt may explain these results. However, the participation of other NADPH-dependent TR activity(ies) that can complement that of Gnd cannot be ruled out. Overall, the metabolic conditions described above assume that the tellurite-modified redox status results in the activation of this metabolic pathway as a detoxification response for the oxyanion. These results are in agreement with the current model of metabolic module activation during the cell's antioxidant response (Mailloux *et al.*, 2007; Singh *et al.*, 2008; Lemire *et al.*, 2010).

5   Concluding Remarks

Results from this work can be summarized in a model showing the multiple functions of NADPH in the cell antioxidant response to tellurite (Scheme 1).

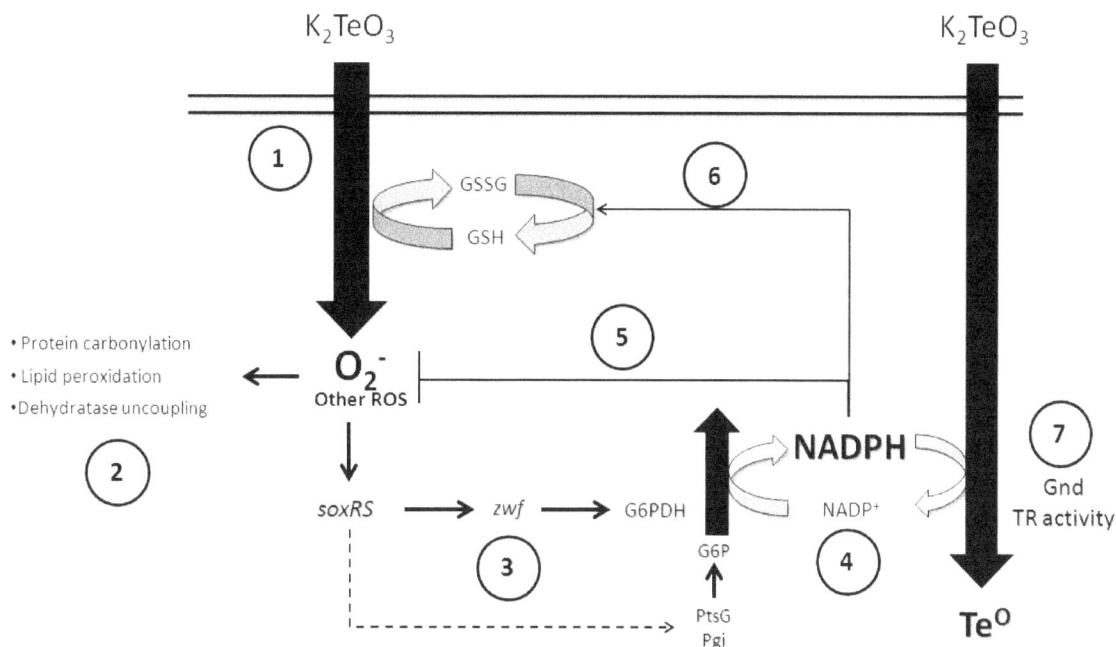

Scheme 1: The role of G6PDH and NADPH in the *E. coli* response to tellurite. K_2TeO_3 (potassium tellurite), GSH (reduced glutathione), GSSG (oxidized glutathione), *soxRS* (*soxRS* regulon), $O_2^{\cdot-}$ (superoxide anion), *zwf* (glucose-6-phosphate dehydrogenase gene), G6PDH (glucose-6-phosphate dehydrogenase), ICDH (isocitrate dehydrogenase), GDH (glutamate dehydrogenase), PtsG (specific glucose permease), Pgi (phosphoglucose isomerase), G6P (glucose-6-phosphate), Gnd (6-phosphogluconate dehydrogenase).

After cell entry, tellurite is reduced by cellular thiols or NADPH-dependent tellurite reductase enzymes (1). Increased ROS content then causes oxidative damage to many cell targets (2). In response to oxidative stress establishment, the *soxRS* regulon is induced (3), which in turn activates different genes involved in the generation of NADPH that is probably used in toxicant reduction. Activation of PtsG, Pgi and G6PDH activities lead to metabolic flux redistribution towards the pentose phosphate shunt, with a concomitant increase of intracellular NADPH (4). In turn, this nucleotide could act directly by decreasing intracellular ROS levels (5) or in regenerating the GSH pool (6) thus decreasing the overall oxidative status. Our results suggest that the increase of G6PDH activity, and hence NADPH concentration, induces the NADPH-dependent tellurite reductase activity of the Gnd enzyme (7).

Acknowledgements

This work was supported by grants # 1090097 from Fondecyt and Dicyt-USACH, to C.C.V. J.M.S was supported by a doctoral fellowship from MECESUP UCH407 and Becas Chile, Chile. F.A.S was supported by Fondecyt Postdoctoral # 3120049.

References

Arenas FA, Díaz WA, Leal CA, Pérez-Donoso JM, Imlay JA, Vásquez CC. (2010) The Escherichia coli btuE gene, encodes a glutathione peroxidase that is induced under oxidative stress conditions. Biochem Biophys Res Commun 398: 690-694.

Avazéri C, Turner RJ, Pommier J, Weiner JH, Giordano G, Verméglio A. (1997) Tellurite reductase activity of nitrate reductase is responsible for the basal resistance of Escherichia coli to tellurite. Microbiology 143: 1181-1189.

Blanchard JL, Wholey WY, Conlon EM, Pomposiello PJ. (2007) Rapid changes in gene expression dynamics in response to superoxide reveal SoxRS-dependent and independent transcriptional networks. PLoS ONE 2: e1186.

Borghese R, Borsetti F, Foladori P, Ziglio G, Zannoni D. (2004) Effects of the metalloid oxyanion tellurite (TeO$_3^{2-}$) on growth characteristics of the phototrophic bacterium Rhodobacter capsulatus. Appl Environ Microbiol 70: 6595-6602.

Borsetti F, Tremaroli V, Michelacci F, Borghese R, Winterstein C, Daldal F, Zannoni D. (2005) Tellurite effects on Rhodobacter capsulatus cell viability and superoxide dismutase activity under oxidative stress conditions. Res Microbiol 156: 807-813.

Brumaghim JL, Li Y, Henle E, and Linn S. (2007) Effects of hydrogen peroxide upon nicotinamide nucleotide metabolism in Escherichia coli: changes in enzyme levels and nicotinamide nucleotide pools and studies of the oxidation of NAD(P)H by Fe(III). J Biol Chem 278: 42495-42504.

Calderón IL, Arenas FA, Pérez JM, Fuentes DE, Araya MA, Saavedra CP, Tantaleán JC, Pichuantes SE, Youderian PA, Vásquez CC. (2006) Catalases are NAD(P)H-dependent tellurite reductases. PLoS ONE 1: e70.

Calderón IL, Elías AO, Fuentes EL, Pradenas GA, Castro ME, Arenas FA, Pérez JM, Vásquez CC. (2009) Tellurite-mediated disabling of [4Fe-4S] clusters of Escherichia coli dehydratases. Microbiology 155: 1840-1846.

Castro ME, Molina R, Díaz W, Pichuantes SE, Vásquez CC. (2008) The dihydrolipoamide dehydrogenase of Aeromonas caviae ST exhibits NADH dependent tellurite reductase activity. Biochem Biophys Res Commun 375: 91-94.

Chasteen TG, Fuentes DE, Tantaleán JC, Vásquez CC. (2009) Tellurite: history, oxidative stress, and molecular mechanisms of resistance. FEMS Microbiol Rev 33: 820-832.

Giró M, Carrillo N, Krapp AR. (2006) Glucose-6-phosphate dehydrogenase and ferredoxin-NADP(H) reductase contribute to damage repair during the soxRS response of Escherichia coli. Microbiology 152: 1119-1128.

Kirsch M, De Groot H. (2001) NAD(P)H, a directly operating antioxidant? FASEB J 15: 1569-1574.

Krapp AR, Humbert MV, Carrillo N. (2011) The soxRS response of Escherichia coli can be induced in the absence of oxidative stress and oxygen by modulation of NADPH content. Microbiology 157: 957-965.

Lemire J, Mailloux R, Auger C, Whalen D, Appanna VD. (2010) Pseudomonas fluorescens orchestrates a fine metabolic-balancing act to counter aluminium toxicity. Environ Microbiol 12: 1384-1390.

Mailloux RJ, Bériault R, Lemire J, Singh R, Chénier DR, Hamel RD, Appanna VD. (2007) The tricarboxylic acid cycle, an ancient metabolic network with a novel twist. PLoS ONE 2: e690.

Moscoso H, Saavedra C, Loyola C, Pichuantes S, Vásquez C. (1998) Biochemical characterization of tellurite-reducing activities of Bacillus stearothermophilus V. Res Microbiol 149: 389-397.

Nasoff MS, Baker HV, Wolf RE. (1984) DNA sequence of the Escherichia coli gene, gnd, for 6-phosphogluconate dehydrogenase. Gene 27: 253-264.

Nicolas C, Kiefer P, Letisse F, Krömer J, Massou S, Soucaille P, Wittmann C, Lindley ND, Portais JC. (2007) Response of the central metabolism of Escherichia coli to modified expression of the gene encoding the glucose-6-phosphate dehydrogenase. FEBS Lett 581: 3771-3776.

Pérez JM, Arenas FA, Pradenas GA, Sandoval JM, Vásquez CC. (2008) Escherichia coli YqhD exhibits aldehyde reductase activity and protects from the harmful effect of lipid peroxidation-derived aldehydes. J Biol Chem 283: 7346-7353.

Pérez JM, Calderón IL, Arenas FA, Fuentes DE, Pradenas GA, Fuentes E, Sandoval JM, Castro ME, Elías AO, Vásquez CC. (2007) Bacterial toxicity of potassium tellurite: unveiling an ancient enigma. PLoS ONE 2: e211.

Pomposiello PJ, Bennik MH, Demple B. (2001) Genome-wide transcriptional profiling of the Escherichia coli responses to superoxide stress and sodium salicylate. J Bacteriol 183: 3890-3902.

Ralser M, Wamelink MM, Kowald A, Gerisch B, Heeren G, Struys EA, Klipp E, Jakobs C, Breitenbach M, Lehrach H, Krobitsch S. (2007) Dynamic rerouting of the carbohydrate flux is key to counteracting oxidative stress. J Biol 6: 10.

Reinoso CA, Auger C, Appanna VD, Vásquez CC. (2012) Tellurite-exposed Escherichia coli exhibits increased intracellular α-ketoglutarate. Biochem Biophys Res Commun 421: 721-726.

Rowley DL, Fawcet WP, Wolf RE. (1992) Molecular characterization of mutations affecting expression level and growth rate-dependent regulation of the Escherichia coli zwf gene. J Bacteriol 174: 623-626.

Rowley DL, Wolf RE. (1991). Molecular characterization of the Escherichia coli K-12 zwf gene encoding glucose 6-phosphate dehydrogenase. J Bacteriol 173: 968-977.

Rui B, Shen T, Zhou H, Liu J, Chen J, Pan X, Liu H, Wu J, Zheng H, Shi Y. (2010) A systematic investigation of Escherichia coli central carbon metabolism in response to superoxide stress. BMC Syst Biol 4: 122.

Rungrassamee W, Liu X, Pomposiello PJ. (2008) Activation of glucose transport under oxidative stress in Escherichia coli. Arch Microbiol 190: 41-49.

Sandoval JM, Levêque P, Gallez B, Vásquez CC, Buc Calderón P. (2010) Tellurite-induced oxidative stress leads to cell death of murine hepatocarcinoma cells. Biometals 23: 623-632.

Sandoval JM, Arenas FA, Vásquez CC. (2011) Glucose-6-phosphate dehydrogenase protects Escherichia coli from tellurite-mediated oxidative stress. PLoS ONE 6: e25573.

Siliprandi D, De Meio RH, Toninello A, Zoccarato F. (1971) The action of tellurite, a reagent for thiol groups, on mito-chondria oxidative processes. Biochem Biophys Res Commun 45: 1071-1075.

Siliprandi D, Storey DT. (1973) Interaction of tellurite with the respiratory chain in rat liver mitochondria. FEBS Lett 29: 101-104.

Silver S. (1998) Genes for all metals - a bacterial view of the periodic table. J Ind Microbiol Biotechnol 1: 1-12.

Silver S, Phung L. (1996) Bacterial heavy metal resistance: new surprises. Annu Rev Microbiol 50: 753-789.

Singh R, Lemire J, Mailloux RJ, Appanna VD. (2008) A novel strategy involved in anti-oxidative defense: the conversion of NADH into NADPH by a metabolic network. PLoS ONE 3:e2682.

Singh R, Mailloux RJ, Puiseux-Dao S, Appanna VD. (2007) Oxidative stress evokes a metabolic adaptation that favors increased NADPH synthesis and decreased NADH production in Pseudomonas fluorescens. J Bacteriol 189: 6665-6675.

Taylor DE. (1999) Bacterial tellurite resistance. Trends Microbiol 7: 111-115.

Tremaroli V, Fedi S, Zannoni D. (2007) Evidence for a tellurite-dependent generation of reactive oxygen species and absence of a tellurite-mediated adaptive response to oxidative stress in cells of Pseudomonas pseudoalcaligenes KF707. Arch Microbiol 187: 127-135.

Trutko SM, Akimenko VK, Suzina NE, Anisimova LA, Shlyapnikov MG, Baskunov BP, Duda VI, Boronin AM. (2000) Involvement of the respiratory chain of Gram-negative bacteria in the reduction of tellurite. Arch Microbiol 173: 178-186.

Turner RJ, Aharonowitz Y, Weiner JH, Taylor DE. (2001) Glutathione is a target in tellurite toxicity and is protected by tellurite resistance determinants in Escherichia coli. Can J Microbiol 47: 33-40.

Turner RJ, Weiner JH, Taylor DE. (1999) Tellurite-mediated thiol oxidation in Escherichia coli. Microbiology 145: 2549-2557.

Ying W. (2008) NAD+/NADH and NADP+/NADPH in cellular functions and cell death: regulation and biological conse-quences. Antioxid Redox Signal 10: 179-206.

Zannoni D, Borsetti F, Harrison JJ, Turner RJ. (2008) The bacterial response to the chalcogen metalloids Se and Te. Adv Microb Physiol 53: 1-72.

Gene Introduction by Electrospraying

Kazuto Ikemoto
Niigata Research Laboratory
Mitsubishi Gas Chemical Company Inc., Japan

1   Introduction

Gene introduction is a basic biotechnology technique that is essential for protein production and analysis. Typically, in such techniques, a chemical carrier component forms molecular complexes or particles with DNA that are then transported into cells by endocytosis. Electroporation, gene guns, and lasers are used to introduce genes. One of the problems with such techniques is that they can induce marked changes in cells and may be cytotoxic. In addition, although these methods increase energy in only a limited region of the cell, the stimulation is strong and therefore the energy output is high. We aimed at introducing genetic material into a living cell by using a physical-stimulation technique that would have high efficiency, but no cytotoxicity. Electrospray ionization (ESI) is frequently used in mass spectrometry (MS) analysis, and we used this method for transfection and paid careful attention to prevent the electrospray-induced destruction of the genetic material by using a soft ionization approach. We succeeded in using a mixture of cells and DNA for electrospraying. Physical analysis showed that the collisions of millimeter-sized droplets with cells activated the intracellular uptake of DNA. The size of the droplets was much larger than that of the cells. The mechanism for electrospraying is different from that for a gene gun. Electrostatic charges on the droplets are necessary for bacteria, but not for animal cells. Electrospraying can be used for the minimally destructive transfection of cell lines, bacteria, and chicken embryos. The advantages of this method are the simple structure of the device, simple protocol, low cell damage, and low running costs. In this article, we describe the principle of, devices used for, protocols, and mechanisms underlying gene introduction.

2   Electrospraying

The electrospray event is performed by applying a high voltage at a capillary tip. The liquid becomes spherical because of surface tension at the capillary tip. When a high voltage is applied, the liquid changes its shape into a form called the Taylor cone because the charged liquid is pulled toward the counter electrode. When the charged repulsion of the surface is greater than the surface tension, the liquid is separated into smaller droplets and these droplets fly toward the counter electrode. A highly charged droplet at the capillary tip splits into micro- or nano-scale droplets, and the charged fine liquid aerosol is accelerated by the high voltage electric field. Figure 1 shows the scheme and photographs of the electrospray technique. No voltage is applied in the left image, while a high voltage is applied in the right image.

ESI is frequently used in MS analysis. This method has been used for the soft ionization of macromolecules and biomaterials (Fenn et al., 1989). The ionized material is contained in the liquid for ESI. Moreover, in desorption electrospray ionization (DESI) for MS analysis, the electrically charged droplet hits the surface molecule and is ionized under ambient conditions (Cooks et al., 2006). The substance is ionized by bombarding charged droplets during DESI. Electrospraying is also used for the production of nanofibers (Loscertales et al., 2004) and nanoparticles (Chen et al., 2008). Because ESI is widely used, the conditions for electrospraying are widely known. It is difficult to charge nonpolar liquids, e.g., hexane, with electricity and they are not suitable for use in ESI. In addition, because pure water has a high surface tension, it is difficult to use in electrospraying. Therefore, in MS, an organic solvent and a few ionic materials are added. Solutions with high transmission characteristics, such as the electrolytes, are difficult to charge with electricity. However, it has been reported that a highly conductive solution is not suitable for ESI because solutions with conductivity greater than 10^{-3} S/cm cannot be dispersed (Kebarle *et al.*, 1993; Drozin, 1955). Electrospraying is an important technique in science and it can be performed with a simple device. In addition, electrospraying uses a simple and basic technique that is used for the dispersal of pesticides and the application of cosmetics. A very similar technique to electrospraying is the electrostatic application of paint, which is widely used in the automotive industry.

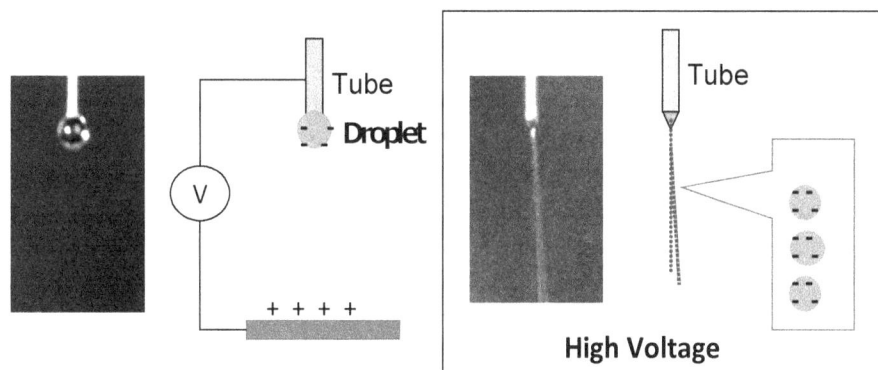

Figure 1: No voltage is applied in the left photograph. The liquid at the tip of the nozzle is spherical. The droplet surface is charged when the voltage is applied to the nozzle. High voltage (kV) is applied in the right photograph. The liquid at the tip of the nozzle forms a Taylor cone. The small droplets appear like a straight thread when sprayed at high speed.

3   Transfection

The delivery of foreign nucleic acids into a living cell is an important technique in molecular biology and medical research. The introduction of a gene into a microbes, animal cells, and plant cells is carried out by different methods. *Escherichia coli*, as a representative microbial species, is widely used as a transfection-competent cell. In addition, *Agrobacterium* is widely used for the transfection of plant cells. The word "transfection" is commonly used for the introduction of nucleic acids into animal cells. Animal cells are more difficult to transfect than *E. coli*. The transfection of animal cells is performed using three methods: viruses, reagents, and devices. Viruses are highly efficient; however, given the different legislation related to their use in many countries, they are not discussed here. Reagents are widely used to transfect cells, e.g., cationic polymers (Boussif *et al.*, 1995) and cationic liposomes (lipofection) (Nyunt *et al.*, 2009). Typically, a chemical carrier forms molecular complexes or particles with DNA that are then transported into cells by endocytosis. The reagent and DNA complex make farther than a cell the small particle formation. These molecules hybridize with the nucleic acid and then liberate it in the cell. These reagents are generally cytotoxic; therefore, efforts to reduce their toxicity have been conducted. This method of transfection requires a complicated operation in which the culture medium is changed after treating the cells with the DNA-chemical reagent mixture in serum-free medium. In addition, the chemical structure of the reagents is complicated and they are very expensive.

Transfection techniques using devices rely upon the physical stimulation of the target cells such as electroporation, gene gun, microinjection, and laser. Electroporation is a popular method that applies a high voltage pulse to a cell for gene introduction. However, adherent cells need to be in a floating state for electroporation. Unfortunately, the usual culture medium produces a spark (towing) when a high voltage pulse is applied, and it must be replaced with a low conductivity solution during electroporation. A gene gun fires a projectile (gold particle) that is coated with DNA into the cell (Klein *et al.*, 1987). This method is effective in plant cells, which have a cell wall. This method introduces many copies of the gene into one cell; however, as the average number of transfected cells is small, this technique is not used very often in animal cells. Microinjection is the injection of material into a cell using a small needle. It is a valid method for large cells such as egg cells. However, this method requires advanced training. The introduction of DNA using a laser has tremendous potential (Stevenson *et al.*, 2010). However, further development is needed to reduce the price of the devices and protocols for this approach. A problem with such techniques is that they can induce marked changes in cells and may be cytotoxic. In addition, although these methods increase energy in only a limited part of the cell, the stimulation is strong and, thus, the energy output is high. These techniques sometimes cause severe damage to cells, especially mammalian cells, or need complex and expensive devices. It has been thought that gene introduction methods require a very small particle and a special technique.

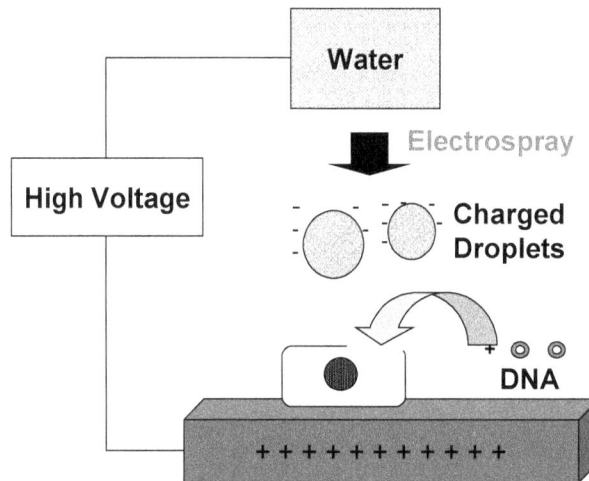

Figure 2: Scheme of droplet impact transfection by electrospraying. A mixture of cells and DNA are sprayed with the charged droplets.

We hypothesized that the impact of the liquid droplets during electrospraying would transport nucleic acid into a cell through transient channels that are created by mild damage on the cell surface (Ikemoto *et al.*, 2011; Okubo *et al.*, 2008). A mixture of cells and nucleic acid is sprayed with charged droplets, and the gene is introduced into the cells. The spray liquid consists of water; therefore, the running costs are low. This approach could have applications as a technique for the minimally destructive transfection of cell lines, bacteria, and chicken embryos. This method was named "droplet impact" Previously, a gene gun-type device used electrospraying for particle acceleration (Pui *et al.*, 2000); therefore, in this approach, it was not necessary to make the DNA-coated particles that are used with a normal gene gun. However, gene gun-type devices have a lower transfection efficiency than droplet impact, and use a different mechanism to introduce the nucleic acid.

The characteristics of representative gene introduction methods are shown in Table 1. This electrospray approach minimized the faults associated with the methods using a device.

Method	Reagent	Device	Device	Device
	Liposome Cationic Polymer	Electroporation	Gene Gun	Electrospray (Droplet Impact)
Running Cost	High	Low	High	Low
Protocol	Easy	Easy	Difficult	Very Easy
Efficiency	High	High	Low	High
Cell Type	Difficult for Floating Cells	Difficult for Adhesive cells	Difficult for Floating Cells	Good for Adhesive and Floating cells

Table 1: The characteristics of gene introduction methods

4   Electrospray Transfection

4.1   Device for Gene Introduction

The electrospray device appears to be special, and the MS and electrospinning devices also appear to be very expensive. However, the electrospray device that is used for the application of makeup or pesticide dispersion is cheap. The electrospray device is a simple structure that is comprised of a high voltage power supply, a nozzle, and a pump. An electrospray device for transfection will require the structure to the cells shed spray.

The structure of our device is shown in Figure 3a. The Petri dish containing the cells and DNA is electrosprayed. The dish is placed on the counter electrode that forms the ground potential. The pump supplies the liquid to the nozzle, which is wired to the high voltage power supply. The inside of the dish is wired to the opposite electrode with a metal ribbon to form the ground potential when the dish is plastic or glass. The high voltage power supply can be the same device used for electrostatic painting, a light electron tube, and electrophoresis. We use a capillary electrophoresis power supply. The pump can consist of a tube pump or a syringe pump. Electrospraying is performed by applying a high voltage to the metal nozzle through which the solution is propelled. A charged drop at the tip of the nozzle splits the stream into small droplets, and the charged aerosol is accelerated by the high voltage electric field toward the cells. For transfection, the liquid droplets are sprayed onto a mixture of cells and plasmid DNA. In this way, a basic device with a fixed nozzle can be made easily.

To construct a device enabling higher efficiency requires some remodeling of the basic design (Figure 3a). The range of the spray from a fixed nozzle at a height of 2 cm is ca. 1 cm in diameter. Therefore, contraptions are necessary to produce a uniform spray. A multi-nozzle cannot make an overlapped range of the spray because of the presence of electrostatic repulsion. We selected a nozzle that can be moved in order to spray the entire surface of the dish (Figure 3b, right). We used a robot dispenser (Shotmini; Musashi Engineering Inc.) and a capillary electrophoresis power supply (HCZE-30PN; Matsusada Precision Inc.) for the scanning device. A factor that needs to be considered with electrospraying is electric discharge. The metal nozzle becomes the needle-plate electrode and is easy to create a discharge. The needle electrode produces a corona discharge, and higher voltages can form a spark discharge from this arrangement. An electrolyte that is nontoxic to the cells is suitable for spraying; however, a highly conductive solution is not suitable for electrospraying.

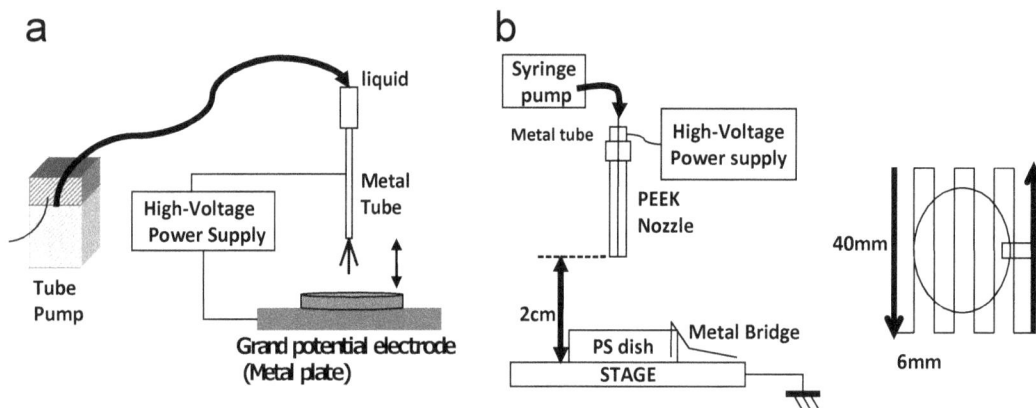

Figure 3: a: The electrospray device consists of a high voltage power supply, a metal nozzle, and a pump. b: The structure of the moving nozzle prevents an electric discharge with an insulator nozzle (PEEK). The nozzle sprays the whole dish by using a scanning pattern. The dish is connected to the ground potential by a metal bridge.

It is assumed that the electrical discharge from the flowing liquid and metal nozzle diminishes the intensity of the electric field. Moreover, it was found that using a metallic nozzle for electrospraying, either with or without a liquid medium, generated an electric current (60 µA, -15 kV) that flowed as a discharge, and this discharge caused damage to the plasmid DNA. The damage to supercoiled plasmids was the same as that reported for ESI-MS of DNA (Cheng *et al.*, 1996). To overcome this problem, we employed an insulated nozzle that separates the droplets from the edge of the electrode, thereby preventing electrostatic breakdown. The insulated nozzle did not cause DNA damage, and the electric current of its discharge dropped by half. In addition, it is thought that the lower discharge level would improve cell viability. This device enables electrospraying with a high concentration of electrolyte (electric conductivity over 100 mS/cm) and also enables electrospraying of a high conductivity solution, which was previously impossible.

4.2   Transfection of Animal Cells

The transfection of animal cells is used for scientific research or industrial purposes, for example, the production of pharmaceutical products such as antibodies, vaccines, and induced pluripotent stem cells. Research of animal cells is conducted mainly on cultured cells *in vitro*. Cultured cells either float in a nutrient medium or are attached to the culture dish. Electrospraying can be used to introduce a gene into adhesive cell cultures. It can also be used to transfect floating cell cultures by temporarily converting the cultures to the adhesive type (e.g., by using coated dishes).

Firstly, the fixed nozzle device was used for transfection. Adhesive Chinese hamster ovary cells (CHO-DHFR cells) and human cancer cells (HeLa cells) were tested as model cells, and almost the same results were obtained. The culture medium was removed from the culture dish (diameter of 35 mm), and a water solution containing the plasmid vector pEGFP-N1, which expressed green fluorescence protein (GFP), was added to the culture dish. The water was electrosprayed onto the cells from a height of 2 cm at -10 kV, and culture medium was then added to the dish. After 24 h of cultivation, many cells showed intense green fluorescence, and the number of cells showing fluorescence increased as the applied voltage was increased, indicating that the kinetic energy of the droplets is an important factor for this method. The application of voltage between the capillary and culture dish without water spraying caused almost the same current as that during electrospraying, suggesting that corona discharge occurs only with the application of voltage, but corona discharge alone without water spraying failed to introduce the plasmid into the cells.

We studied the parameters that affect transfection efficiency and found that increasing the volume of the added solution significantly decreased transfection efficiency. Moreover, transfected cells were found in the region in which the sprayed aerosol had collided, and the proportion of GFP-positive cells increased with increasing cell density. These results clearly indicate that contact between the droplets and the cells is important for gene introduction by electrospraying.

Another important factor affecting the transfection efficiency of electrospraying is the swelling of the cell caused by the intracellular pressure generated by the hypotonic environment. Using water instead of phosphate-buffered saline (PBS) for pre-incubation before electrospraying resulted in a significant increase in the number of GFP-positive cells. Moreover, incubation with water for approximately 10 min resulted in the highest transfection efficiency in this study, suggesting that high osmotic pressure was induced by the swollen state of the cells. The charged microdroplets generated by electrospraying collide with the highly tensioned plasma membrane and easily penetrate the membrane by momentum transfer from the high-speed droplets. After making a small hole in the cell membrane, DNA may enter the cell through this hole by diffusion. However, the possibility of the plasmid being moved by osmotic pressure cannot be ruled out because a relatively high pressure force, 750 kPa (calculated by the van't Hoff equation), is generated in CHO cells. The efficiency of transfection was also affected by the timing of the addition of DNA and electrospraying; the addition of DNA prior to electrospraying resulted in a high transfection efficiency, while the addition of DNA soon after electrospraying resulted in a significant decrease in efficiency, suggesting that the holes persist for 1 min.

Unfortunately, the fixed nozzle device was not effective for transfection. Therefore, we used the improved device with the moving insulator nozzle for transfection (Ikemoto et al., 2012), and we assessed the spray liquid and incubation conditions of the cells for efficient gene transfer.

Pre-incubation of the cells is very important for all gene introduction methods. For the electrospray method, the following approach is used. The surface of the dish has a large influence; a dish coated with poly-Lys increases the transfection efficiency in CHO cells to almost twice that for non-coated dishes. Cell adhesion is important because it is related to the mechanism of electrospraying, and culturing the cells in a coated dish is effective. The cells also need time to attach to the dish before electrospraying, e.g., CHO cells require more than 12 h. In addition, adhesion is expected to increase the tolerance of the cells to the stress from the change in osmolarity and from the spray. Therefore, cell viability increases the efficiency of gene introduction. In addition, viability is important for the production of proteins from the introduced nucleic acid following transfection, which is also true for the other gene introduction methods; therefore, optimum cell culture conditions are important in all in vitro experiment.

CHO cells preincubated with the plasmid pEGFP-N1 were electrosprayed with the solution by moving the nozzle at 5 mm/s and with less than a 6-mm interval between the scans, at a liquid flow rate of 6 mL/h (Figure 3b).

The effect on transfection efficiency of various spray media, such as water, nutrient media, normal and high-concentration PBS, dissolved sugar, and solutions of specific electrolytes, e.g., organic cations, salt, and phosphates, was examined for electrospraying at -12 kV. The results of this examination are shown in Table 2. Nonionic 20% (w/w) sucrose resulted in an efficiency of 1%; monosaccharides (glucose and fructose), sugar alcohols (sorbitol and xylitol), and organic solvents (DMSO, methoxyethanol, and propylene glycol) gave similar results. An amino sugar electrolyte solution of 5% (w/w) glucosamine and alpha-MEM resulted in an efficiency of 25%. In contrast, high concentrations of sodium chloride and phosphate yielded an efficiency of >60% (Figure 4a). After electrospraying, most of the cells survived and maintained 100% confluence. The efficiency of many gene-introduction methods is lowered because of the interference caused by serum; however, serum interference does not affect electrospraying. We compared the efficiency of electrospraying with that of other transfection methods. Transfection efficiency was 0.2% for the calcium phosphate method and 11.4% for the liposome method (Lipofectamine, Invitrogen). The electrospray method showed higher efficiency (25–69%) than other gene-introduction approaches did under the same conditions.

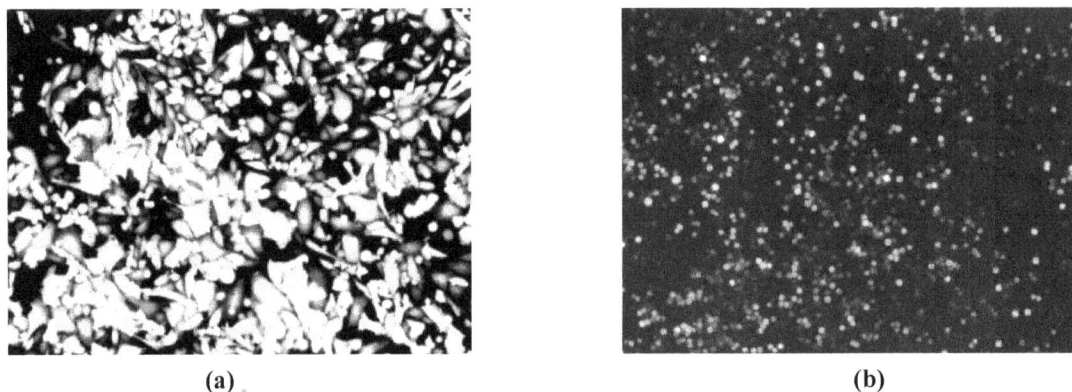

(a)   (b)

Figure 4: a: Microphotograph of GFP expression in CHO cells induced by electrospraying (5× PBS, -12 kV). b: Microphotograph of GFP expression in Jurkat cells induced by electrospraying (5× PBS, -12 kV). The cells were attached to a polyethylenimine-coated dish.

This high efficiency was not restricted to CHO cells, as Jurkat cells were also transfected at a relatively high efficiency (45%) by electrospraying with 5× PBS at -12 kV (Figure 4b). Jurkat cells normally grow unattached in culture medium; however, for this experiment, the cells were attached using a polyethylenimine coating on the surface of the culture dishes. It was found that unattached and floating cells were not transfected by the electrospray method.

No.		Efficiency (%)	No.		Efficiency (%)
1	Water	0.8	6	2.5% NaH_2PO_4 + 2.5% Na_2HPO_4	61
2	20% Sucrose	1.3	7	4.5% NaCl	67
3	a-MEM	25	8	3× PBS	68
4	5% Glucosamine HCl	25	9	5× PBS	69
5	PBS	48	10	10× PBS	42

Table 2: Transfection efficiency by liquid electrospraying at -12 kV

4.3   Protein Transport into Cells

We were also able to demonstrate high efficiency transfection with protein. Approximately 50% of the cells preincubated with an FITC-IgG antibody (150 µg/mL) and 93% preincubated with an FITC-insulin antibody (2.5 mg/mL) were detectable by fluorescence microscopy after electrospraying with 3× PBS at -12 kV (Figure 5). Some cells included FITC-insulin following mixing because insulin is a small molecule; however, the electrospray process made it possible to transport insulin into more cells. Highly concentrated insulin was introduced into cells at a high efficiency. If the cells are incubated in IgG at a high concentration, the efficiency will be higher. Apparently, proteins such as insulin (6 kDa) and IgG (15 kDa), which are both approximately 2 orders of magnitude smaller than the test plasmid DNA (2.8 MDa), could also be transported relatively efficiently into cells by the electrospray method.

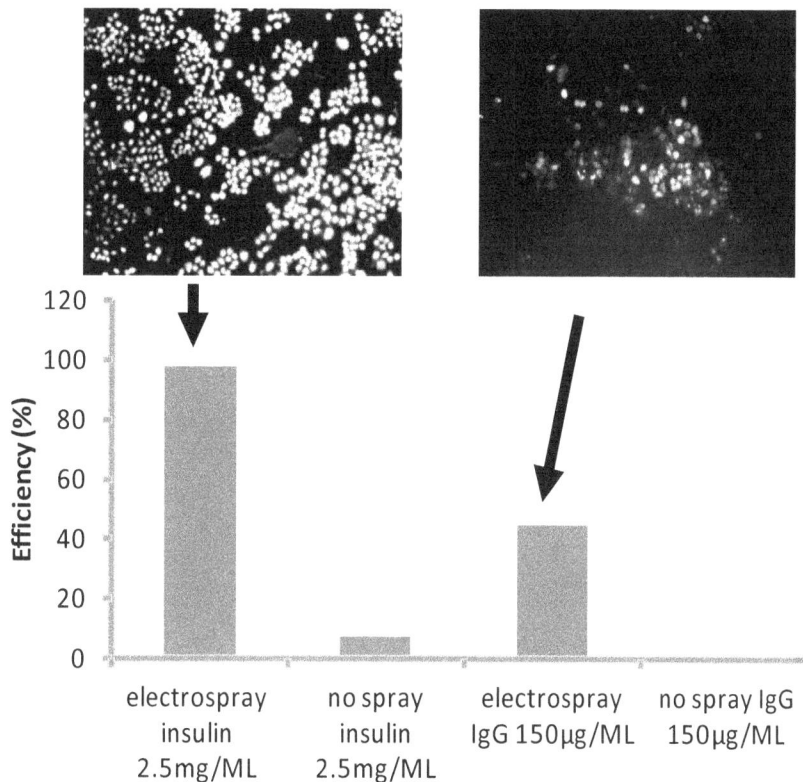

Figure 5: Efficiency of transporting insulin into CHO cells by electrospraying (3× PBS -12 kV) and with no spray (2.5 mg/mL). Similarly, IgG (H+L) VEC b1-1488 was conjugated with FITC and redissolved at a concentration of 150 µg/mL. The photographs show fluorescent cells containing FITC-insulin (left) and FITC-IgG (right).

4.4   Embryo

Furthermore, using a chicken embryo, we also demonstrated that this method could be applied to a developmental specimen *in vitro*. The plasmid vector pEGFP-N1 was put on the target region of the chicken embryo and PBS was electrosprayed onto the embryo from a height of 10 cm at +10 kV. The results of gene transduction in the embryo are shown in Figure 6.

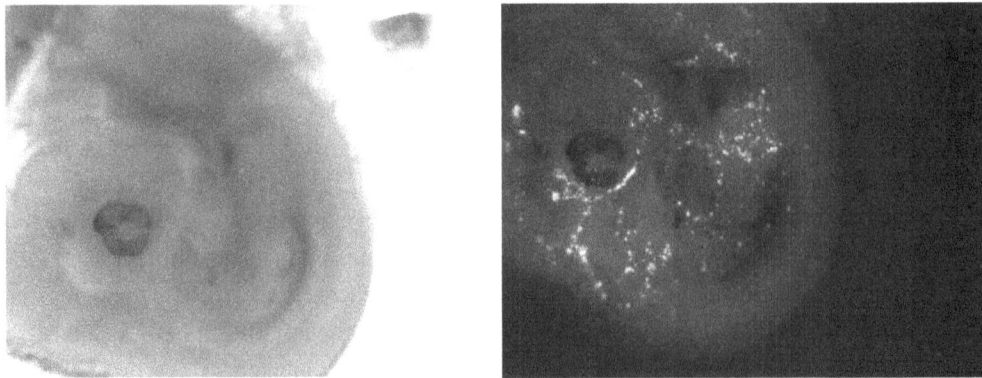

Figure 6: The photograph on the left is of the embryo in a normal light field. The photograph on the right is a fluorescent image. Cells expressing GFP are observed in the embryo.

5   Gene Introduction Mechanism

Apparently, ionic solutes in the electrospray medium favor a higher transfection efficiency than nonionic solutes; therefore, we focused on conductivity as the primary electrophysical factor that is associated with ionic materials. The relationship between conductivity and gene transfection efficiency is displayed in Figure 7. The results showed that the efficiency for water was low (0.8%). The transfection efficiency increased dramatically to higher than 60%, with maximum efficiency obtained between 40–80 mS/cm conductivity. Conversely, 10× PBS, which had the highest conductivity (132 mS/cm), caused an unstable spray by spark discharge. The unstable spray resulted in low transfection efficiency. In contrast to the sizable influence of conductivity on the success of transfection, we were able to identify factors that do not appreciably influence transfection. Among these are molecular weight, type of cations and anions in the spray solution, and osmotic pressure. Next, the diameter of the droplets was measured microscopically to study the relationship between increasing conductivity and efficiency. The average diameter of the droplets rapidly increased (more than 0.5 mm) until a conductivity of 15 mS/cm was reached, after which it tended to reach a plateau (Figure 7).

The diameter of all liquid droplets was 5 mm at 0 V (data not shown). Subsequently, the droplet charged by the application of high voltage was dispersed by the surface electrostatic force, but high conductivity liquids were difficult to charge and were converted into larger droplets. The graph pertaining to efficiency and diameter shows that gene introduction depended on the size of the droplets (Figure 7), and 70% of the cells were transfected when the droplet diameter was 0.5–1.2 mm. These results indicate that the actual diameter of the droplets was larger than that of the cells, and larger droplets were associated with relatively higher transfection efficiency. Furthermore, we performed a detailed analysis of the applied voltage, droplet size, and transfection efficiency in varying ionic electrospray solutions. Water and solutions containing high concentrations of PBS (Hi-PBS) were compared. The transfection efficiency of most liquids depended on the applied voltage. The relationship between the applied voltage and droplet size was small between -8 and -12kV in Hi-PBS. In solutions with high electric conductivity, such as 5× and 10× PBS, the efficiency was higher at low voltages because the size of the droplets was larger (Figure 8).

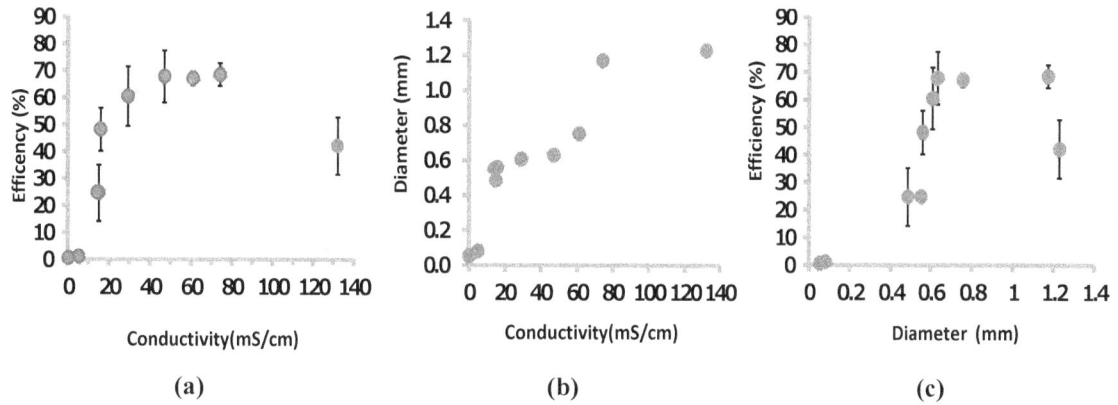

Figure 7: a) The transfection efficiency in CHO cells electrosprayed at -12 kV depends on conductivity. b) Average diameter of the droplets at -12 kV vs. conductivity of the electrospray liquids. c) Transfection efficiency vs. the diameter of the droplets.

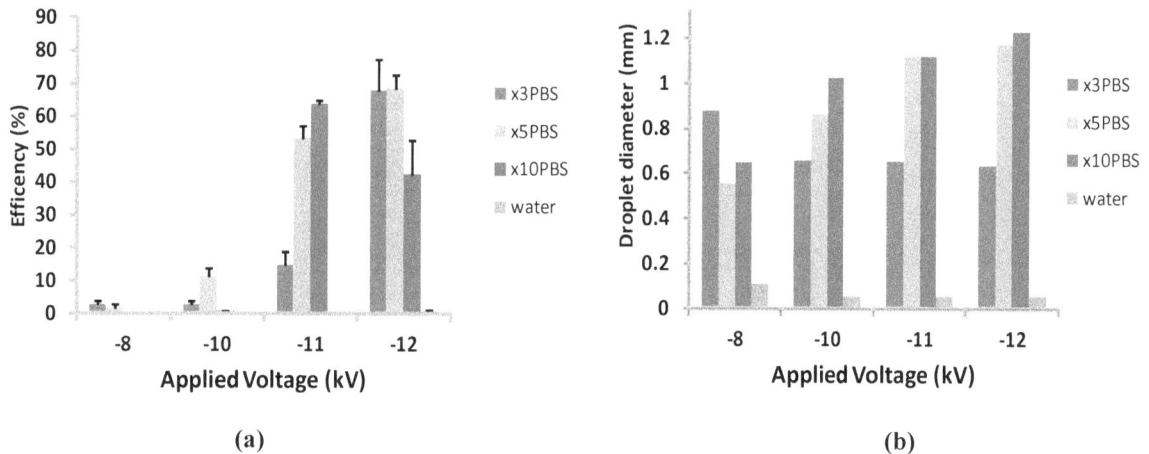

Figure 8: a) Transfection efficiency in CHO cells depends on voltage. Transfection efficiency is high at -11 and -12 kV in Hi-PBS, and a maximum efficiency of 0.8% is attained at -12 kV in water. b)

We measured the average velocity of the electrosprayed droplets using high-speed photography. The mean velocity was measured to be approximately 2 m/s lower than that reported for DESI and ESI-MS (0.1 km/s) (Nemes *et al.*, 2007; Venter *et al.*, 2006). Our method cannot be used to measure the individual size and velocity of droplets; however, it is thought that the mean values reflect individual velocity and size because the typical size distribution curve of the electrosprayed droplets is very sharp. For the distribution of droplet diameter at -12 kV, the effective size is 0.1–1 mm, and gene introduction is difficult with droplets smaller than this. Before beginning the analysis of electrospray transfection, we speculated that the electrosprayed droplets would be very small compared with the size of a cell, and that the micro-droplets would perforate the cell membrane by causing mechanical damage. However, the actual diameter of the droplets is approximately 10^2 times larger than that of the cells. The finding that larger droplets result in higher transfection efficiency leads to the hypothesis that the most critical parameter for transfection is the impact energy generated by the collision of large droplets. Possibly related to this observation is the fact that a large projectile is effective at ionization in secondary ion MS (Hiraoka *et al.*, 2006; Cornett *et al.*, 1994). The total energy density associated with spraying cells is calculated from the spray volume and droplet velocity. Water and 10× PBS have the same energy density (6.0×10^{-2} Jm^{-2}) at -12 kV; however, it is not the resulting total energy that is important, but rather the energy of each droplet. We think that contact time, i.e., the time required for the transfer of the collision energy, is an important factor for the simple mechanism of energy transfer. The contact time that delivers a good transfection rate is between 10^{-5} and 10^{-6} s, depending on the diameter of the droplet. Our current interpretation would be that small droplets are not capable of delivering sufficient transfer energy for efficient transfection, but rather large droplets are effective conduits for energy transfer once they have contacted the cells. Furthermore, the function of the droplets was examined using a fluorescent dye (FITC-glucosamine) that does not pass through the cell membrane. We compared electrospraying the dye versus simply incubating the cells in it, using 3× PBS as the solute. Although strong cellular fluorescence was seen with the electrosprayed dye, only slight fluorescence was seen when the cells were incubated in the dye (Figure 9).

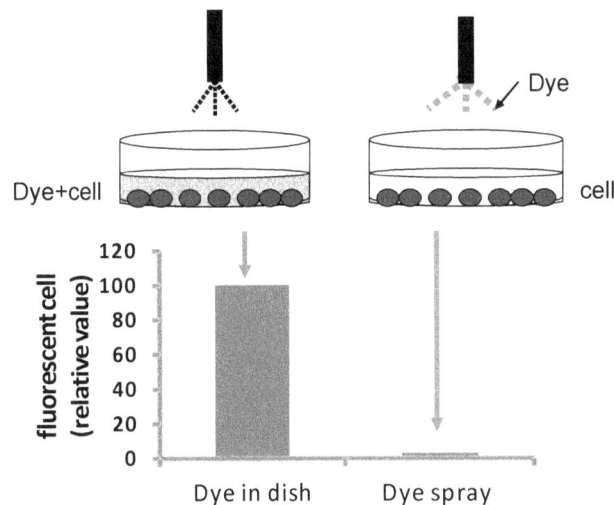

Figure 9: Study of the transfection mechanism using dye. The efficiency for the droplet impact method (dye in dish) is high, but the efficiency for gene gun-type transfection (dye spray) is low.

We conclude that the droplets generated by electrospraying greatly enhanced the uptake of the dye. The collision of a droplet with a cell indirectly makes the cell permeable; therefore, the droplet promotes the cellular uptake of DNA. Electrospraying with a gene gun has been reported, but this method has a different mechanism than that described here. The pressure accompanying droplet impact is approximately 10^3–10^4 Pa; however, this is too low to induce gene transfection. We postulate that a vertical collision induces a change of the cell's shape, and this somehow raises its permeability for gene transport. In addition, the experiment with the dye shows the differences between the droplet impact method (dye in dish) and the efficiency of the gene gun-type approach (dye spray). When electrospraying was used, the droplet impact method becomes highly efficient. Because the gene gun-type must pass through two barrier layers, i.e., the aqueous layer covering the cells and the cell membrane, its efficiency is low. The electric charge per volume is small in large droplets. Similar characteristics can be produced easily by other spraying methods. Hence, we conclude that the electrical charge on a droplet is not important for transfection by this method in mammalian cells. As an interesting side observation, the velocity and diameter of the droplets are similar to those of rain droplets (terminal velocity of 0.7 – 4 m/s; diameter from 0.2 – 1 mm) (Ahrens, 2007), and thunderclouds can impart an electrical charge to the rain droplets (Ceremonie *et al.*, 2004). From the results of our electrospray experiments, one could even speculate that thunder showers may be involved in some way with horizontal gene transfer in nature. The electrospray method described here is very different from other techniques of gene delivery. It is very surprising that cellular DNA or protein uptake would be facilitated by such a macroscale event, i.e., collision with a droplet much larger than the target cell (Figure 10). This macroscale method for transfection may offer a much more efficient, simpler, and more rapid technique for many types of cells.

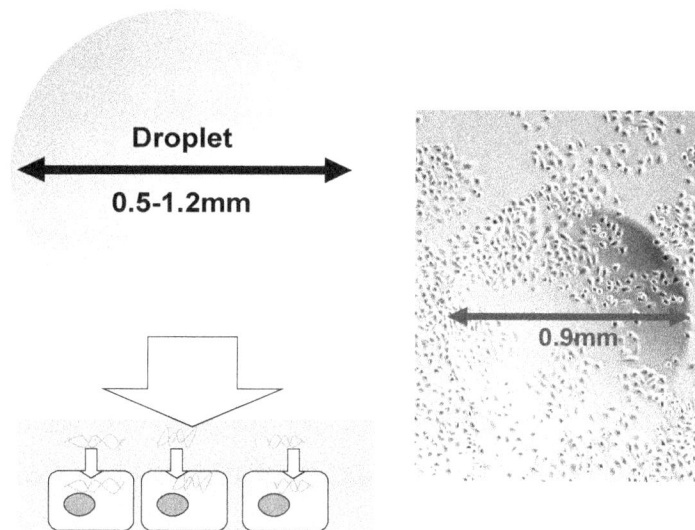

Figure 10: Scheme: Transfection mechanism of droplet strike. Large droplets strike the solution and nucleic acids are pushed into the cells. The photograph on the right compares the size of the droplet and to the size of the cells. Effective droplets for gene transport are significantly larger than the cells.

6   Other Spray Methods

In gene transfection using electrospraying, the size of an effective droplet was in the millimeter scale. This same characteristic can be produced by other spraying methods, such as those involving the use of a fragrance atomizer. Thus, we examined whether transfection using a fragrance atomizer or free-falling droplets could introduce DNA into cells (Figure 11). Surprisingly, the GFP plasmid was transfected into mammalian cells using a fragrance atomizer and free-falling droplets, despite the lack of a charge on the droplets, and we confirmed GFP expression in CHO cells (Table 3). This method works using gas rather than liquid as the spray "medium." We tested air, carbon dioxide, and dimethyl ether with our device. The cells sprayed with gas took up the DNA. This result shows that the electric charge is not important for gene introduction in animal cells, and this supports the mechanism that we suggest.

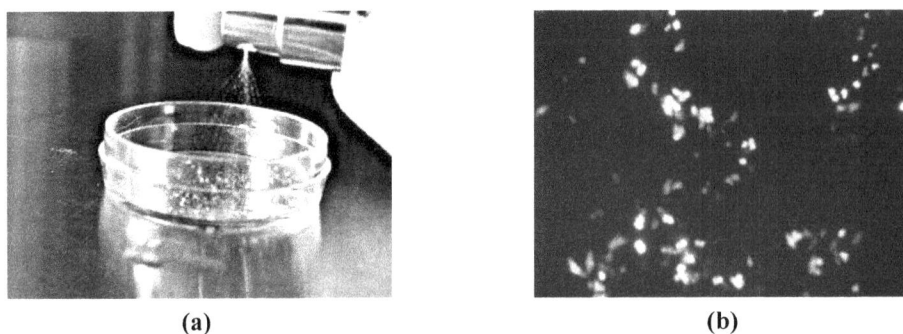

(a)   **(b)**

Figure 11: a) Spray transfection using a fragrance atomizer. b) GFP-expressing cells follow-ing transfection using a PBS spray from a fragrance atomizer.

	Electrospray	Atomizer	Free-falling	Gas Flow
Droplet Size (mm)	0.1–1.2	0.12	5.0	-
Spray Volume	30 µL	50–60 µL	300 µL	0.4 L
Droplet Velocity (m·s^{-1})	1.8–2.1	5–8	1.5 m height	136–380
Efficiency (CHO)	40–80%	1.80%	0.30%	8.1%
Efficiency (*E. coli*)	10^4–10^5 cells/µg	1–3 cells/µg	1–3 cells/µg	-

Table 3: Comparison of the introduction of nucleic acid into cell using different forms of spraying.

7   Bacteria (Transformation)

E. coli was used as a representative bacterial species. The competent cell method, in which cells are pro-cessed with calcium ions, establishes the transformation of *E. coli*. Therefore, the advantage of a new method is small. However, this study is useful as a model experiment because there are bacteria for which this method is not established.

This method was also applicable to the non-competent *E. coli* strain k12 (Figure 12). A pUC19 plasmid encoding an ampicillin-resistant gene was mixed with an *E. coli* colony on an agarose dish, and ampicillin-resistant *E. coli* cells were obtained after carrying out electrospraying with water at more than -7 kV. Electrophoretic analysis also demonstrated that the antibiotic-resistant colonies carried the plasmid. The gene introduction efficiency was 10^4 – 10^5 cells/µg. We also performed an experiment using a gene gun-type approach. A plasmid-water solution was sprayed onto a lawn of *E. coli*. Then, gene introduction required plus or minus 18 kV. We found that the droplet impact method can be used with the low voltage approach rather than a gene gun-type approach. A fragrance atomizer and free-falling transformation had a very low efficiency in *E. coli*; therefore, electrical effects may be important in the transformation of bacteria and there may also be other important mechanisms. *E. coli* are 1 – 2 µm in size, i.e., much small-er than animal cells. Therefore, the droplets are bigger than the cells. This shows that the electrospray mechanism is not the same in bacterial cells as it is in animal cells. Interestingly, gene introduction was not successful with the other spray methods; therefore, an electric charge is necessary in bacteria. Elec-troporation or DESI may function by the same mechanism in these cells. Recently, gene gun-type DNA transfer has progressed; a high efficiency of 10^6 cells/μg was accomplished using gold nanoparticles and calcium chloride (Lee *et al.*, 2011). Future developments of this approach are expected.

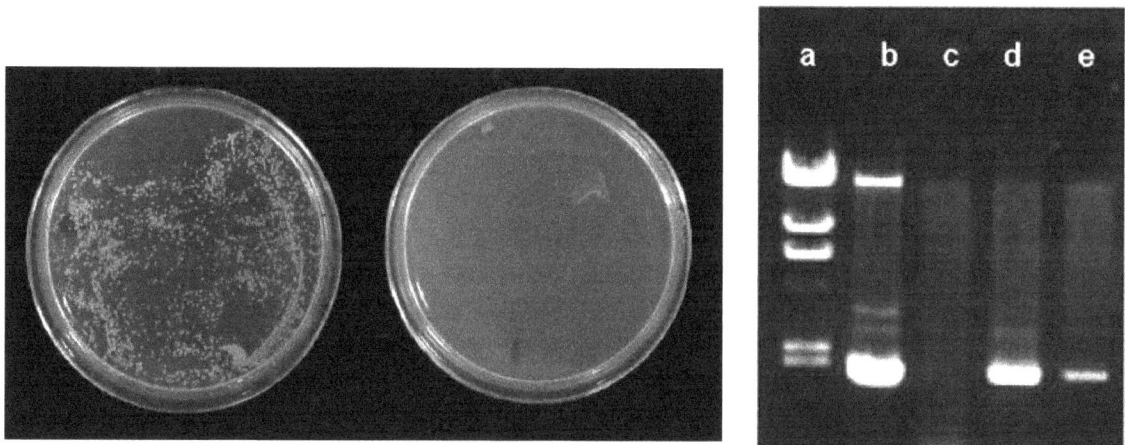

Figure 12: The left dish containing an antibiotic shows *E. coli* treated with electrospraying and an antibiotic-resistance plasmid. The right dish is the control experiment of untreated *E. coli*. The right photograph shows the result from electrophoretic analysis. a: size marker, b: plasmid DNA, c: control *E. coli*, d: -7 kV electrospraying, and e: -12 kV electrospraying.

8   Protocol (CHO cell)

We introduced the electrospray gene in the introduction using CHO cells as the basic protocol. The protocol of this method is very simple (Table 4).

Step	Operation		Material
1	Pre-incubation	Plate CHO cells in a dish (10000 cells/dish, 2 mL medium) 20–48 h, 37°C, 5% CO_2	Poly-L-lysine-coated dish (35 mm) a-MEM + 10% FBS
2	Before Spray	Remove the medium Mix with 100 μL plasmid Room temperature, 5–10 min incubation.	Plasmid DNA in pure water (100 μg/mL)
3	Electrospray	Pump: 6 mL/h, -10 kV Scanning (5 mm/s, 6 mm interval)	3× PBS Device (see device section)
4	After Spray	Add 2 mL medium, mix 20–48 h, 37°C, 5% CO_2	a-MEM + 10% FBS
5	Detect	Fluorescent microscopy	Microscopy

Table 4: Transfection protocol for CHO cells using droplet impact with electrospraying

9   Conclusion

The electrospray method described here is very different from other techniques of gene delivery. Most of the commonly used transfection methods require the use of technologies smaller than the cells themselves, in which artificial nanometer-scale materials and technologies (known as nanotechnologies) are employed. It is very surprising that cellular DNA or protein uptake would be facilitated by a macroscale event, i.e., collision with a droplet much larger than the target cells. This macroscale method for transfection may offer a much more efficient, simpler, and more rapid technique for many types of cells. In summary, we achieved very high transfection efficiencies for genes and proteins using our electrospray method. Both a normal liquid spray and gas flow successfully induced the transfection of cells. We obtained surprising results showing that oversized droplets, approximately 100-times larger than the cells, gave the highest transfection activity. This method is enhanced by increasing the size of droplets and raising the applied voltage, and it does not require any special reagents. In addition, the underlying mechanisms may have some relevance for horizontal gene transfer during evolution. We expect the following advances from these results. It will be proved that spray technology can be used for gene introduction. Printer technology, in particular, is expected. In addition, more simple techniques will be developed, such as the use of a bottle, because small drops are not necessary for gene introduction. Hybrids of chemical and physical stimulation will be developed.

References

Boussif, O. et al. (1995). A versatile vector for gene and oligonucleotide transfer into cells in culture and in vivo: polyethylenimine. Proc. Natl. Acad. Sci. U.S.A., 92, 7297–7301.

Nyunt, M. T. et al. (2009). Physico-chemical characterization of polylipid nanoparticles for gene delivery to the liver. Bioconjug. Chem., 20, 2047–2054.

Klein, T. M., Wolf, E. D., Wu, R. & Sanford J. C. (1987). High-velocity microprojectiles for delivering nucleic acids into living cells. Nature, 327, 70–73.

Stevenson, D. J., Gunn-Moore, F. J., Campbell, P., & Dholakia, K. (2010). Single cell optical transfection. J. R. Soc. Interface, 7, 863–871.

Fenn, J. B., Mann, M., Meng, C. K., Wong, S. F. & Whitehouse, C. M. (1989). Electrospray ionization for mass spectrometry of large biomolecule. Science, 246, 64–71.

Cooks, R. G., Ouyang, Z., Takats, Z. & Wiseman, J. M. (2006). Ambient mass spectrometry. Science, 311, 1566–1570.

Chen, H., Zhao, Y., Song, Y. & Jiang, L. (2008). One-step multicomponent encapsulation by compound-fluidic electrospray. J. Am. Chem. Soc., 130, 7800–7801.

Loscertales, I. G., Barrero, A., Márquez, M., Spretz, R., Velarde-Ortiz, R. & Larsen, G. (2004). Electrically forced coaxial nanojets for one-step hollow nanofiber design. J. Am. Chem. Soc., 126, 5376–5377.

Ikemoto K. et al. (2011). Method of transferring substance into cell. United States patent 7,927,874.

Okubo, Y. Ikemoto, K. Koike, K. Tsutsui, C. Sakata, I. Takei, O. Adachi, A. Sakai T. (2008). DNA introduction into living cells by water droplet impact with electrospray process. Angew. Chem. Int. Ed., 47, 1429–1431.

Kebarle, P. & Tang, L. (1993). From ions in solution to ions in the gas phase-the mechanism of electrospray mass spectrometry. Anal. Chem., 65, 972–986.

Drozin, V. G. (1955). The electrical dispersion of liquids as aerosols. J. Colloid. Sci., 10, 158–164.

Ikemoto K., Sakata I., and Sakai T. (2012). *Collision of millimetre droplets induces DNA and protein transfection into cells. Sci Rep., 2: 289. doi: 10.1038/srep00289.*

Cheng, X. et al. (1996). *Molecular weight determination of plasmid DNA using electrospray ionization mass spectrometry. Nucl. Acids Res., 24, 2183–2189.*

Nemes, P., Marginean, I. & Vertes, A. (2007). *Spraying mode effect on droplet formation and ion chemistry in electrospray. Anal. Chem., 79, 3105–3116.*

Venter, A., Sojka, P. E. & Cooks, R. G. (2006). *Droplet dynamics and ionization mechanisms in desorption electrospray ionization mass spectrometry. Anal. Chem., 78, 8549–8555.*

Hiraoka, K., Asakawa, D., Fujimaki, S., Takamizawa, A. & Mori, K. (2006). *Electrosprayed droplet impact/secondary ion mass spectrometry. Eur. Phys. J. D., 38, 255–229.*

Cornett, D. S., Lee, T. D. & Mahoney, J. F. (1994). *Matrix-free desorption of biomolecules using massive cluster impact. Rapid Commun. Mass Spectrom., 8, 996–1000.*

Chen, D., Wendt, C. H. & Pui, D. Y. H. (2000). *A novel approach for introducing bio-materials into cells. J. Nanoparticle Res., 2, 133–139.*

Ahrens, C.D. (2007). *Meteorology Today. 8th Edition, Japanese version. Tokyo: Maruzen Co., Ltd.*

Ceremonie, H., Buret, F., Simonet, P. & Vogel, T. M. (2004). *Isolation of lightning-competent soil bacteria. Appl. Environ. Microbiol., 70, 6342–6346.*

Lee Y., Wu B., Zhuang W., Chen D., Tang, Y. (2011). *Nanoparticles facilitate gene delivery to microorganisms via an electrospray process. J. Microbiological Methods, 84, 228–233.*

DNA Aptamers: Discovery and Affinity Purification of Proteins

Jeffrey A. DeGrasse
Office of Regulatory Science, Center for Food Safety and Applied Nutrition
US Food and Drug Administration, USA

Stacey L. DeGrasse
Office of Regulatory Science, Center for Food Safety and Applied Nutrition
US Food and Drug Administration, USA

1   Introduction

Current immuno-affinity chromatographic methods enable target proteins to be isolated, purified, detected, identified, and quantified. However, the success of these methods depends upon the availability of a high quality antibody, the development of which is non-trivial and costly. An aptamer is a functional nucleic acid that exhibits high affinity and specificity to its target (Bunka & Stockley, 2006; Ellington & Szostak, 1990; Robertson & Joyce, 1990; Tuerk & Gold, 1990). In contrast to antibodies, aptamers are discovered and developed without the extensive time and financial investments or ethical concerns of animal husbandry (Iliuk *et al.*, 2011; Tombelli *et al.*, 2005). In this chapter, the discovery of an aptamer by a systematic evolution of ligands by exponential enrichment (SELEX) method used in our laboratory (DeGrasse, 2012) is detailed. Further, a method to utilize the successful aptamer in an aptamer isolation protocol is provided. Finally, using an aptamer (APT^{SEB1}) specific to staphylococcal enterotoxin B (SEB), the general aptamer isolation protocol is applied to the isolation of SEB from a mixture of closely related enterotoxins using non-fat dry milk as a representative food matrix.

2   Methodology

2.1   Preparation of Target-Coupled Paramagnetic Beads

2.1.1   Coupling the Target Protein to Paramagnetic Beads Using the Dynabeads® Antibody Coupling Kit

1. Suspend 60 mg of freeze dried Dynal M-270 epoxy coated paramagnetic beads in 2 ml dimethyl formamide.

2. Transfer 100 µl of M-270 epoxy coated beads (30 mg/ml) to a screw cap vial.

3. Place the vial onto a magnet (e.g., DynaMag™-2 Magnet, Life Technologies) and allow beads to collect to the side of tube (about 1 minute). Aspirate the supernatant.

4. Wash the beads by adding 1 ml buffer C1 (buffers C1, C2, HB, LB, and SB are components of the Dynabeads antibody coupling kit; Life Technologies). Mix by gentle pipetting.

5. Place the vial onto a magnet and allow beads to collect to the side of tube. Aspirate the supernatant.

6. To the beads, add 120 µl of buffer C1 and mix.

7. Add 30 µg of target protein.

8. Add 150 µl of buffer C2 and mix.

9. Incubate with end-over-end rotation overnight at 37 °C.

10. The next day, spin down the solution briefly, and then place the vial onto a magnet and allow beads to collect to the side of tube. Aspirate the supernatant.

11. Wash the beads sequentially with the following buffers:

    a.   800 µl of buffer HB

b.   800 μl of buffer LB

c.   800 μl of buffer SB

d.   800 μl of buffer SB

e.   800 μl of buffer SB. Incubate with end-over-end rotation for 15 minutes.

f.   Note: After each wash, place the vial onto a magnet and allow beads to collect to the side of tube. Aspirate the supernatant.

12. Resuspend the beads in 300 μl PBS-T (10 mM phosphate buffer, 2.7 mM KCl, 140 mM NaCl, 0.05% Tween, pH 7.4, Sigma, St. Louis, MO) and store at 4 °C. The final concentration of beads is 10 μg/μl, or 6.7 x 10^5 beads/μl.

13. Note: Uncoupled beads for counter-selection are produced in a similar manner, but without a ligand.

2.1.2   Preparation of Uncoupled Paramagnetic Beads Using the Dynabeads® Antibody Coupling Kit

1. Suspend 60 mg of freeze dried Dynal M-270 epoxy coated paramagnetic beads in 2 ml dimethyl formamide.

2. Transfer 100 μl of M-270 epoxy coated beads (30 mg/ml) to a screw cap vial.

3. Place the vial onto a magnet (e.g., DynaMag™-2 Magnet, Life Technologies) and allow beads to collect to the side of tube (about 1 minute). Aspirate the supernatant.

4. Wash the beads by adding 1 ml buffer C1 (buffers C1, C2, HB, LB, and SB are components of the Dynabeads antibody coupling kit; Life Technologies). Mix by gentle pipetting.

5. Place the vial onto a magnet and allow beads to collect to the side of tube. Aspirate the supernatant.

6. To the beads, add 150 μl of buffer C1 and mix.

7. Add 150 μl of buffer C2 and mix.

8. Incubate with end-over-end rotation overnight at 37 °C.

9. The next day, spin down the solution briefly, and then place the vial onto a magnet and allow beads to collect to the side of tube. Aspirate the supernatant.

10. Wash the beads sequentially with the following buffers:

a.   800 μl of buffer HB

b.   800 μl of buffer LB

c.   800 μl of buffer SB

d.   800 μl of buffer SB

e.   800 μl of buffer SB. Incubate with end-over-end rotation for 15 minutes.

    f.   Note: After each wash, place the vial onto a magnet and allow beads to collect to the side of tube. Aspirate the supernatant.

11. Resuspend the beads in 300 µl PBS-T (10 mM phosphate buffer, 2.7 mM KCl, 140 mM NaCl, 0.05% Tween, pH 7.4, Sigma, St. Louis, MO) and store at 4 °C. The final concentration of beads is 10 µg/µl, or 6.7 x 10^5 beads/µl.

2.1.3   Bead Coupling Validation via Mass Spectrometry

1. Simultaneously analyze pure standard (positive control), uncoupled beads (negative control), and coupled beads for comparison.

2. Transfer 40 µl of coupled beads and uncoupled beads into separate vials.

    a.   Wash the beads three times with 100 µl of 50 mM ammonium bicarbonate.

3. Transfer 1 µl of 1 µg/µl standard to another vial.

4. To each vial, add 25 µl of 50 mM ammonium bicarbonate, heat at 99 °C for 5 minutes, and then cool on ice. Spin down.

5. Add 25 µl of 50 mM ammonium bicarbonate/18% acetonitrile.

6. Add 2 µl of 0.5 µg/µl trypsin (Promega, Madison, WI).

7. Incubate for 4 hours at 60 °C with agitation.

8. Quench the proteolysis with 5.2 µl of 10% acetic acid.

9. Analyze via any appropriate LC-MS/MS method.

2.2   SELEX

The general schematic of the SELEX protocol is outlined in Figure 1. The DNA used for the SELEX protocol is listed in Table 1.

2.2.1   Round 1

1. Prepare the library by diluting 50 µl of 100 µM library stock (5 nmoles) into 450 µL PBS-T. Incubate at 95 °C for 5 minutes and then cool on ice until needed.

2. Prepare target-coupled Dynabeads. Transfer 20 µl of the protein-coupled beads to a microcentrifuge vial and remove the supernatant. Wash the beads twice in 500 µl PBS-T and resuspend the beads in 1 ml PBS-T.

3. Mix in a 50 ml centrifuge tube in the following order:

    a.   48.5 ml of PBS-T,

    b.   1 ml of washed protein-conjugated beads in PBS-T,

    c.   50 µl of 1 mg/ml bovine serum albumin (Sigma-Aldrich),

    d.   5 µl of 1 mg/ml poly(deoxyinosinic-deoxycytidylic) acid (Sigma-Aldrich), mix the solution, and

    e.   500 µl of heated/cooled library solution.

Library	5' – GGT ATT GAG GGT CGC ATC N$_{40}$ GAT GGC TCT AAC TCT CCT CT
Forward Primer	5' – GGT ATT GAG GGT CGC ATC
Reverse Primer	5' – AGA GGA GAG TTA GAG CCA TC
Biotinylated Reverse Primer	5' – [Biotin]AGA GGA GAG TTA GAG CCA TC

Table 1: DNA used for SELEX

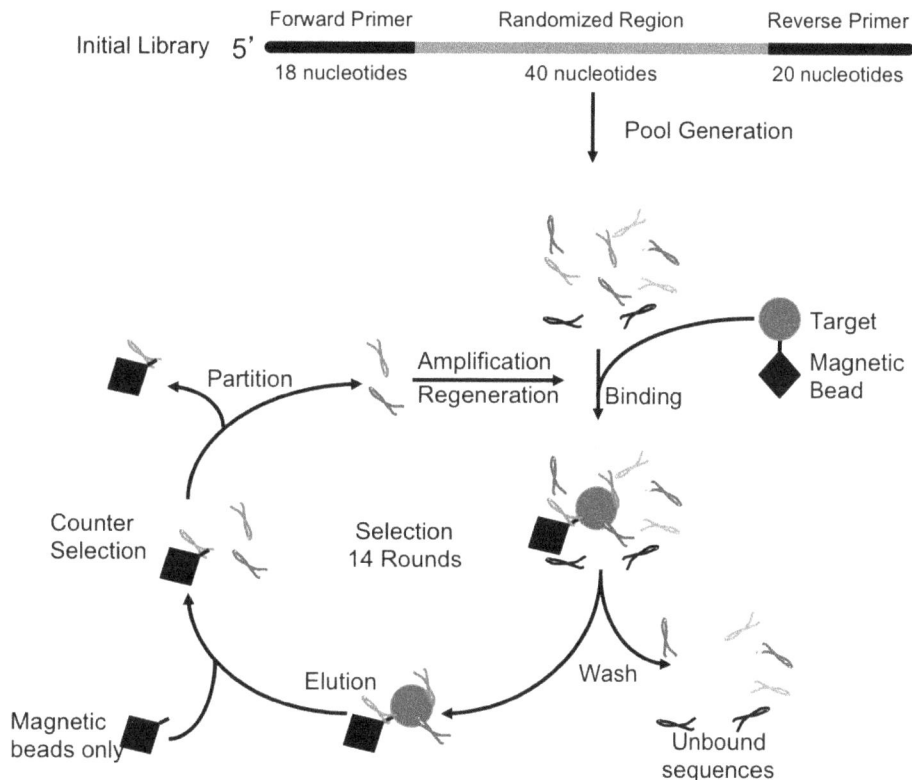

Figure 1: Schematic outlining the SELEX protocol.

4. Selection: Incubate with rotation at room temperature for 30 minutes.

5. Collect beads by placing the centrifuge tube onto a large magnet for 20 minutes and remove all but ~1.0 ml of supernatant.

6. Resuspend the beads and transfer the mixture to a microcentrifuge tube, place onto a magnet, and then remove the remaining supernatant.

7. Wash the beads once with 1 ml of PBS-T and remove the supernatant.

8. PCR amplification step 1. Add:

   a. 22.5 µl of nuclease-free water to beads in microcentrifuge tube and transfer entire volume to PCR tube,

b. 2.5 µl of 10 µM forward and biotinylated reverse primer mix,

c. 25 µl of AmpliTaq Gold Fast PCR Master Mix (Life Technologies),

d. PCR reaction:

    i. 95 ˚C for 10 minutes

    ii. 15 cycles of

        1. 96 °C for 3 seconds

        2. 56 °C for 3 seconds

        3. 68 °C for 5 seconds

    iii. 72 ˚C for 10 seconds

    iv. Hold at 4 ˚C.

9. Transfer the supernatant (not the beads) to a fresh PCR tube.

10. PCR amplification step 2. Add to four PCR tubes:

a. 21.5 µl of nuclease-free water,

b. 1 µl of PCR product from step 1,

c. 2.5 µl of 10 µM forward and biotinylated reverse primer mix,

d. 25 µl of AmpliTaq Gold Fast PCR Master Mix (Life Technologies),

e. PCR reaction:

    i. 95 ˚C for 10 minutes

    ii. 35 cycles of

        1. 96 °C for 3 seconds

        2. 56 °C for 3 seconds

        3. 68 °C for 5 seconds

    iii. 72 ˚C for 10 seconds

    iv. Hold at 4 ˚C.

f. Pool the contents of the four PCR tubes.

g. Test product on an agarose gel (e.g., E-Gel® 4% pre-cast high-resolution agarose gel, Life Technologies) for size and quality.

11. Purify and denature dsDNA

a. Transfer 100 µl of streptavidin-coupled Dynabeads (Life Technologies, 1 mg) to a micro-centrifuge tube and remove supernatant. Wash twice with 1 ml of PBS-T and remove the final wash.

    b.   To 135 µl PCR product, add 34.5 µl of 5 M NaCl and mix. Freeze remainder of PCR products as an archive.

    c.   Add the DNA to the streptavidin-coupled Dynabeads and incubate for 10 minutes, with rotation at room temperature.

    d.   Remove the supernatant and then wash the beads three times with 1 ml PBS-T and then remove the supernatant.

    e.   Denature the dsDNA to liberate ssDNA aptamer candidates by adding 50 µl of freshly prepared 100 mM NaOH to the washed beads.

    f.   Incubate for 5 minutes, place onto a magnet and retain the supernatant.

12. Transfer supernatant to a fresh vial containing 850 µl of PBS-T and 100 µl of 0.1 M monobasic phosphate buffer (Test pH beforehand to ensure a solution pH of ~7.5).

13. Heat the mixture to 95 °C for 5 minutes, then cool on ice.

2.2.2   Round 2

1. Prepare target-coupled Dynabeads. Transfer 20 µl of the protein-coupled beads to a microcentrifuge vial and remove the supernatant. Wash the beads twice in 500 µl of PBS-T and resuspend the beads in 1 ml of PBS-T.

2. Add the ssDNA product from Section 2.2.1, step 13, to the coupled beads.

3. Selection: Incubate with rotation at room temperature for 10 minutes.

4. Wash the beads three times with 1 ml of PBS-T and remove the supernatant.

5. PCR amplification. Add:

    a.   22.5 µl of nuclease-free water to beads in microcentrifuge tube and transfer entire volume to PCR tube,

    b.   2.5 µl of 10 µM forward and biotinylated reverse primer mix,

    c.   25 µl of AmpliTaq Gold Fast PCR Master Mix (Life Technologies),

    d.   PCR reaction:

        i.   95 °C for 10 minutes

        ii.   35 cycles of

            1.   96 °C for 3 seconds

            2.   56 °C for 3 seconds

            3.   68 °C for 5 seconds

        iii.   72 °C for 10 seconds

        iv.   Hold at 4 °C.

    e.   Test product on an agarose gel for size and quality.

6. Purify and denature dsDNA

    a. Transfer 100 µl of streptavidin-coupled Dynabeads (1 mg) to a microcentrifuge tube and remove supernatant. Wash twice with 1 ml of PBS-T and remove the final wash.

    b. To 45 µl PCR product, add 11.5 µl of 5 M NaCl and mix. Freeze remainder of PCR products as an archive.

    c. Add the DNA to the streptavidin-coupled Dynabeads and incubate for 10 minutes, with rotation at room temperature.

    d. Remove the supernatant and then wash the beads three times with 1 ml of PBS-T and then remove the supernatant.

    e. Denature the dsDNA to liberate ssDNA aptamer candidates by adding 50 µl of freshly prepared 100 mM NaOH to the washed beads.

    f. Incubate for 5 minutes, place onto a magnet and retain the supernatant.

7. Transfer supernatant to a fresh vial containing 850 µl of PBS-T and 100 µl of 0.1 M monobasic phosphate buffer (Test pH beforehand to ensure a solution pH of ~7.5).

8. Heat the mixture to 95 °C for 5 minutes, then cool on ice.

2.2.3   Rounds 3-14

Round	Counter Selection	Protein-conjugated Selection Beads	Incubation Time
3	0	20 µl	10 min
4-6	50 µl	10 µl	10 min
7-9	50 µl	3 µl	10 min
10-11	50 µl	1 µl	10 min
12-14	50 µl	1 µl	None

Table 2: The amount of selection beads and incubation is reduced as SELEX progresses in order to the increase selection constraints.

1. Prepare the coupled beads:

    a. Selection beads: transfer X µl of protein-conjugated beads to DNA microcentrifuge tube and remove supernatant (See Table 2, where X is the volume indicated in the column entitled "Protein-conjugated Selection Beads"). Wash the beads twice in 500 µl of PBS-T.

    b. Counter Selection: transfer 50 µl of blank/negative conjugated (Counter Selection) beads to DNA microcentrifuge tube and remove supernatant. Wash the beads twice in 500 µl of PBS-T.

2. Add the ssDNA product from the previous round to the counter-selection beads.

3. Selection: Incubate with rotation at room temperature for 10 minutes.

4. Transfer supernatant to protein-conjugated beads and incubate for the appropriate amount of time (see Table 2) at room temperature.

5. Wash the beads five times with 1 ml of PBS-T and remove the supernatant.

6. PCR amplification. Add:

    a.   22.5 µl of nuclease-free water to beads in microcentrifuge tube and transfer entire volume to PCR tube,

    b.   2.5 µl of 10 µM forward and biotinylated reverse primer mix,

    c.   25 µl of AmpliTaq Gold Fast PCR Master Mix (Life Technologies),

    d.   PCR reaction:

        i.   95 °C for 10 minutes

        ii.   35 cycles of

            1.   96 °C for 3 seconds

            2.   56 °C for 3 seconds

            3.   68 °C for 5 seconds

        iii.   72 °C for 10 seconds

        iv.   Hold at 4 °C.

    e.   Test product on a gel for size and quality.

7. Purify and denature dsDNA

    a.   Transfer 100 µl of streptavidin-coupled Dynabeads (1 mg) to a microcentrifuge tube and remove supernatant. Wash twice with 1 ml PBS-T and remove the final wash.

    b.   To 45 µl PCR product, add 11.5 µl of 5 M NaCl and mix. Freeze remainder of PCR products as an archive.

    c.   Add the DNA to the streptavidin-coupled Dynabeads and incubate for 10 minutes, with rotation at room temperature.

    d.   Remove the supernatant and then wash the beads three times with 1 ml of PBS-T and then remove the supernatant.

    e.   Denature the dsDNA to liberate ssDNA aptamer candidates by adding 50 µl of fresh 100 mM NaOH to the washed beads.

    f.   Incubate for 5 minutes, place onto a magnet and retain the supernatant.

8. Transfer supernatant to a fresh vial containing 850 µl of PBS-T and 100 µl of 0.1 M monobasic phosphate buffer (Test pH beforehand to ensure a solution pH of ~7.5).

9. Heat the mixture to 95 °C for 5 minutes, then cool on ice.

2.2.4   DNA Sequencing

1. After the final round, insert the PCR product into a cloning plasmid, such as the TOPO® TA cloning vector (Life Technologies) according to manufacturer instructions.

2. Insert the cloning plasmid into a suitable strain of *E. coli*, such as One Shot® Top10 *E. coli* (Life Technologies) using the appropriate transformation protocol.

3. Plate the transformed bacteria and grow overnight on pre-warmed (37 °C) LB agar plates containing the appropriate antibiotics.

4. At least 50 individual colonies should be selected for sequencing. In this work, the bacterial colonies were submitted for rolling circle amplification and Sanger sequencing (GENEWIZ, South Plainfield, NJ).

5. The returned sequences should be edited to remove known plasmid and primer regions, assessed for quality (i.e., proper length and sequence confidence), and then aligned with Geneious 5.5 and ClustalW2.

6. Correctly-sized sequences with the greatest number of copies should be assessed for binding using the aptamer isolation assay described in Section 2.3.

2.3   Aptamer Isolation Assay

Following the selection of an aptamer, the goal is to then use the aptamer to isolate the target from a complex mixture.

1. For each experiment, generate 1 μg of modified (5' NH$_3$-C6 linker) aptamer using PCR (same reaction conditions as above).

2. Purify the PCR product by ethanol precipitation:

    a. Transfer the PCR product to a microcentrifuge tube.

    b. Adjust the MgCl$_2$ concentration to 0.01 M.

    c. Add ammonium acetate to a final concentration of 2.5 M.

    d. Add 2 volumes of ice-cold ethanol.

    e. Incubate the solution at – 20 °C for one hour.

    f. Recover the DNA by centrifugation at maximum speed for 30 minutes at 4 °C.

    g. Remove supernatant.

    h. Carefully add 800 μl of 70% ethanol and centrifuge for 5 minutes at 4 °C.

    i. Remove supernatant and allow the pellet to dry.

    j. Resuspend in 30 μl of 10 mM Tris, pH 7.5.

3. Couple the dsDNA to Dynal M-270 epoxy coated paramagnetic beads:

    a. Suspend 60 mg of freeze dried Dynal M-270 epoxy coated paramagnetic beads in 2 ml dimethyl formamide.

b. Transfer 10 µl of M-270 epoxy coated beads (30 mg/ml) into a screw cap vial.

c. Place vial onto a magnet (e.g., DynaMag™-2 Magnet, Life Technologies) and allow beads to collect to the side of tube (about 1 minute). Then aspirate supernatant.

d. Wash beads by adding 500 µl of buffer C1 (buffers C1, C2, HB, LB, and SB are components of the Dynabeads antibody coupling kit; Life Technologies). Mix by pipetting.

e. Place vial onto a magnet and allow beads to collect to the side of tube (about 1 minute). Then aspirate supernatant.

f. To the beads, 120 µl of buffer C1 and mix.

g. Add 30 µl of purified 5' modified aptamer.

h. Add 150 µl of buffer C2 and mix.

i. Incubate with end-over-end rotation overnight at 37 °C.

j. The next day, spin the vials and then place vial onto a magnet and allow beads to collect to the side of tube (about 1 minute). Then aspirate supernatant.

k. Wash the beads with the following buffers:

   i. 800 µl of buffer HB
   ii. 800 µl of buffer LB
   iii. 800 µl of buffer SB
   iv. 800 µl of buffer SB
   v. 800 µl of buffer SB. Incubate for 15 minutes.
   vi. Note: After each wash, place vial onto a magnet and allow beads to collect to the side of tube (about 1 minute). Then aspirate supernatant.

l. Resuspend the beads in 100 µl of PBS-T (10 mM phosphate buffer, 2.7 mM KCl, 140 mM NaCl, 0.05% Tween, pH 7.4, Sigma, St. Louis, MO).

m. Heat the DNA coupled beads to 95 °C for 2 minutes. Then rapidly collect the beads and remove the supernatant. Suspend the beads in 100 µl of fresh PBS-T then place on ice.

4. Resuspend the aptamer-coated beads in 1 ml of an appropriate sample matrix (e.g., 1 µg/µl target protein in PBS-T).

5. Incubate the solutions for 10 minutes at room temperature.

6. Afterwards, wash the beads 3 times with 500 µl of PBS-T.

7. After the final wash is removed, the eluate can be analyzed by a number of readouts. In this work, polyacrylamide gel electrophoresis was employed.

   a. To the beads, add 50 µl of 1X lithium dodecyl sulfate (LDS) sample buffer (Life Technologies) on top of the coated beads, and incubate the mixture at 70 °C with agitation for 10 minutes. For a positive control, add standards of BSA and SEB (200 ng, each) to 50 µl of 1x LDS loading buffer (Life Technologies).

b.   Load 25 µl each of the samples and standards, as well as 5 µl of the molecular weight ladder (SeeBlue Plus2 Pre-Stained Standard, Life Technologies), onto a NuPAGE® 4-12% Bis-Tris pre-cast polyacrylamide gel (Life Technologies) with 3-(N-morpholino)propanesulfonic acid (MOPS) as the running buffer. Conduct electrophoresis at 125 V for the initial 5 minutes and then at 200 V for approximately 30 minutes. Visualize the proteins with silver stain according to manufacturer's instructions (Thermo Fisher Scientific).

3   Results

The above protocol was applied to the discovery of an ssDNA aptamer with affinity and specificity to *Staphylococcal* enterotoxin B. That aptamer, APT[SEB1], was then used to purify SEB from a mixture of closely related enterotoxins in non-fat dry milk.

3.1   Bead Coupling Validation via Mass Spectrometry

Thirty micrograms of highly purified SEB (Toxin Technology, Sarasota, FL; 1 µg/µl) were coupled to Dynal M-270 epoxy coated paramagnetic beads. The success of the SEB-bead coupling reaction was determined by LC-MS (see Section 2.1.3). Ten microliters of the tryptic peptide mixture was injected onto a 0.15 x 100 mm C18 column (nanoAcquity HPLC, Waters, Billerica, MA). Mobile phase A (0.1 M acetic acid) was washed over the column for 5 minutes at a flow rate of 1 µl/min. The peptides were eluted over a 10-minute linear gradient from 0% to 70% of mobile phase B (0.1 M acetic acid in acetonitrile). The eluate was analyzed by an LTQ mass spectrometer (Thermo Fisher Scientific, Waltham, MA). After conducting an initial MS survey scan, the top 9 parent ions (by relative intensity) were further analyzed by collision induced dissociation (CID) fragmentation (MS/MS).

Figure 2A shows a characteristic standard SEB MS peak (m/z 655.8 Da) which is consistent with the known tryptic peptide VTAQELDYLTR. The retention time window is from 5 to 10 minutes, and the mass range is filtered to show those ions with a mass-to-charge ratio between 655 and 656 Da. This signature MS peak is present in panel B (SEB-coupled beads) but not in panel C (beads alone). To confirm the presence of SEB, the peptide that comprises the peak in Figure 2A was further fragmented via CID MS/MS analysis; that fragmentation pattern is shown in Figure 2D. The MS/MS spectrum is consistent with the known sequence of the peptide (VTAQELDYLTR). This fragmentation pattern is also present in the analysis of the SEB-coupled beads (Figure 2E). This observation confirms the presence of SEB coupled to the paramagnetic beads.

3.2   SELEX

The SELEX method outlined in section 2.2 was used to discover an aptamer to SEB, which we designated as APT[SEB1]. At the conclusion of the method, the vast majority (98%) of the sequences returned from the sequence reaction were identical. The sequence of APT[SEB1] was identified as 5'-GGT ATT GAG GGT CGC ATC **CAC TGG TCG TTG TTG TCT GTT GTC TGT TAT GTT GTT TCG T**GA TGG CTC TAA CTC TCC TCT.

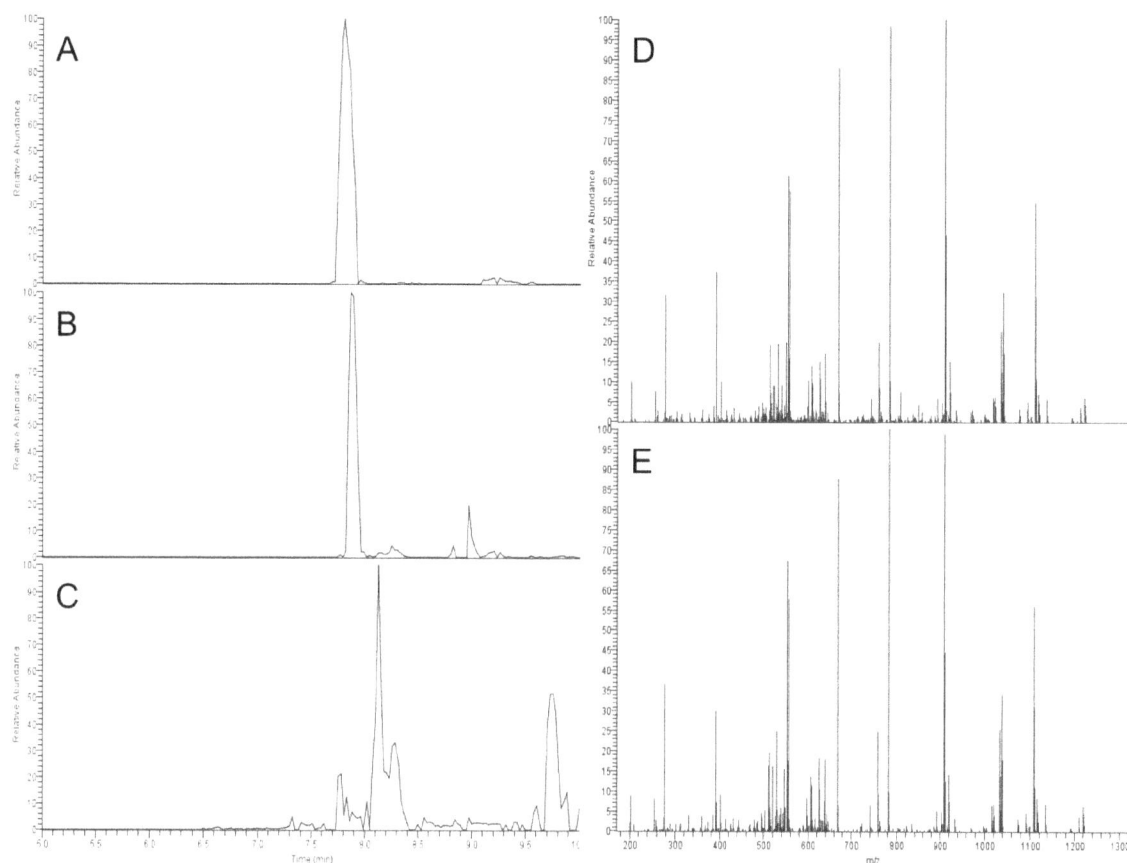

Figure 2: LC-MS confirmation of the paramagnetic bead-SEB coupling reaction. Panels A-C are the extracted ion chromatograms (655-656 Da) within a retention time window from 5 to 10 minutes. Panel A shows the signature MS peak (m/z 655.8 Da) from standard SEB. That peak is present in the SEB-bead coupling reaction (Panel B) but not with the beads alone (Panel C). The peptide detected in Panel A was fragmented by CID (MS/MS), and the resultant fragmentation pattern is shown in Panel D. That same characteristic pattern is present when the SEB-coupled beads are similarly analyzed (Panel E).

3.3 Aptamer Isolation Assay

The method described in section 2.3 was applied to the isolation of SEB from skimmed milk using the aptamer APT^{SEB1} (Figure 3). We incubated the SEB-coupled beads with two different sample matrices. The first sample matrix consisted of 1 ml of 50% w/v non-fat dry milk (Safeway, Inc. Pleasanton, CA) in PBS-T incurred with 1 µg each of the following proteins: Bovine Serum Albumin (Sigma), SEA, SEB, SEC_1, SEC_2, SEC_3, SED, SEE (Toxin Technologies, Figure 3, Lane 4). The second sample matrix was similar to the first sample, but without the addition of 1 µg of SEB (Figure 3, Lane 5).

The presence of a band in lane 4 (Figure 3), demonstrates the ability of APT^{SEB1} to bind to SEB in a complex protein matrix (e.g., milk proteins, bovine serum albumin, SEA, SEC_1, SEC_2, SEC_3, SED, and SEE). The presence of a very faint band in lane 5 (Figure 3) shows the selectivity of the aptamer to predominantly bind to SEB in the presence of other enterotoxins, BSA and milk proteins (compare lane 4 to lane 5). The cross-reaction is minor, despite the high similarity shared amongst the enterotoxins (e.g., the primary structure of SEC_1 is ~70% identical to that of SEB).

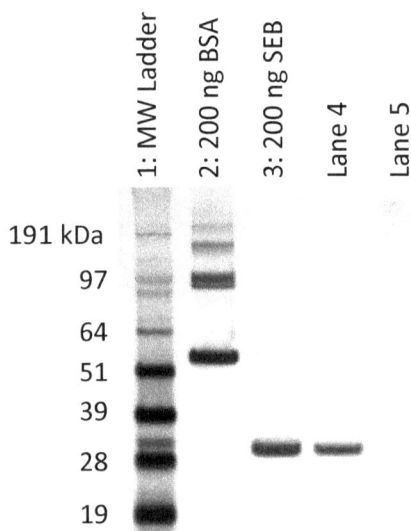

Figure 3: Aptamer isolation assay. Lanes 1-3 are standards. Fifty percent non-fat dry milk was incurred with bovine serum albumin, SEA, SEC_1, SEC_2, SEC_3, SED, and SEE (lanes 4 & 5) and also SEB (lane 4 only). Apt^{SEB1} successfully isolated SEB from the complex mixture (lane 4), but due to its high specificity, APT^{SEB1} did not isolate other proteins (lane 5).

4   Conclusion

The work outlined in this chapter demonstrates that aptamers can be efficiently developed to proteins. Moreover, aptamers possess binding properties similar to receptors or antibodies, without the ethical concerns of animal use. The ability of aptamers to bind and isolate their targets from a complex mixture suggests that aptamers could provide alternatives to commercial antibodies for the generation of aptamer-affinity assays. These assays would be lower in cost and could be widely distributed.

Acknowledgements

The authors thank John Callahan for his critical review of this manuscript.

References

Bunka, D. H. J. & Stockley, P. G. (2006). Aptamers come of age - at last. Nature Reviews Microbiology, 4(8), 588-596.

DeGrasse, J. A. (2012). A Single-Stranded DNA Aptamer That Selectively Binds to Staphylococcus aureus Enterotoxin B. Plos One, 7(3).

Ellington, A. D. & Szostak, J. W. (1990). In vitro selection of RNA molecules that bind specific ligands. Nature, 346(6287), 818-822.

Iliuk, A. B., Hu, L., & Tao, W. A. (2011). Aptamer in bioanalytical applications. Analytical Chemistry, 83(12), 4440-4452.

Robertson, D. L. & Joyce, G. F. (1990). Selection in vitro of an RNA enzyme that specifically cleaves single-stranded DNA. Nature, 344(6265), 467-468.

Tombelli, S., Minunni, A., & Mascini, A. (2005). Analytical applications of aptamers. Biosensors & Bioelectronics, 20(12), 2424-2434.

Tuerk, C. & Gold, L. (1990). Systematic evolution of ligands by exponential enrichment: RNA ligands to bacteriophage T4 DNA polymerase. Science, 249(4968), 505-510.

Investigation of an Efflux Pump Membrane Protein: A Roadmap

Alice Verchère, Manuela Dezi, Isabelle Broutin, Martin Picard

Laboratoire de Cristallographie et RMN Biologiques

CNRS UMR 8015 & Université Paris Descartes, Sorbonne Paris Cité, France

1   Introduction

In bacteria, efflux pumps are divided into five families: the major facilitator superfamily (MFS), the multidrug and toxic compound extrusion (MATE) family, the small multidrug resistance (SMR) family, the resistance-nodulation-division (RND) superfamily, and the ATP binding cassette (ABC) superfamily.

MFS members are the most numerous pump proteins found in bacteria. They are found in all organisms and are able to extrude various substrates using the proton motive force to drive their active transport. They can be either substrate-specific or multi-specific. These transporters have been reviewed in (Fluman and Bibi, 2009). Efflux pumps belonging to the SMR family extrude cationic compounds and are the smallest transport proteins known. EmrE is a paradigm of this protein family. This transporter has been studied intensively (for a review see, *e.g.,* (Schuldiner, 2009)). Transporters belonging to the MATE family have been characterized recently and are thought to play a prominent role in the acquisition of resistance phenotypes by bacteria. They are driven by an electrochemical gradient of cations. For instance, NorM of *Vibrio parahaemolyticus* was the first characterized member of the MATE family, and it pumps fluoroquinolones and ethidium in exchange for the influx of Na^+ (Kuroda and Tsuchiya, 2009).

The emergence of resistance against therapeutics is of utmost concern in public health. Active efflux often leads to a so-called 'Multi-Drug Resistance phenotype' that leads more or less inexorably to therapeutic failures. Although the pumps described above play important roles in drug resistance, we will focus on ABC transporters and RND pumps in detail in this work.

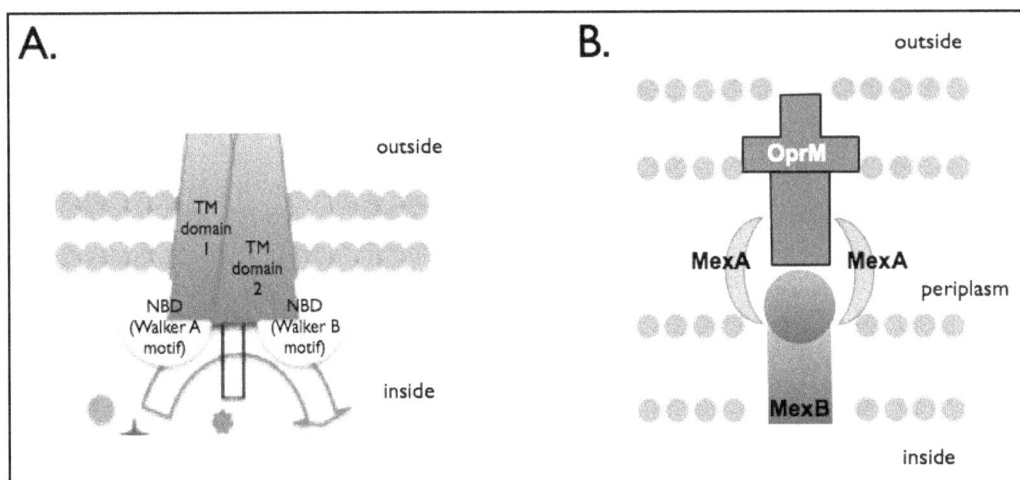

Figure 1: Schematic representation of an ABC transporter (A) and an RND efflux pump (B)

ABC (ATP-binding cassette) proteins constitute one of the largest protein families and are widely distributed in all living organisms from microbes to humans. The fundamental role played by these proteins, highlighted by their relatively conserved structure, is the energy-dependent transport of substrates across the lipid bilayer (Locher, 2009). ABC transporters have diverged into two classes, as characterized by the direction of transport: importers, which are almost unique to bacteria; and, exporters, which exist in both prokaryotes and eukaryotes.

ABC proteins consist of two soluble nucleotide-binding domains (NBD) and two transmembrane domains. The NBDs contain conserved motifs, the Walker A and B motifs, which are also present in many other ATPases, as well as a specific ABC family motif that has permitted the identification of approximately 48 ABC genes in humans. The NBD and transmembrane domains can be present in a single polypeptide chain (full transporter) or can be present in a single transporter as a result of homo- or heterooligomerization of two polypeptides (half transporter). These latter 'half transporters' become functionally competent after specific dimerization that allows close interaction of the two NBDs at the interface of the two ATP binding sites.

Among human ABC transporters, Pgp, ABCG2 and MRP1/2 belong to the so-called MDR (multi-drug resistant) subgroup because their overexpression confers resistance to anticancer treatments. The generally accepted mechanism of multi-drug resistance is that MDR proteins actively pump the cytotoxic drugs out of the cells, maintaining the drug concentration within the cells below the toxic level (Szakacs et al., 2008). Indeed, some cancer cells show a primary resistance to chemotherapy because of the presence of MDR proteins. Drug treatment can also induce overexpression of these transporters, resulting in cells becoming increasingly less sensitive to diverse substrates.

Because the key physiological role of MDR-ABC is to provide general xenobiotic resistance, it is not surprising that MDR proteins can pump a wide range of chemically unrelated substrates, mainly hydrophobic compounds as well as a variety of amphipathic anions and cations. Owing to the capacity to provide a kind of "chemoimmunity" (Sarkadi et al., 2006), this complex network of multidrug transporters is a class of proteins of outstanding medical importance. Thus, a more detailed understanding of the structure of these transporters and the molecular mechanisms of their substrate translocation is needed. Despite advances in structural analysis, much work remains to be done to obtain structures of the transporters in the presence of their substrates in order to complete the fine description of the transport coupled to the hydrolysis of the nucleotides.

In Gram-negative bacteria, which are protected by an outer membrane, efflux transporters are often organized as multicomponent systems in which the efflux pump located in the inner membrane works in conjunction with a periplasmic fusion protein and an outer membrane protein (Nikaido, 2009). Transport is made possible by the reversible assembly of a tripartite protein complex consisting of the following: i) a membrane protein of the RND family (Resistance, Nodulation, Cell Division), which is embedded in the inner membrane and is responsible for the active transport (driven by the proton motive force); ii) a periplasmic protein, whose putative role is to stabilize the entire complex; and iii) an exit channel composed of a ß-barrel inserted in the outer membrane and a bundle of α-helices protruding into the periplasmic space. The complete sequencing of the genome of the Gram-negative bacterium *Pseudomonas aeruginosa* allowed the identification of 12 RND pumps, four of which have been shown to be involved in antibiotic resistance. The four pumps display different resistance phenotypes, and only the MexAB-OprM system is expressed constitutively; the others are expressed under special circumstances. In this bacterium, efflux transporters are organized as systems within which MexB acts as an energy-dependent pump with broad substrate specificity, OprM acts as a porin, and MexA is thought to stabilize the whole complex. Much of the structural and functional information available concerning these pumps comes from the homologous AcrAB-TolC system of *Escherichia coli*. It has been demonstrated that inhibition of MDR pumps increases antibiotic susceptibility (Lomovskaya et al., 2007) and reduces the probability of emergence of antibiotic-resistant mutants (Markham and Neyfakh, 1996).

However, in spite of the efforts that have been made to develop useful inhibitors of these pumps, no inhibitors are yet available for treatment (Markham and Neyfakh, 1996).

In the context of the foregoing, it becomes urgent to obtain a deeper understanding of the molecular basis of transport by ABC proteins and efflux pumps. This goal is clearly complicated by the fact that the transporters involved are membrane proteins. In the following paragraphs, we will first discuss the methodologies employed for the manipulation of membrane proteins of this type. We will then give a brief overview of the existing assays for investigating transporter activity, highlighting the respective pitfalls and caveats. Lastly, we will present an original approach we recently developed for the functional study of MexB, an RND pump. This protocol provides the technical information and methods necessary to design an efficient *in vitro* functional test for membrane protein transporters, including: i) the reconstitution of the protein in a membranous environment; ii) the creation of a closed compartment necessary for the vectorial transport of substrate; and iii) the choice of a fluorescent dye that avoids any artifactual effect due to the hydrophobic nature of the substrate. Although they were specifically designed for an RND transporter, the described methods could potentially be adapted for use with any other membrane protein transporter.

2   Membrane Protein Overexpression and Stabilization

Up to 30% of the genes in each genome encode integral membrane proteins. These proteins share crucial roles such as gatekeeping (receptors), transport of nutrients, ions and noxious compounds (transporters), and maintenance of permeability across membrane bilayers (channels). Hence, the biochemical and biophysical community has directed much effort toward understanding these important and ubiquitous molecules. Unfortunately, the manipulation of integral membrane proteins remains a very difficult task because of their intrinsic instability after they are removed from their natural environment, the lipid bilayer. This makes them particularly difficult to manipulate during the processes of protein expression and purification. Fortunately, a wide variety of state-of-the-art techniques and methodologies for working with integral membrane proteins have been developed and published.

In the following paragraphs, we will first focus on the progress that has been made regarding heterologous prokaryotic overexpression in the Gram-negative bacterium *E. coli*. We will then give a brief overview of the methods available for maintaining membrane protein stability in solution.

2.1   Heterologous Overexpression in *E. coli*

Escherichia coli is the most popular host system for overexpressing recombinant proteins. Thanks to the wealth of information that has been published since the 1960's regarding the genetics and physiology of this bacterium, its use in the expression of soluble proteins appears rather straightforward. Indeed, recombinant expression in *E. coli* is convenient because of the simplicity of genetic manipulation of this bacterium (Terpe, 2006). By contrast, it is clear that membrane proteins are still very difficult to overproduce in the *E. coli* system. The two major pitfalls are membrane protein targeting to the membrane and finding a suitable compromise between high-level expression and production of toxic heterologous protein (Wagner *et al.*, 2006). Thus, designing an overexpression protocol often involves screening of a multitude of conditions, including a variety of affinity tags and distinct expression hosts.

2.1.1   Folding

Of crucial importance, the machinery of the host cell must be adapted to the protein to be produced. The rate of elongation of the nascent polypeptide chain on the ribosome must match the rate required for adequate folding of the protein. For successful protein expression, the rates of these processes must be balanced; a fair compromise must be found between the growth conditions and the quality of the overexpressed protein (Narayanan *et al.*, 2010; Schlinkmann *et al.*, 2012). In fact, the best growth conditions are not necessarily the best conditions as far as protein folding is concerned. Hence, optimizing protein overexpression often requires decreasing the growth rate (and consequently the protein production rate) by lowering the growth temperature. Exceeding the capacity of the cell to process the nascent membrane protein correctly may reduce the yield of well-folded material. This is especially true for *E. coli* because membrane protein production in this host is regularly accompanied by inclusion body formation.

Folding has been shown to be assisted by membrane protein chaperones that differ from those for soluble proteins (Makrides, 1996). The expression of these chaperones often results in a significant gain in production. The addition of natural ligands or prosthetic groups necessary for the functioning of the protein can also significantly improve the yield of overproduced protein. Another promising approach consists of screening thermostable mutants of the targeted protein (Tate and Schertler, 2009).

2.1.2   Toxicity

Overproduction of a foreign membrane protein at non-physiological levels may reveal toxicity of the protein (cell death, inclusion body formation) for *E. coli*. A major breakthrough has been achieved with the isolation of *E. coli* strains that are able to sustain overexpression of membrane proteins that are extremely toxic to standard strains. One example of this is the so-called C43 strain derived from the classical BL21 (DE3) strain; this strain retains its ability to induce expression via T7 polymerase (Miroux and Walker, 1996). It has also been shown that overproduction of the b subunit of the FoF1 ATP synthase in the C43 strain is associated with proliferation of the intracellular membranes. Hence, overexpressing a toxic membrane protein together with the b subunit of the ATP synthase might be an additional option. The C43 (DE3) strain is definitely a must-have production strain for any membrane protein laboratory.

2.1.3   Targeting Proteins to the Membrane

As an alternative to the use of dedicated protein production strains or the modification of growth conditions, the protein itself can be modified. A very promising approach relies on the fusion of the target protein with a model membrane protein that is inserted in the membrane or that crosses the membrane to reach the periplasm or the outer membrane. This approach aids the traffic of the membrane protein to the membrane. In addition, the resulting chimera may allow better expression of poorly expressed proteins, better solubility and better refolding. Protein fusion partners such as glutathione-S-transferase, NusA and green fluorescent protein (GFP) can be tested for their ability to improve the expression of poorly expressed membrane proteins (Peti and Page, 2007). The use of green fluorescent protein (GFP) fused to the C-terminus of the target protein provides an additional asset by permitting easy *in vivo* optical detection of the location of the expressed protein in the cell. Mistic is an amphipathic membrane-associated protein from *Bacillus subtilis* that has been shown to increase the expression of 'difficult' membrane proteins (e.g., eukaryotic proteins) in *E. coli*. Although the exact mechanism of action of this protein is unknown, it is speculated to help refold the membrane protein into the lipid membrane (Midgett and Madden, 2007).

2.1.4   New Strategies

Recent breakthroughs in membrane protein biochemistry have been achieved by exploring new creative methodologies. For instance, the first high-resolution structure of a mammalian GPCR was made possible by expressing the GPCR as a chimera with T4 lysozyme, thereby increasing the solvent-exposed receptor area (Rosenbaum *et al.*, 2007). A similar strategy relies on the stabilization of membrane proteins by antibodies; this method can be used to increase the polar region of the protein from which crystal packing intermolecular interactions originate. "Alternative scaffold proteins" have been developed to overcome the limits of antibodies (poor expression); the concept is to engineer new artificial proteins based on the principles naturally found in repeat-containing proteins such as ankyrin (Kawe *et al.*, 2006) and the HEAT repeat proteins (Urvoas *et al.*, 2010).

2.2   Detergent Stabilization

The hydrophobic properties inherent to membrane proteins make them impossible to manipulate in solution unless a hydrophobic mimic is added to replace the membrane bilayer. Hence, detergents are widely used to extract membrane proteins out of their lipidic environment and, hopefully, to maintain them in solution. The major concern relies on the fact that detergents may affect the protein's folding and/or function. A wealth of commercial detergents are available; these detergents have a wide range of chemical properties due to variability in the size, charge and chemical nature of their head groups and in their aliphatic chain lengths.

2.2.1   General Features

Detergents exhibit great chemical variability; the head group of a detergent may be large, small, zwitterionic or singly charged, whereas its hydrophobic tail size may range from polyaromatic to short or long alkyl chains. Detergents exist in solution either as monomers or, as their concentration increases, as micelles. The concentration of detergent above which micelles form is called the critical micellar concentration (CMC). It is essential to know the CMC of a detergent being used to purify a membrane protein because the membrane protein will be kept stable in solution when the detergent concentration is above the CMC. The CMC varies depending on the type of detergent and is very dependent on the physicochemical environment of the protein, including the temperature, ionic strength, and pH of the solution.

2.2.2   Preferred Detergents

The most widely used detergents display sugar-based headgroups. Dodecylmaltoside, DDM, is considered to be one of the best detergents for use with membrane proteins because it is an efficient membrane solubilizer and because it preserves the integrity of most membrane proteins. Recently, a new detergent, MNG (maltose neo-pentyl glycol), has been described as a promising tool for obtaining higher protein stabilization and favoring the crystallization process (Chae *et al.*). Octyl-glucopyranoside, ßOG, is also a first-choice detergent because of its general mildness. This detergent is also convenient to work with due to its high CMC, which makes it easy to exchange for other detergents or for lipidic membranes.

Digitonin has been shown to preserve weak interactions between integral membrane proteins; however, it is unfortunately a poor solubilizer.

2.2.3   Promising New Tools

Detergents have the major drawback that they tend to destabilize membrane proteins, leading to their more or less inevitable inactivation. One attempt at alleviating this problem involves the use of amphipols (Popot *et al.*, 2011; Tribet *et al.*, 1996). Amphipols are polymers that can substitute for detergents in keeping membrane proteins water-soluble. They consist of a soluble polyacrylic acid backbone to which octylamine and isopropylamine are attached. The many alkyl chains carried by amphipol bind non-covalently to the hydrophobic transmembrane surface of the protein, providing multiple attachments points and rendering the association quasi-irreversible, while polar groups keep the membrane protein / amphipol complexes water-soluble.

3   Design of Functional Assays for Membrane Protein Transporters

Information on intrinsic mechanisms of antibiotic resistance is still partial and fragmentary. As stated above, the obstacles to membrane protein investigation are numerous. Fortunately, publications have recently appeared concerning some of the constituents of an *E. coli* efflux pump system. The structures of TolC (Koronakis *et al.*, 2000) and AcrB (Murakami *et al.*, 2006; Seeger *et al.,* 2006) were solved by X-ray crystallography. Our current understanding of ABC structure is based on a small number of X-ray crystal structures of bacterial exporters and importers; the structures of only a few full-length exporters (Dawson and Locher, 2006; Hollenstein *et al.*, 2007; Locher *et al.*, 2002; Oldham *et al.*, 2007; Pinkett *et al.*, 2007; Ward *et al.*, 2007) and only one eukaryotic MDR (Aller *et al.*, 2009) have been reported. The latter, the P-glycoprotein, is of particular interest as a relevant pharmacological target. These great advances have allowed the molecular mechanisms of assembly of these proteins to be understood in more detail. Nevertheless, many questions still remain on the actual mechanism of transport.

   Although structural data give significant information about the possible mechanism of action of these proteins, it is important to couple this information with dynamic and kinetic data. To that end, investigations can be realized either *in vivo* or *in vitro*. *In vivo* methods are rather straightforward and have the advantage that they are obtained in a native environment. However, in this context, information ascribable to a given transporter must be extracted from the complexity of the cellular system. For that purpose, controls must be performed to discriminate between active efflux and passive diffusion, and many mutants must be tested in parallel to assess the contribution of the protein under study compared to those of its numerous possible partners. Finally, in order to understand the transport mechanism of a protein, it is essential to know its kinetic constants. In intact cells, it is not possible to let the substrate and the inhibitor diffuse across the outer membrane to reach the transporter (Nikaido and Takatsuka, 2009). Thus, kinetic constants are much more easily accessible using an *in vitro* approach. Nevertheless, very valuable information has been obtained from *in vivo* studies employing two main strategies, the efflux of fluorescent dyes from cells in suspension (ref. (Blair *et al.*, 2009; Bohnert *et al.*)) and the investigation of the effect of mutations on the MIC (minimal inhibitory concentration) of antibiotics (ref. (Guan and Nakae, 2001; Mao *et al.*, 2002; Middlemiss and Poole, 2004; Tikhonova *et al.*, 2002)).

   In vitro functional studies offer the possibility of studying purified proteins isolated from the complexity of *in vivo* systems. As stated above, *in vitro* studies make it possible to estimate kinetic constants (Zgurskaya and Nikaido, 1999), as well as to depict the individual catalytic steps of the reaction or to focus on conformational changes linked to transport activity (Mehmood *et al.*; Seeger *et al.*; Seeger and van Veen, 2009). These features cannot easily be studied in a native environment because of the strong influence of protein-protein and protein-lipid interactions. Thus, *in vitro* systems allow for more tunable activity studies that do not substitute for but definitively complete the *in vivo* approach. This is particularly true for membrane protein transporters for which designing a functional assay is a real challenge. Indeed, one has to keep in mind that the purified membrane protein has to be stabilized in a hydrophobic environment consisting of either a surfactant or, more often, a membrane-mimicking environment. Experimental bilayers have been studied for decades, and several types of experimentally useful bilayers, including black lipid membranes (BLM), sponge phase, nanodiscs, bicelles, and lipodiscs, have been described to date (Alvarez *et al.*, 2010; Janshoff and Steinem, 2006; Kawai *et al.*, 2012; Rigaud and Levy, 2003; Serebryany *et al.*, 2012; Ujwal and Bowie, 2011). Transport assays usually involve the use of liposomes because compartmentation is necessary for vectorial substrate translocation. In the following, we will give a brief overview of methodologies that have been designed for the study of ABC and RND transporters reconstituted in liposomes.

3.1   ABC Transporter Assays

ABC importers and exporters have common features: i) they show high conformational flexibility; and ii) they adopt two main conformations, outward-facing during ATP hydrolysis and inward-facing in the resting state. Drugs are translocated by way of conformational changes in the transmembrane domains, which switch from an open to a closed conformation in response to the hydrolysis of ATP in the soluble domains (Figure 2A). A great variety of assays that allow measurement of these proteins' activity have been developed, although the results can be affected by artifacts that result from the hydrophobic nature of the substrates and the relatively loose coupling of transport and ATP hydrolysis (Locher, 2009; Poolman *et al.*, 2005).

Two practical approaches have been proposed to study *in vitro* substrate transport: in cells, for which the monolayer transport assay is the best example, and using proteins reconstituted in artificial or native liposomes that support drug-stimulated ATPase activity, nucleotide and drug binding (reviewed in (Poolman *et al.*, 2005; Sarkadi *et al.*, 2006; Szakacs *et al.*, 2008)). The monolayer transport assay is based on the fact that substrates cross cell membranes via vectorial transcellular movement (Figure 2B). Polarized cells are seeded at confluence on a membrane surface, and the substrate is added to the solution on the basolateral side of the cells; to analyze transport rates, the amount of substrate in both the basolateral and apical compartments is evaluated. Membrane vesicles with transporters inserted in the bilayer permit both direct and indirect functional assays; this method has been used successfully with several ABC transporters (Poolman *et al.*, 2005; Sarkadi *et al.*, 2006; Szakacs *et al.*, 2008). In this case, both native membranes obtained from overexpressing cells (mammalian, insect or bacterial) and reconstituted proteins in artificial membranes can be used. When artificial membranes are used, detergent screening and the large choice of lipids available allow the reconstitution of the proteins at high efficiency. Moreover, artificial liposomes can be filled with substrates or nucleotides in cases in which the protein is reconstituted in a right side-in position (NBD inside), while they are added in the external medium for proteins reconstituted in inside-out orientation (NBD outside) (Figure 2C).

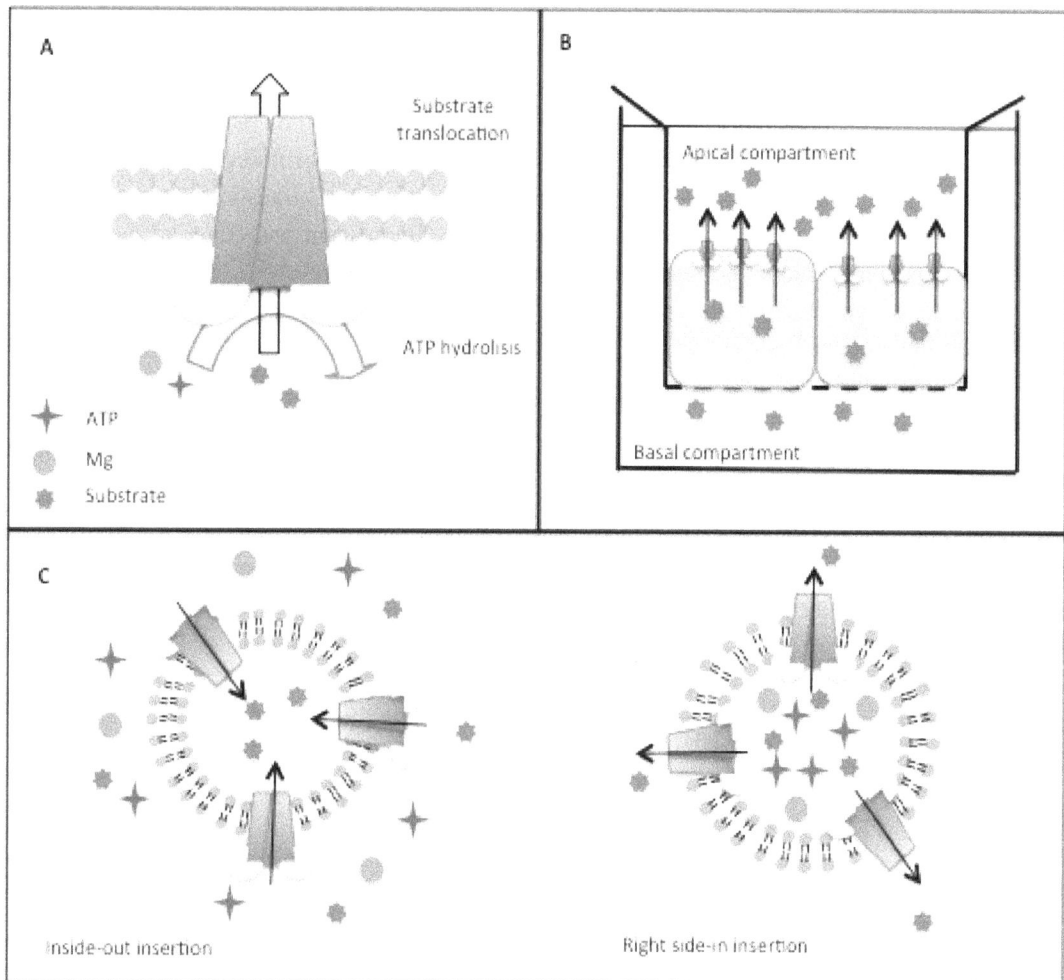

Figure 2: ABC transporter functional assays. A) ABC transporters are composed of a transmembrane domain (in blue) and a soluble domain (NBD) (in yellow); translocation of the substrate (red star) through the transmembrane domain is driven by ATP hydrolysis in the presence of magnesium (orange circle) at the NBD side. B) Monolayer transport assay in cells seeded on a filter well; substrate is translocated vectorially from the basal compartment and accumulates in the supernatant on the apical side. C) Reconstitution of ABC transporters in liposomes can lead to inside-out and right-side-in insertion of the proteins; in both cases, direct or indirect measurement of protein activity can be performed by measuring the accumulation of fluorescent or radiolabeled substrate inside the vesicle or the ATP hydrolysis rate, respectively.

Indirect functional assays rely on the measurement of ATPase activity and nucleotide binding at the NBD side. As explained above, the substrate is translocated using energy derived from ATP hydrolysis; thus, the ATP hydrolysis rate is a simplified measure of the transport activity of these proteins. Moreover, a specific ABC transporter inhibitor, vanadate, provides a fundamental and reliable control. Another indirect way to prove functionality of the protein is the nucleotide trapping assay. Because ABC proteins possess a nucleotide binding domain, the use of non-hydrolysable, radiolabeled nucleotide offers a rapid way to screen for the ability of the protein to actively translocate a substrate. These ATP or ADP analogs bind covalently to the NBD, are easily detectable and allow the investigator to achieve a detailed understanding of the ATP hydrolysis steps (Orelle *et al.*, 2008).

Direct transport of substrates can be deduced from the distribution of radiolabeled or fluorescent substrates. For ABC transporters involved in lipid transport, the flip-flop of fluorescent lipids between the inner and the outer leaflet is indicative of protein activity. For other ABC transporters, Hoechst 33342 or ethidium bromide are powerful substrates that become highly fluorescent once intercalated within DNA molecules that can be included in the inner compartment of the vesicles.

A more recent approach to the study of ABC transporters is based on the reconstitution of the protein in giant unilamellar vesicles (GUVs) that, due to their size (20-100 μm), offer an opportunity to monitor fluorescent substrate translocation to the lumen of the vesicles by fluorescence microscopy (Geertsma *et al.*, 2008). Reconstitution of ABC transporters in GUVs also opens the way to the analysis of protein diffusion within the membrane connected to transport and/or to the ATP hydrolytic cycle.

At the same time, assays relying on vesicular transport are subject to strong limitations as a result of several possible artifacts: i) the hydrophobic nature of the compounds potentially transported; ii) the tendency of the substrate to non-specifically bind to the membrane or to leak out of the vesicles; and iii) the weak coupling between transport and ATPase activity. In the latter case in particular, the assay shows that the protein can actively bind and hydrolyze ATP, but it does not prove the translocation of the substrate. Indeed, most of the transporters show basal ATPase activity, probably related to endogenous stimulation due to the lipid environment or to experimental conditions. As a consequence, the exact stoichiometry of ATP hydrolysis and substrate transport is unknown.

3.2   RND Transporter Assays

The same limitations as those described above for ABC transporters hold for RND pumps. In addition, it is necessary to generate the proton gradient needed by the RND to extrude its substrate, and several strategies have been developed for that purpose.

Zgurskaya and Nikaido achieved the first successful functional reconstitution of AcrB in 1999 (Zgurskaya and Nikaido, 1999). When proteoliposomes containing AcrB in their membranes are subjected to a ΔpH (outside acid), the protein catalyzes the extrusion of fluorescent phospholipids. Extruded fluorescent phospholipids are then trapped by protein-free acceptor vesicles. When known substrates of AcrB are added to the test buffer, the efflux of fluorescent phospholipid is inhibited. This efflux is massively catalyzed by the addition of AcrA and also by addition of Mg^{2+}.

In a second assay carried out in this study, the pH inside the liposome was monitored. To that end, pyranine is encapsulated in the liposomes, and its fluorescence is measured as a function of time. Pyranine is a pH-dependent fluorescent probe; when the pH of the pyranine environment decreases, its fluorescence decreases. The fluorescence of entrapped pyranine in AcrB proteoliposomes is measured; substrates of AcrB are then added to the buffer and a ΔpH (inside acidic, see below) is imposed. In this case, a proton efflux is observed (see Figure 3). This study proves that AcrB is a proton antiporter and that AcrB activity is catalyzed by the presence of AcrA and Mg^{2+}.

In this study, the proton gradient is generated using two strategies. The first strategy involves diluting vesicles containing a buffer at pH = 7 into a buffer at lower pH. The second strategy involves the use of valinomycin, a potassium-selective ionophore. Liposomes containing KCl are diluted into a buffer containing NaCl. When valinomycin is added, it partitions into the liposome membrane, allowing potassium

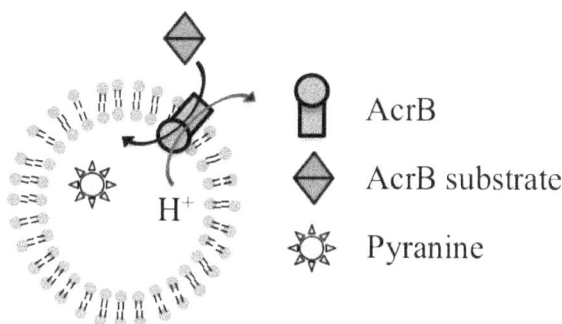

Figure 3: AcrB reconstitution in liposomes. Cartoon representation of proteoliposomes reconstituted with AcrB in the presence of a proton gradient, together with an AcrB substrate and a pH variation reporter, pyranine.

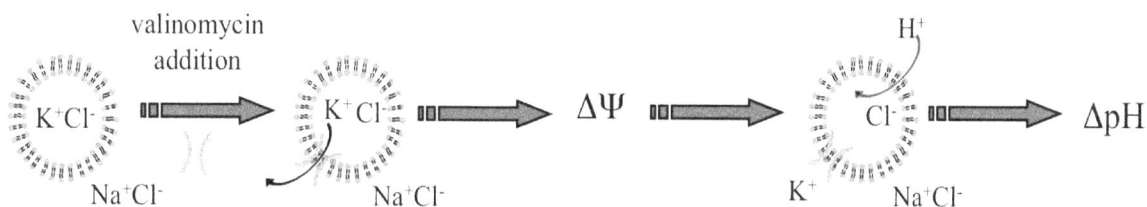

Figure 4: Valinomycin-mediated acidification of a liposome.

to leak out of the vesicle. This creates a charge difference between the inside and the outside of the vesicles. This charge difference is compensated by an influx of protons, which induces a ΔpH (see Figure 4).

Soon afterwards, the successful reconstitution of another RND, CzcA, was reported. CzcA is the RND of the efflux pump $CzcB_2A$ and is responsible for heavy metal resistance in *Ralstonia sp* (Goldberg et al., 1999). In that study, a pH gradient was imposed, and radiolabeled substrates of the pump ($^{65}Zn^{2+}$, $^{57}Co^{2+}$ or $^{109}Cd^{2+}$) were added to the reaction mixture. After incubation, the samples were filtered through membrane filters, and the radioactivity remaining on the membrane was quantified. In this case, the substrate could not diffuse spontaneously across the membrane bilayer, allowing accurate measurement of transport activity. This study determined the kinetics of heavy metal extrusion by CzcA. The RND pump was reconstituted in proteoliposomes containing NH_4Cl; the proton gradient was generated by diluting those liposomes in a buffer containing NH_3, which induced acidification of the liposome. Such a gradient was shown to be stable over tens of minutes, *i.e.,* significantly longer than had been previously described.

Reconstitution of another multidrug efflux RND from *E. coli*, AcrD, was achieved in 2005 (Aires and Nikaido, 2005). AcrD belongs to the AcrAD-TolC complex, which is homologous to the AcrAB-TolC complex; it extrudes aminoglycosides, which are hydrophilic antibiotics. In this study, the proton gradient (acidic inside) was generated using the valinomycin method, and the pH inside the liposomes was monitored using pyranine as described above. In this case, the hydrophilic nature of the substrates is an advantage because these substrates do not diffuse spontaneously across the lipid bilayer. Hence, it is possible to investigate their path of transport ("cytosolic" or "periplasmic"). AcrD can capture its substrate from the external medium, which corresponds to the cytosol in the bacteria. Efflux of protons is also observed when aminoglycosides are present inside the liposomes, suggesting that aminoglycosides can be captured from both sides; this transport is improved by the presence of AcrA.

In 2010, a functional test for the RND MexB was designed (Welch *et al.*, 2010). In this study, the substrate of the pump is Hoechst 33342, a DNA intercalating agent that has a low fluorescence in aqueous medium and a high fluorescence when intercalated in DNA. Here, the proton gradient is generated by diluting proteoliposomes containing potassium acetate in a potassium acetate-free buffer. Upon dilution, a proton gradient (alkaline inside, see Figure 5) is generated. Hoechst 33342 fluorescence is monitored as a function of time. In the presence of a ΔpH, liposomes that are devoid of MexB or that have been reconstituted with a non-functional MexB mutant exhibit an increase in fluorescence upon addition of Hoechst 33342. This is attributed to Hoechst 33342 intercalation in DNA after spontaneous diffusion of the dye across the lipid bilayer. In contrast, when functional MexB is present, Hoechst 33342 is pumped out of the liposome and the fluorescence remains unchanged. In this study, the addition of MexA did not seem to have an influence on MexB activity. Thus, the role that MexA plays when MexB transports its substrate is still controversial.

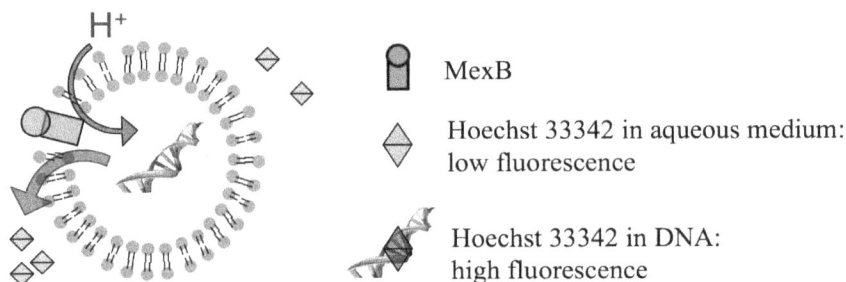

Figure 5: MexB reconstitution into liposomes. Representation of proteoliposomes reconstituted with MexB, its substrate in the presence of a proton gradient

Functional tests give relevant information when they are performed in parallel with structural studies. In *E. coli*, the efflux pump CusCBA is responsible for extruding biocidal Cu(I) and Ag(I) ions. In 2010, Yu et al. described a high-resolution structure of the RND CusA (Long *et al.*, 2010). They also designed a functional assay for obtaining experimental evidence regarding the proton pathway suggested by the X-ray crystal structure. In this study, CusA was reconstituted in liposomes containing the fluorescent indicator Phen Green SK, which quenches in the presence of Ag^+. A proton gradient (acidic inside) was generated by dilution of liposomes containing HEPES KOH at pH 6.6 in a buffer containing HEPES KOH at pH 7.1. This experiment was performed on a stopped-flow apparatus. In CusA proteoliposomes in the presence of a proton gradient, Phen Green SK fluorescence decreased, indicating that CusA transports Ag^+. When CusA was mutated at residues involved in the proton pathway (these were identified based on the crystal structure), Phen Green SK fluorescence was steady. This result indicates that the proton pathway described by these authors is relevant.

As stated above, functional *in vitro* assays have been shown to be an excellent and tunable tool for the characterization of transport activity at the molecular level. The active reconstitution of a protein in a membrane-like environment and the necessity of vectorial substrate translocation, which are essential features of these assays, at the same time represent the bottle-neck step in developing functional *in vitro* assays for membrane protein transporters. To contribute to improvement of the existing protocols, we decided to focus on the detailed description of a functional assay we designed for MexB, a member of the RND family. In this specific case, the co-reconstitution of two membrane proteins and an accurate preparation of liposomes filled with a specific content are required.

4   Photo-induced Proton Gradient for the *in vitro* Investigation of a Bacterial Efflux Pump

Very recently, we designed a functional test for MexB (Verchère *et al.*, 2012). This assay will be described in detail, and the description should permit adaptation of this test to any RND or membrane protein driven by the proton motive force. Indeed, the strength of our assay is the method used to generate the proton gradient needed for MexB to function.

As described earlier, there are many ways to generate a proton gradient, including dilution of liposomes prepared at a known pH with buffer at a different pH and addition of valinocymin to liposomes containing potassium ions. The valinomycin technique has been widely used, although it is somewhat tedious to perform (Picard *et al.*, 2012). Although both of these strategies are efficient, they have two main drawbacks: they are not reproducible, and they are irreversible. Therefore, we attempted to find a way to generate a proton gradient that is reproducible, tunable and reversible. To do so, we have adapted a method known for decades but not heretofore used as an RND functional test (Racker and Stoeckenius, 1974).

4.1   Rationale of the Assay

To create a ΔpH, we co-reconstitute bacteriorhodopsin (BR) with RND in the liposome membrane. BR is a membrane protein that can be purified from the purple membrane of *Halobacter salinarium,* a halophilic marine Gram-negative obligate aerobic archaeon. This protein absorbs light because of the presence of a chromophore, retinal, and uses this light energy to actively transport protons. In terms of its structure and function, BR is one of the best-described membrane proteins, because it can easily be obtained from bacteria in large quantities.

Upon illumination by white polychromatic light, BR pumps protons. Therefore, if BR is reconstituted in liposome membranes, illumination of the liposomes will create a ΔpH (acidic inside) because of the pumping of protons inside the liposomes by BR.

In our method, RNDs are reconstituted in liposomes in which pyranine is encapsulated. As explained in paragraph 2 ("RND functional assay"), the presence of the fluorescent probe pyranine inside liposomes allows us to instantly monitor the intravesicular pH.

4.2   Road Map

4.2.1   Protein Overexpression and Purification

In this method, MexA and MexB are heterologously expressed from pBAD-mexA or pET-mexB (pBAD33-GFPuv, Invitrogen; pET22b vector, Novagen) in E. *coli* (strain C43 DE3). Induction is performed for 2-3 hours in cells that have reached the exponential phase. Cells are then harvested and disrupted using a French press. After membrane preparation and solubilization, the target protein is purified on a nickel column. The yield of homogeneously purified MexA and MexB are about 6–7 mg and 0.5 mg per liter of culture, respectively. The purified proteins are concentrated using Vivaspin (VivaScience) concentrators with cutoff 30 kDa or 100 kDa, respectively.

For the preparation of bacteriorhodopsin, *Halobacter halobium* cells are grown under illumination at 37°C in a liquid growth medium containing NaCl 4 M, MgSO$_4$ 150 mM, trisodium citrate 10 mM, KCl 30 mM, yeast extract 5 g/L, and peptone 5 g/L. Purple membrane is isolated on a sucrose gradient and solubilized as follows: a membrane suspension containing 15–20 mg BR at 7 g.L^{-1} is sonicated for 5 min and incubated for 40 h with 100 mM octylthioglucoside (OTG). The concentration of solubilized BR is estimated using $\varepsilon_{570\,nm} = 54000$ M^{-1}cm^{-1} and ε (280 nm) = 1080000 M^{-1}cm^{-1}.

4.2.2   Liposome Preparation

The first step in this protocol is the formation of liposomes. This step involves handling of phospholipids. Because they are very sensitive to oxidation, they should be stored in organic solvent (usually chloroform) and dried just before manipulation under a steam of nitrogen or vacuum for at least one hour in a glass beaker.

After drying, lipids form a film that can be hydrated with suitable buffers. The choice of buffer is a key step in designing a functional assay. The following considerations apply:

-     Buffer needed by the protein (HEPES 25 mM, K$_2$SO$_4$ 100 mM, MgCl$_2$ 1.5 mM).

-     Depending on the substrate pathway through the RND, the substrate can either be encapsulated in liposomes or added to the external medium during the functional test. In our case, the substrate is Hoechst 33342; it is encapsulated at 140 µM.

-     Pyranine 2 mM.

Hydration of the lipid film with the buffer leads to the formation of multilamellar vesicles (MLV). This step must be performed gently using a pipette. The liposome suspension is then incubated 10 minutes at 37°C; the suspension should appear turbid at this stage. To add enough energy to form the phospholipid vesicles, the suspension is sonicated for 10 minutes at 40 W with 30'' pulse, 30'' off cycles at room temperature. The liposome suspension should appear much more limpid than before sonication because the sonication converts the MLV into large unilamellar vesicles (LUV). The extrusion procedure is carried out following the manufacturer's protocol (Avanti Polar Lipids Inc, Alabaster, Alabama, USA). To obtain a monodisperse population of liposomes, the LUVs must be extruded through nitrocellulose membranes with pores of known diameter. Two cycles of extrusion should be performed; for each cycle, the liposome suspension should be passed through the filter at least 11 times. For the first cycle, the membrane pores should measure twice the final liposome diameter (in our case, 200 nm pore size). For the second cycle, the pores should measure the final desired liposome diameter (100 nm in our case). At this point, the liposome suspension should be limpid.

4.2.3   Incorporation of Membrane Proteins in Liposomes

Membrane proteins can be reconstituted in liposomes (Rigaud and Levy, 2003) because of the solubilizing effects of detergents at a defined concentration.

Solubilization of liposomes with detergent

Liposome solubilization by detergents can be monitored by turbidimetry. To determine the lipid-to-detergent ratio required for solubilization, we take a given amount of liposome (from 1.5 mM to 8 mM lipid in suspension) and add increasing amounts of detergent (0 to 10 times the CMC; in our case, 0 to 50 mM of detergent). We then measure the turbidity of each solution. By plotting turbidity as a function of the detergent-to-lipid ratio, three phases can be described.

Phase I corresponds to detergent partitioning into the liposome membrane. We can add detergent up to a given threshold corresponding to the point at which membranes are saturated with detergent ("Rsat" in Figure 6). During phase II, detergent is no longer incorporated into the liposomes; instead, it is found as free monomers in solution. The concentration of free detergent increases until the formation of detergent micelles and lipid / detergent mixed micelles occurs (see Figure 6). Phase III corresponds to the situation in which liposomes no longer exist and the solution consists of mixed micelles only ("Rsol" in Figure 6). Rsat and Rsol, which depend on the type of lipid and detergent used, should be measured before any membrane protein reconstitution assay.

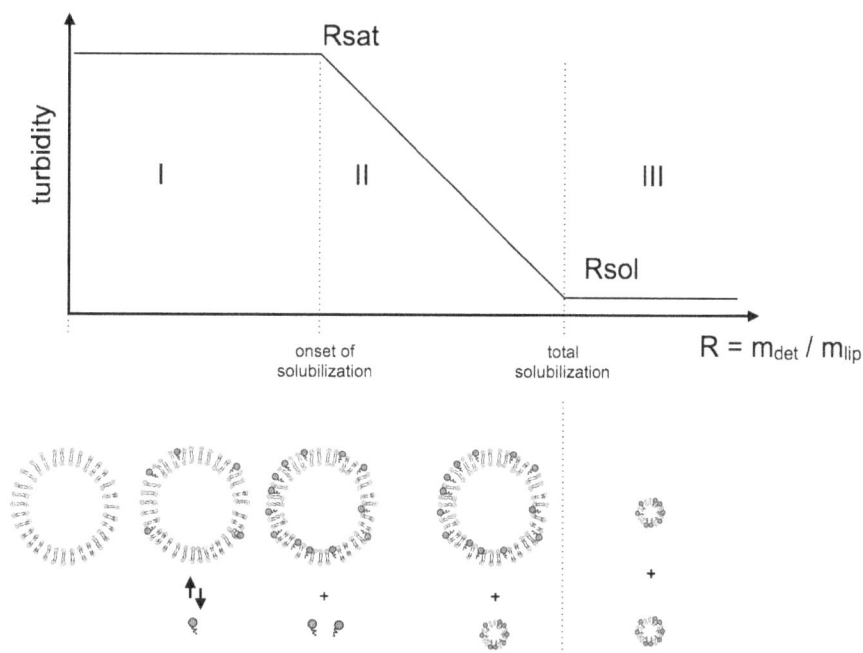

Figure 6: The liposome solubilization three-stage model. Liposome solubilization occurs in the presence of increasing concentration of detergent, as monitored by the resulting turbidity of the liposome suspension. Adapted from (Rigaud and Levy, 2003)).

Protein incorporation

Liposomes are solubilized using a suitable amount of detergent overnight at 4°C (the reconstitution temperature can be adapted to the protein). The detergent-solubilized RND protein is then added to the solubilized liposomes, and the detergent is removed using bio-beads. Bio-beads are porous polystyrene hydrophobic beads on which lipophilic molecules, in our case the detergent, will adsorb. In the presence of bio-beads, membrane proteins lose their detergent coating and spontaneously enter the hydrophobic environment provided by the detergent-destabilized liposome membrane.

It is possible to control the orientation of the protein in the liposomes. If the liposomes have been solubilized at a detergent concentration corresponding to the Rsat, the proteins will insert their hydrophobic domains first and thus will all have the same orientation in the liposomes. If the liposomes have been solubilized at a detergent concentration corresponding to the Rsol, the proteins will insert randomly. Under these conditions, the proteins will have a 50 / 50 orientation in the liposomes. Depending on the desired orientation of the studied RND, liposomes can be solubilized at Rsat or Rsol. In both conditions, the BR will have an optimal orientation: 100% at Rsat, 75% at Rsol. We add BioBeads at a 30:1 BioBead:detergent ratio (w/w) and incubate 5 h in the dark at 4°C with gentle stirring.

4.2.4   Purification of the Liposomes

To remove untrapped pyranine and substrate, the suspension is purified using a desalting column. Before loading liposomes on the column, the column should be washed four volumes of water and equilibrated with the liposome buffer.

4.2.5   Controlling Membrane Protein Insertion in Liposomes

To check that both the RND and the BR have been reconstituted in liposomes, the proteoliposome suspension can be purified on a discontinuous sucrose gradient. Ultracentrifugation of liposomes on a sucrose gradient overnight at 100,000 g permits the separation of liposomes, proteoliposomes and non-incorporated membrane proteins. After ultracentrifugation, non-incorporated proteins are found at the bottom of the tube, while proteoliposomes are trapped at a sucrose interface that corresponds to their intrinsic density. Empty liposomes are recovered at the top of the gradient. Different gradient fractions should be collected gently and analyzed on SDS-PAGE using Coomassie staining or Western blotting. If the protein appears in the middle of the gradient, it means that its reconstitution succeeded. If it appears at the bottom of the gradient, the reconstitution has failed. In such a case, one should change the detergent-to-lipid ratio or the liposome solubilization or incubation time. Usually, sucrose gradients with five layers (60%, 20%, 10%, 5% and 2.5% sucrose) are used.

4.2.6   Fluorescence Assay

Pyranine, which can be entrapped in liposomes, is a pH-dependent probe. Its fluorescence decreases when the pH decreases. Using this probe allows us to monitor the pH within proteoliposomes. As can be seen in Figure 7, pyranine fluorescence is linear between pH 5.7 and pH 7.1. The principle of our assay is to monitor pH changes within the liposome instead of detecting substrate transport through the RND. Indeed, transport of the substrate can be artifactual; for instance, because of their hydrophobic nature, many substrates of RND pumps can passively cross bilayers. Pyranine fluorescence provides secondary information on the activity of the RND proton antiporter; however, because it is directly linked to the activity of the pump, it cannot be artifactual.

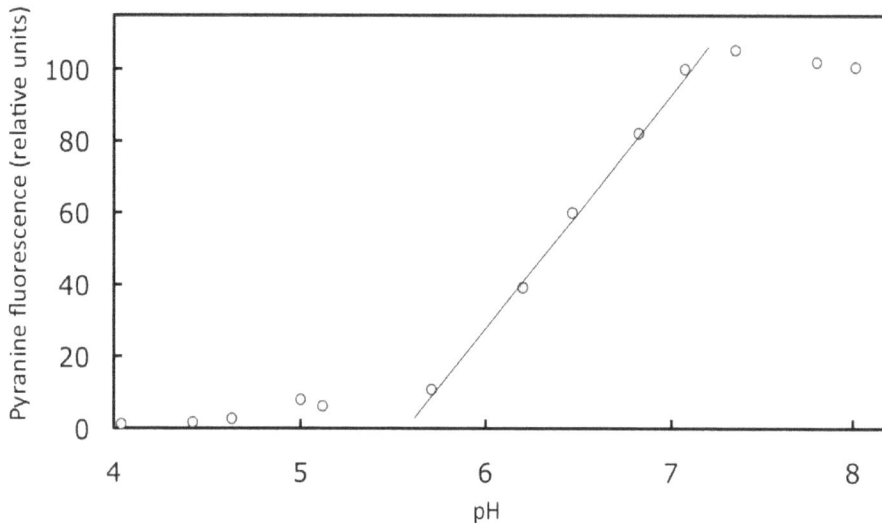

Figure 7: Pyranine fluorescence (λ_{ex}= 455nm, λ_{em}= 509nm) as a function of pH. The following linear regression was calculated between pH = 6 and pH = 7. Dfluorescence (%)=65,9 ΔpH-368 (R^2=0.9946). Adapted from (Verchère *et al.*, 2012)

The assay consists of measuring pyranine fluorescence (λ_{ex}=455 nm and λ_{em}=509 nm) as a function of time while samples are excited at λ_{ex}=550 nm to activate the BR during 50 cycles of 20 seconds each. Because the pH inside the liposomes and pyranine fluorescence are linearly proportional, the pH in the intravesicular part of liposomes can be deduced from the pyranine fluorescence values.

Figure 8 shows the results obtained with our assay. Trace 1 corresponds to the pH inside control liposomes that are free of any membrane protein. As expected, the pH is constant upon illumination. Trace 2 shows the pH inside proteoliposomes containing BR in their membranes. Upon illumination, a proton gradient is created within these proteoliposomes as a result of the BR that pumps protons inside the liposome; thus, the pH inside the liposome decreases. Traces 3 and 4 correspond to proteoliposomes in whose membranes both BR and MexB are reconstituted. We observe that, in both cases, the proton gradient generated by the BR is partially reduced by the activity of MexB. This is true whether the substrate Hoechst 33342 is present (trace 3) or not (trace 4). Because this activity is not substrate-dependent, we interpret it as a basal activity of MexB. Trace 5 was obtained using proteoliposomes containing BR, MexB and MexA in their membranes. In this case, the proton gradient generated by the BR is totally compensated by an activity of MexB. That this activity is substrate-dependent is shown by the fact that when BR/MexAB liposomes are prepared without substrate, we observe basal activity (trace 6).

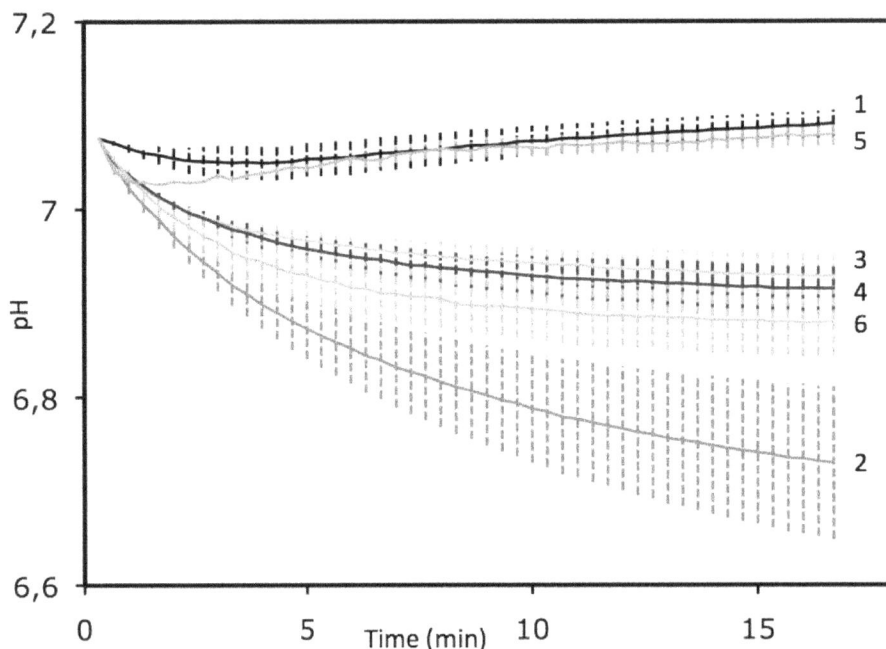

Figure 8: Results of the assay: pyranine fluorescence is measured (λ_{ex}=455 nm and λ_{em}=509 nm) as a function of time, while samples are excited at λ_{ex}=550 nm to activate BR. Pyranine fluorescence variations measured as a function of time for control liposomes (trace a) and proteoliposomes (traces b to f). BR is an efficient way to create a proton gradient within a liposome (trace b); MexB has a basal activity when reconstituted without MexA and/or without substrate (traces c, d and f); MexB has a specific activity when reconstituted with MexA and in the presence of a substrate. Adapted from (Verchère *et al.*, 2012)

Co-reconstitution of BR and an RND in proteoliposomes provides optimal conditions for the RND to be functional: a membrane, thanks to the liposome, and the proton gradient generated by the BR upon illumination.

As mentioned in the Introduction, the use of BR to generate a proton gradient within a liposome permits tuning of the gradient. Indeed, depending on the concentration of buffer present in the liposome, the ΔpH reaches different values, as shown in Figure 9.

In addition to being tunable, the proton gradient generated by the BR is reversible. It is known that BR is activated by light and that protons can diffuse slowly and passively across lipid bilayers. Therefore, if a proteoliposome sample is kept in the dark for 30 minutes, BR stops pumping protons, and the latter protons equilibrate between the outside and the inside of the liposomes. After this recovery time, BR is still functional, and the proteoliposomes can be used again. Owing to the presence of pyranine in the liposomes, we can monitor the intravesicular pH of the liposomes and follow the recovery (see Figure 10). Liposomes can be used for up to 10 cycles of illumination/incubation in the dark.

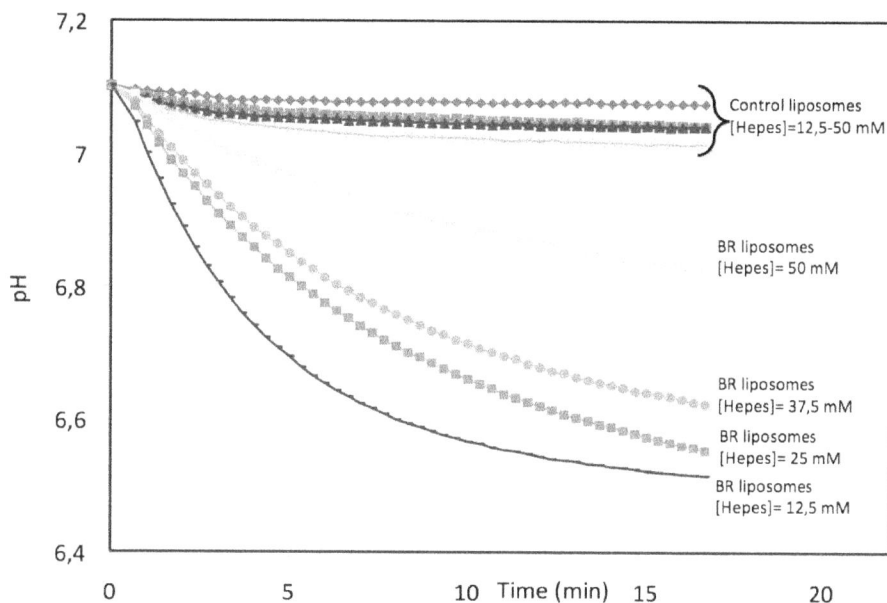

Figure 9: Adaptability of the assay: Pyranine fluorescence variations, measured as a function of time, were normalized to the corresponding pH variations based on the titration presented in Figure 7. Depending on the Hepes concentration, the ΔpH reaches values between 0.25 and 0.55 pH units.

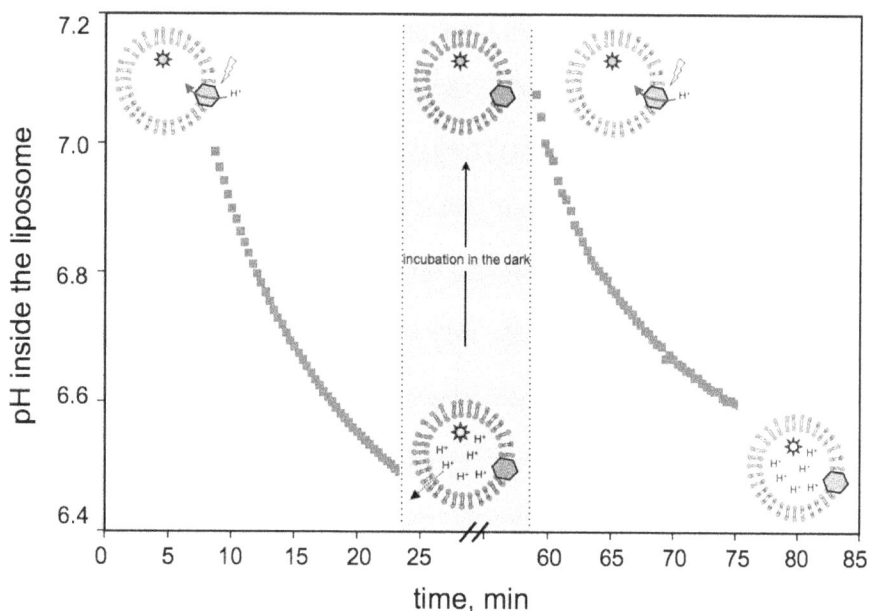

Figure 10: Reversibility of the assay: Pyranine fluorescence of BR proteoliposomes measured as a function of time. From 0' to 25', BR pumps protons as a result of light activation. From 25' to 60', proteoliposomes are incubated in the dark; during this time, protons passively move out of the liposomes until the intravesicular and extravesicular pH are equal. From 60' to 85', BR is still functional and pumps protons upon illumination.

5   Conclusions

There is an urgent need for more reliable *in vitro* activity tests for membrane protein transporters that overcome the pitfalls and limitations of existing tests . Indeed, the availability of better functional assays would make it possible to achieve new insight into the molecular mechanisms of transport and would facilitate the pharmacological screening of new inhibitor candidates. Our protocol may have clear practical applications, in part because it can easily be scaled down. In the context of our assay, the use of BR as a switch for triggering the measurement is an asset because it eliminates the need for second-hand manipulation of the suspension and hence facilitates the automation and parallelization of the system.

Bibliography

Aires, J.R., and Nikaido, H. (2005). Aminoglycosides are captured from both periplasm and cytoplasm by the AcrD multidrug efflux transporter of Escherichia coli. J Bacteriol 187, 1923-1929.

Aller, S.G., Yu, J., Ward, A., Weng, Y., Chittaboina, S., Zhuo, R., Harrell, P.M., Trinh, Y.T., Zhang, Q., Urbatsch, I.L., and Chang, G. (2009). Structure of P-glycoprotein reveals a molecular basis for poly-specific drug binding. Science 323, 1718-1722.

Alvarez, F.J., Orelle, C., and Davidson, A.L. (2010). Functional reconstitution of an ABC transporter in nanodiscs for use in electron paramagnetic resonance spectroscopy. J Am Chem Soc 132, 9513-9515.

Blair, J.M., La Ragione, R.M., Woodward, M.J., and Piddock, L.J. (2009). Periplasmic adaptor protein AcrA has a distinct role in the antibiotic resistance and virulence of Salmonella enterica serovar Typhimurium. J Antimicrob Chemother 64, 965-972.

Bohnert, J.A., Karamian, B., and Nikaido, H. Optimized Nile Red efflux assay of AcrAB-TolC multidrug efflux system shows competition between substrates. Antimicrob Agents Chemother 54, 3770-3775.

Chae, P.S., Rasmussen, S.G., Rana, R.R., Gotfryd, K., Chandra, R., Goren, M.A., Kruse, A.C., Nurva, S., Loland, C.J., Pierre, Y., et al. Maltose-neopentyl glycol (MNG) amphiphiles for solubilization, stabilization and crystallization of membrane proteins. Nat Methods 7, 1003-1008.

Dawson, R.J., and Locher, K.P. (2006). Structure of a bacterial multidrug ABC transporter. Nature 443, 180-185.

Fluman, N., and Bibi, E. (2009). Bacterial multidrug transport through the lens of the major facilitator superfamily. Biochim Biophys Acta 1794, 738-747.

Geertsma, E.R., Nik Mahmood, N.A., Schuurman-Wolters, G.K., and Poolman, B. (2008). Membrane reconstitution of ABC transporters and assays of translocator function. Nat Protoc 3, 256-266.

Goldberg, M., Pribyl, T., Juhnke, S., and Nies, D.H. (1999). Energetics and topology of CzcA, a cation/proton antiporter of the resistance-nodulation-cell division protein family. J Biol Chem 274, 26065-26070.

Guan, L., and Nakae, T. (2001). Identification of essential charged residues in transmembrane segments of the multidrug transporter MexB of Pseudomonas aeruginosa. J Bacteriol 183, 1734-1739.

Hollenstein, K., Frei, D.C., and Locher, K.P. (2007). Structure of an ABC transporter in complex with its binding protein. Nature 446, 213-216.

Janshoff, A., and Steinem, C. (2006). Transport across artificial membranes-an analytical perspective. Anal Bioanal Chem 385, 433-451.

Kawai, T., Caaveiro, J.M., Abe, R., Katagiri, T., and Tsumoto, K. (2012). Catalytic activity of MsbA reconstituted in nanodisc particles is modulated by remote interactions with the bilayer. FEBS Lett 585, 3533-3537.

Kawe, M., Forrer, P., Amstutz, P., and Pluckthun, A. (2006). Isolation of intracellular proteinase inhibitors derived from designed ankyrin repeat proteins by genetic screening. J Biol Chem 281, 40252-40263.

Koronakis, V., Sharff, A., Koronakis, E., Luisi, B., and Hughes, C. (2000). Crystal structure of the bacterial membrane protein TolC central to multidrug efflux and protein export. Nature 405, 914-919.

Kuroda, T., and Tsuchiya, T. (2009). Multidrug efflux transporters in the MATE family. Biochim Biophys Acta 1794, 763-768.

Locher, K.P. (2009). Review. Structure and mechanism of ATP-binding cassette transporters. Philos Trans R Soc Lond B Biol Sci 364, 239-245.

Locher, K.P., Lee, A.T., and Rees, D.C. (2002). The E. coli BtuCD structure: a framework for ABC transporter architecture and mechanism. Science 296, 1091-1098.

Lomovskaya, O., Zgurskaya, H.I., Totrov, M., and Watkins, W.J. (2007). Waltzing transporters and 'the dance macabre' between humans and bacteria. Nat Rev Drug Discov 6, 56-65.

Long, F., Su, C.-C., Zimmermann, M.T., Boyken, S.E., Rajashankar, K.R., Jernigan, R.L., and Yu, E.W. (2010). Crystal structures of the CusA efflux pump suggest methionine-mediated metal transport. Philosophical Transactions of the Royal Society B: Biological Sciences 367, 1047–1058.

Makrides, S.C. (1996). Strategies for achieving high-level expression of genes in Escherichia coli. Microbiol Rev 60, 512-538.

Mao, W., Warren, M.S., Black, D.S., Satou, T., Murata, T., Nishino, T., Gotoh, N., and Lomovskaya, O. (2002). On the mechanism of substrate specificity by resistance nodulation division (RND)-type multidrug resistance pumps: the large periplasmic loops of MexD from Pseudomonas aeruginosa are involved in substrate recognition. Mol Microbiol 46, 889-901.

Markham, P.N., and Neyfakh, A.A. (1996). Inhibition of the multidrug transporter NorA prevents emergence of norfloxacin resistance in Staphylococcus aureus. Antimicrob Agents Chemother 40, 2673-2674.

Mehmood, S., Domene, C., Forest, E., and Jault, J.M. Dynamics of a bacterial multidrug ABC transporter in the inward- and outward-facing conformations. Proc Natl Acad Sci U S A 109, 10832-10836.

Middlemiss, J.K., and Poole, K. (2004). Differential impact of MexB mutations on substrate selectivity of the MexAB-OprM multidrug efflux pump of Pseudomonas aeruginosa. J Bacteriol 186, 1258-1269.

Midgett, C.R., and Madden, D.R. (2007). Breaking the bottleneck: eukaryotic membrane protein expression for high-resolution structural studies. J Struct Biol 160, 265-274.

Miroux, B., and Walker, J.E. (1996). Over-production of proteins in Escherichia coli: mutant hosts that allow synthesis of some membrane proteins and globular proteins at high levels. J Mol Biol 260, 289-298.

Murakami, S., Nakashima, R., Yamashita, E., Matsumoto, T., and Yamaguchi, A. (2006). Crystal structures of a multidrug transporter reveal a functionally rotating mechanism. Nature 443, 173-179.

Narayanan, A., Ridilla, M., and Yernool, D.A. (2010). Restrained expression, a method to overproduce toxic membrane proteins by exploiting operator-repressor interactions. Protein Sci 20, 51-61.

Nikaido, H. (2009). Multidrug resistance in bacteria. Annu Rev Biochem 78, 119-146.

Nikaido, H., and Takatsuka, Y. (2009). Mechanisms of RND multidrug efflux pumps. Biochim Biophys Acta 1794, 769-781.

Oldham, M.L., Khare, D., Quiocho, F.A., Davidson, A.L., and Chen, J. (2007). Crystal structure of a catalytic intermediate of the maltose transporter. Nature 450, 515-521.

Orelle, C., Gubellini, F., Durand, A., Marco, S., Levy, D., Gros, P., Di Pietro, A., and Jault, J.M. (2008). Conformational change induced by ATP binding in the multidrug ATP-binding cassette transporter BmrA. Biochemistry 47, 2404-2412.

Peti, W., and Page, R. (2007). Strategies to maximize heterologous protein expression in Escherichia coli with minimal cost. Protein Expr Purif 51, 1-10.

Picard, M., Verchère, A., and Broutin, I. (2012). Monitoring the active transport of efflux pumps after their reconstitution into proteoliposomes: caveats and keys. Anal Biochem 420, 194-196.

Pinkett, H.W., Lee, A.T., Lum, P., Locher, K.P., and Rees, D.C. (2007). An inward-facing conformation of a putative metal-chelate-type ABC transporter. Science 315, 373-377.

Poolman, B., Doeven, M.K., Geertsma, E.R., Biemans-Oldehinkel, E., Konings, W.N., and Rees, D.C. (2005). Functional analysis of detergent-solubilized and membrane-reconstituted ATP-binding cassette transporters. Methods Enzymol 400, 429-459.

Popot, J.L., Althoff, T., Bagnard, D., Baneres, J.L., Bazzacco, P., Billon-Denis, E., Catoire, L.J., Champeil, P., Charvolin, D., Cocco, M.J., et al. (2011). Amphipols from A to Z. Annu Rev Biophys 40, 379-408.

Racker, E., and Stoeckenius, W. (1974). Reconstitution of purple membrane vesicles catalyzing light-driven proton uptake and adenosine triphosphate formation. J Biol Chem 249, 662-663.

Rigaud, J.L., and Levy, D. (2003). Reconstitution of membrane proteins into liposomes. Methods Enzymol 372, 65-86.

Rosenbaum, D.M., Cherezov, V., Hanson, M.A., Rasmussen, S.G., Thian, F.S., Kobilka, T.S., Choi, H.J., Yao, X.J., Weis, W.I., Stevens, R.C., and Kobilka, B.K. (2007). GPCR engineering yields high-resolution structural insights into beta2-adrenergic receptor function. Science 318, 1266-1273.

Sarkadi, B., Homolya, L., Szakacs, G., and Varadi, A. (2006). Human multidrug resistance ABCB and ABCG transporters: participation in a chemoimmunity defense system. Physiol Rev 86, 1179-1236.

Schlinkmann, K.M., Honegger, A., Tureci, E., Robison, K.E., Lipovsek, D., and Pluckthun, A. (2012). Critical features for biosynthesis, stability, and functionality of a G protein-coupled receptor uncovered by all-versus-all mutations. Proc Natl Acad Sci U S A 109, 9810-9815.

Schuldiner, S. (2009). EmrE, a model for studying evolution and mechanism of ion-coupled transporters. Biochim Biophys Acta 1794, 748-762.

Seeger, M.A., Mittal, A., Velamakanni, S., Hohl, M., Schauer, S., Salaa, I., Grutter, M.G., and van Veen, H.W. Tuning the drug efflux activity of an ABC transporter in vivo by in vitro selected DARPin binders. PLoS One 7, e37845.

Seeger, M.A., Schiefner, A., Eicher, T., Verrey, F., Diederichs, K., and Pos, K.M. (2006). Structural asymmetry of AcrB trimer suggests a peristaltic pump mechanism. Science 313, 1295-1298.

Seeger, M.A., and van Veen, H.W. (2009). Molecular basis of multidrug transport by ABC transporters. Biochim Biophys Acta 1794, 725-737.

Serebryany, E., Zhu, G.A., and Yan, E.C. (2012). Artificial membrane-like environments for in vitro studies of purified G-protein coupled receptors. Biochim Biophys Acta 1818, 225-233.

Szakacs, G., Varadi, A., Ozvegy-Laczka, C., and Sarkadi, B. (2008). The role of ABC transporters in drug absorption, distribution, metabolism, excretion and toxicity (ADME-Tox). Drug Discov Today 13, 379-393.

Tate, C.G., and Schertler, G.F. (2009). Engineering G protein-coupled receptors to facilitate their structure determination. Curr Opin Struct Biol 19, 386-395.

Terpe, K. (2006). Overview of bacterial expression systems for heterologous protein production: from molecular and biochemical fundamentals to commercial systems. Appl Microbiol Biotechnol 72, 211-222.

Tikhonova, E.B., Wang, Q., and Zgurskaya, H.I. (2002). Chimeric analysis of the multicomponent multidrug efflux transporters from gram-negative bacteria. J Bacteriol 184, 6499-6507.

Tribet, C., Audebert, R., and Popot, J.L. (1996). Amphipols: polymers that keep membrane proteins soluble in aqueous solutions. Proc Natl Acad Sci U S A 93, 15047-15050.

Ujwal, R., and Bowie, J.U. (2011). Crystallizing membrane proteins using lipidic bicelles. Methods 55, 337-341.

Urvoas, A., Guellouz, A., Valerio-Lepiniec, M., Graille, M., Durand, D., Desravines, D.C., van Tilbeurgh, H., Desmadril, M., and Minard, P. (2010). Design, production and molecular structure of a new family of artificial alpha-helicoidal repeat proteins (alphaRep) based on thermostable HEAT-like repeats. J Mol Biol 404, 307-327.

Verchère, A., Broutin, I., and Picard, M. (2012). Photo-induced proton gradients for the in vitro investigation of bacterial efflux pumps. Sci Rep 2, 306.

Wagner, S., Bader, M.L., Drew, D., and de Gier, J.W. (2006). Rationalizing membrane protein overexpression. Trends Biotechnol 24, 364-371.

Ward, A., Reyes, C.L., Yu, J., Roth, C.B., and Chang, G. (2007). Flexibility in the ABC transporter MsbA: Alternating access with a twist. Proc Natl Acad Sci U S A 104, 19005-19010.

Welch, A., Awah, C.U., Jing, S., van Veen, H.W., and Venter, H. (2010). Promiscuous partnering and independent activity of MexB, the multidrug transporter protein from Pseudomonas aeruginosa. Biochem J 430, 355-364.

Zgurskaya, H.I., and Nikaido, H. (1999). Bypassing the periplasm: reconstitution of the AcrAB multidrug efflux pump of Escherichia coli. Proc Natl Acad Sci U S A 96, 7190-7195.

Investigation of L/D-Isomerases by Means of Substrate Analogues

Monika Taucher
Institute of Organic Chemistry
University of Innsbruck, Innsbruck, Austria

Verena Gehmayr
Institute for Paper-, Pulp- and Fibre Technology
Graz University of Technology, Styria, Austria

Alexander Jilek
Department of Biotechnology
University of Natural Resources and Life Sciences, Vienna, Austria

1   Introduction

Enzymatic activity intrinsically involves specific substrate binding prior to and during catalysis. It is therefore tempting to utilize the specificity of this interaction for the study and characterization of enzymes. This can be achieved with substrate analogues, which bind to the active site in a substrate-like manner (as opposed to by allosteric regulators, which bind at a different and sometimes even distant site), yet can preferably not be catalytically processed by the enzyme; therefore, they can act as inhibitors of the enzyme reaction. Since these compounds share important structural features with regular substrates, they are readily accessible by rational design strategies based on substrate structure. It is obvious that such experiments contribute to the elucidation of the enzyme mechanism (i.e., mapping of the active site, substrate binding and catalytic mechanism). Moreover, substrate analogues can also be of more general use in the study of the enzymes when integrated in methods such as preparative and analytical affinity chromatography, affinity capillary electrophoresis, affinity gel electrophoresis, affinity labeling or chemical proteomics, or even in prospective medical or biotechnological applications.

In this contribution, the versatility of substrate analogues acting as substrates or by different modes of inhibition (for example, tight binding vs. competitive inhibition) is discussed using the recent example of peptidyl-aminoacyl-L/D-isomerases. In the biosynthesis of some bioactive peptides, these enzymes invert the chirality of an amino acid in peptide linkage. In this contribution, there is a focus on unnatural amino acids because of two facts: (i) Since the isomerase acts on peptides, it is necessary to expand the natural set of proteinogenic amino acids for research purposes; this aspect is discussed in chapter 2, and some possible applications in chapter 3. (ii) On the other hand, the enzyme by itself generates unusual D-amino acids within otherwise all-L-peptides. The possible consequences of this notable exception from the largely homochiral field of peptide and protein biochemistry will also be discussed in chapter 4.

1.1   Peptidyl-Aminoacyl-L/D-Isomerases in the Secretory Pathway

In higher eukaryotes, the majority of bioactive peptides are synthesized as larger precursors. Upon transit through the secretory pathway and in immature secretory granules, these precursors are processed by endo- and exoproteolytic cleavages (Canaff et al., 1999). Formation of the mature products often also includes a variety of additional posttranslational reactions. Examples are the biosynthesis of carboxy-terminal amides, amino-terminal pyroglutamic acids, and the formation of tyrosine sulphate. An intriguing post-translational reaction is the change of chirality of amino acids within the peptide backbone whereby an L-amino acid is converted to the D-isomer (Kreil, 1997).

The first animal peptide which was found to contain a D-amino acid as the second residue was dermorphin, isolated from the skin of a South American tree frog (Montecucchi et al., 1981). This peptide binds with high affinity to µ-opiate receptors. The D-residue in this and related amphibian opioid peptides is essential for the biological function, whereas the all-L-isomers lack activity.

Further studies led to the discovery of additional diastereomeric peptides from numerous sources (Buczek et al., 2005; Fujisawa et al., 1992; Han et al., 2008; Heck et al., 1994; Jimenez et al., 1996; Kreil et al., 1989; Mignogna et al., 1993; Montecucchi et al., 1981; Mor et al., 1989; Ohta et al., 1991), which include two components, a natriuretic peptide and a β-defensin, from the venom of the male platypus, a primitive mammal (Torres et al., 2002; Torres et al., 2005). All of those peptides contain a single D-amino acid substitution in a well-defined position, which is the second residue of the mature product in all vertebrate peptides known to date. Many more diastereomeric peptides possibly exist, but may have gone unnoticed due to the very difficult analytics. In all cases, where the structure of the precursor polypeptides was deduced from cloned cDNAs, a codon for the corresponding L-amino acid is present in the mRNA at the position where a D-residue occurs in the mature form. This fact shows that the D-residue is enzymatically introduced during a posttranslational event by the action of enzymes (Richter *et al.*, 1987), which could be termed peptidyl aminoacyl L/D-isomerases.

1.2   Peptidyl-Aminoacyl-L/D-Isomerases from Various Species

The first enzyme of this class was isolated from the venom of the funnel web spider *Agalychnis aperta* (Heck *et al.*, 1994). It converts Ser-46 of the 48-residue peptide termed ω-agatoxin IV. Both isomers co-exist in this venom. When this enzyme was sequenced, it turned out that it consisted of an 18-residue light chain and a 243-residue heavy chain (Shikata *et al.*, 1995) with a considerable sequence identity to serine proteases interlinked by disulfide bonds. The similarity was highest to thrombin and kallikrein (26% and 35%, respectively), particularly in the region of the conserved catalytic triad. This fact may indicate a common ancestry. However, whether these residues also play an active role as catalytic bases in the isomerase, is as yet unknown.

Another L/D-isomerase has been purified and characterized from the skin secretions of fire-bellied toads (*B. variegata*, *B. bombina* as well as *B. orientalis*) (Jilek *et al.*, 2005). The enzyme catalyses the posttranslational stereo-inversion of bombinins H, peptides with antibacterial and hemolytic properties, which are also present in the skin secretions (Mangoni *et al.*, 2000; Mignogna *et al.*, 1993). Again, both isomers are present in the skin glands. Interestingly, the D-amino acid at the second position affects bio-physical properties and folding propensity of the peptides (Bozzi *et al.*, 2008; Mangoni *et al.*, 2006; Zangger *et al.*, 2008). For the purification of this isomerase, skin secretions from *Bombinae* were collected and processed as described (Mignogna *et al.*, 1996; Simmaco *et al.*, 1991). Several chromatographic techniques had to be combined; these comprised glycoprotein-selective affinity chromatography (ConA-Sepharose, elution with methylmannoside), ion exchange chromatography (SP- and Q-Sepharose) as well as size exclusion chromatography (Sephacryl S-300). At last, a homogeneous protein (as judged by SDS-PAGE) with an apparent molecular mass of 52 kDa was obtained. Based on fragments of the protein sequence, the sequence could be established by a combination of multiple cloning strategies. Surprisingly, the message was of enormous size (> 10kbp) and consisted of repetitive elements. Apparently, this protein is excised from a polyprotein containing several isomerase domains separated by short individual spacer sequences. In several vertebrate and invertebrate species genes are present, which code for related proteins; the most interesting example is the amino-terminal domain H of the human IgG-Fcγ binding protein (Harada *et al.*, 1997), which thus could have isomerase activity. The similarity is highest in a central region, which contains two conserved histidine residues as well as a pair of cysteines.

Intriguingly, an isomerase has been purified from the venom of male platypus, a primitive mammal (Torres *et al.*, 2002; Torres *et al.*, 2005). Its sequence, however, is not known to date. Other isomerases from hylid frogs, conus snails, and crustaceans as well as the isomerase activities, which are likely present in mouse heart and papaya fruit, are not yet studied to considerable detail (Arakawa *et al.*, 2012; Koh *et al.*, 2010; Soyez *et al.*, 2000).

The expression of cRNA coding an *Bombina* isomerase domain in *Xenopus* oocytes yielded tiny amounts of active enzyme, whereas all attempts to express the enzyme in different over-expression systems were unsuccessful to date. Also, the expression of an enzymatically active spider enzyme was not reported to date. Considerable clues concerning the catalytic mechanism could, nevertheless, be gained by studies, where selective derivatisation of certain functional groups led to the inactivation of the enzyme, and by deuterium (or tritium) incorporation experiments, both of which are discussed in the next chapters. See also the compendium in Table 1.

2   Exploring the Active Site and the Reaction Mechanism

The inversion of an L- to a D-amino acid within a peptide linkage was a hitherto new and rather unusual reaction. On the other hand, amino acid racemases were well known to catalyze the formation of free D-amino acids from the corresponding L-isomer. Most of these enzymes act with pyridoxalphosphate as a cofactor and the reaction proceeds via a Schiff base as an intermediate. However, some amino acid racemases do not require a cofactor. This class of racemases comprises, for example, the proline, aspartate, and glutamate racemases from different bacteria (Glavas & Tanner, 1997; Liu *et al.*, 2002; Rudnick & Abeles, 1975). In these enzymes, two cysteine residues act as proton acceptor and donor, respectively, in a deprotonation-protonation reaction acting at the α-carbon of the substrate. Apparently, the isomerization of amino acids in peptides proceeds via a similar mechanism, albeit the involvement of catalytic cysteines has been ruled out by experiments in the presence of thiol-scavengers (N-ethylmaleimide or β-mercaptoethanol); instead, the inactivation by diethylpyrocarbonate favors one or two histidines in the cases of the frog (Jilek *et al.*, 2005) and platypus isomerases (Bansal *et al.*, 2008). This view is furthermore supported by the pH-dependence of the reaction rate catalyzed by the frog enzyme, which shows a steep decline below pH 5.5. However, this mechanism necessarily implies the abstraction of a weakly acidic α-proton by a weakly basic residue of the enzyme, as it is represented by the imidazole group of histidine. Remarkably, the pKa value of an α-proton of an amino acid residue in peptide linkage might be higher than 20 and therefore be close to the upper limit of enzyme-catalyzed proton transfer reactions (Cleland *et al.,* 1998). In order to overcome this catalytical challenge, isomerases and amino acid racemases share important mechanistic features.

2.1   Some Remarks on Kinetics and Substrates Composed of Natural Amino Acids

The interaction within the enzyme-substrate complex is usually non-covalent, albeit the reversible formation of certain high-energy covalent bonds can also be important. For the spider isomerase, for example, it was suggested that the formation of an acyl-enzyme intermediate could be an explanation for the strong sequence similarity with the serine proteases. Thereby, substrate peptide could bind to the serine of the enzyme's conserved catalytic triad in a step that is analogous to the first step of amide hydrolysis. Nevertheless, no experimental evidence for a covalent acyl-enzyme intermediate has been gained thus far. The initial binding step of a ligand (substrate or analogue) to the enzyme is reversible:

$$\text{L} + \text{E} \underset{k_d}{\overset{k_a}{\rightleftharpoons}} \text{LE} \tag{1}$$

Once the equilibrium has been reached, association and dissociation occur at equal speed, and the situation can be described by the "affinity constant" K_{affinity}:

$$K_{\text{affinity}} = k_{\text{association}} / k_{\text{dissociation}} = c_{\text{LE}} / c_{\text{L}} \, c_{\text{E}} \tag{2}$$

Upon the initial binding step, enzymes convert their substrates. The following general reaction equation can be written for an enzyme, which consists of a single active unit and acts on a single substrate:

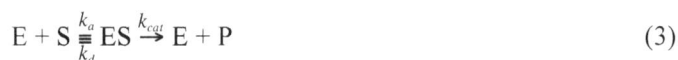

$$\text{E} + \text{S} \underset{k_d}{\overset{k_a}{\rightleftharpoons}} \text{ES} \overset{k_{cat}}{\rightarrow} \text{E} + \text{P} \tag{3}$$

The rate of the enzyme catalyzed reaction v can be expressed by the well-known Michaelis-Menten equation:

$$v = v_{max} \, c_s \, / \, (c_s + K_M) \tag{4}$$

the maximal possible catalytic rate v_{max} is equal to k_{cat} multiplied by the total enzyme concentration in the system c_{enzyme}. The Michaelis-Menten constant combines the reaction constants of substrate binding and its conversion, and, therefore, is obviously not immediately linked to the affinity constant:

$$K_M = (k_{dissociation} + k_{cat}) \, / \, k_{association} \tag{5}$$

For a reversible enzyme reaction, the Michaelis-Menten equation applies solely to the initial reaction velocities in each direction and Michaelis-Menten parameters are different for forward and backward reactions. The isomerization reactions catalyzed by the enzymes from spider, frog and platypus proceed in both directions. A K_M for the spider isomerase has been determined to be 8 mM for the conversion of substrate aceyl-Gly-Leu-Ser-Phe-Ala (Heck *et al.*, 1996); for the frog enzyme, we found a K_M of 700 μM for the isomerization of labeled substrate Ile-Phe-Gly-Pro-Ser-Arg-Cs*-amide[1] (Jilek *et al.*, 2012).

If the enzymatic reaction proceeds to the equilibrium, a constant K_{equ} can be defined (Haldane, 1930):

$$K_{eq} = c_p \, / \, c_s = (k_{cat,forward} \, K_{M,backward}) \, / \, (k_{cat,backward} \, K_{M,forward}) \tag{6}$$

For the spider enzyme acting on the same substrate, K_{eq} was found to be 1.8. For the frog enzyme, K_{equ} range from 2.85 to 0.59 in different substrates, which indicates that the reaction proceeds more efficiently in one direction, either from L to D or *vice versa*, depending on the substrate sequence. We have currently no explanation for this observation. For the standard substrate, K_{eq} is close to 1.

2.1.1 Deuterium Exchange Experiments

When the isomerase reaction has been performed in deuterated (or tritiated) water, selective incorporation of deuterium (or tritium) into the peptide has confirmed that the stereo conversion catalyzed by the spider and the frog enzymes proceeds via a deprotonation-protonation mechanism (Heck *et al.*, 1996; Jilek *et al.*, 2005). Deuterium exchange experiments are a well-approved means in order to distinguish between one-base (one-hydrogen-acceptor) and two-base (two-hydrogen-acceptor) mechanisms (Cardinale & Abeles, 1968). The one-base mechanism is depicted in Figure 1. Substrate and enzyme form an anionic intermediate in which the α^2-hydrogen of the substrate has been transferred to the hydrogen acceptor site of the enzyme, where it is then subject to irreversible exchange (under the experimental conditions) with deuterium of the solvent. Subsequently, the substrate is then re-protonated (in fact deuterated) to give either the deuterio-D-residue or to give the deuterio-L-residue.

The two-base mechanism is also shown in Figure 1. The enzyme contains two catalytic bases, only one of which is protonated (deuterated in D_2O) in the catalytically active form. Upon substrate binding, its α^2-hydrogen is then transferred to the available catalytic base to form the anionic intermediate. The intermediate can either form the product (here the D-isomer) or re-form the substrate. Given that in the presence of the substrate the protons bound to the catalytic bases cannot exchange with solvent protons, deuterium will only be introduced into the product. No deuterium will be introduced into the substrate, regardless of its actual stereochemistry. When the reactions catalyzed by either isomerases from spider or frog were performed in D_2O, mass spectral data indicated that deuterium was solely incorporated into the

---

[1] Abbreviations are listed in the appendix.

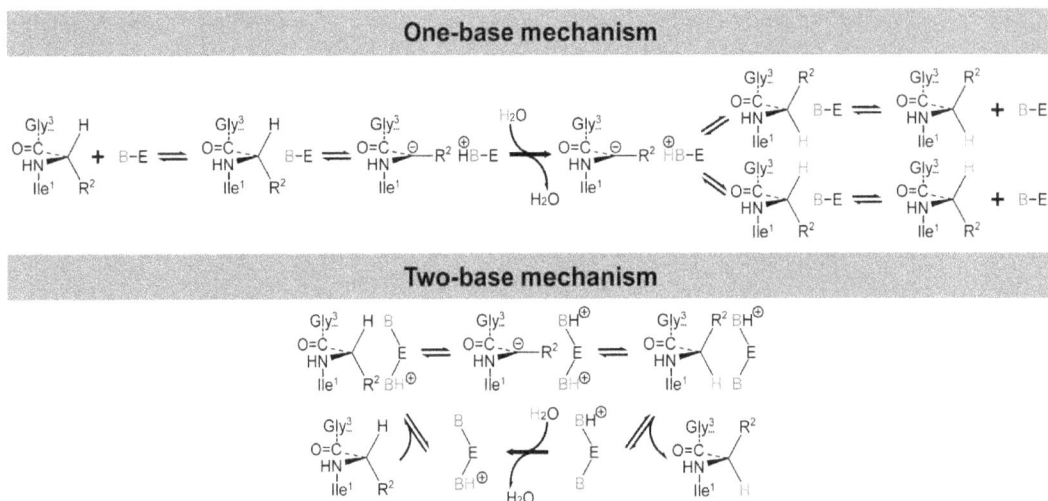

Figure 1: Reaction schemes of hypothetical one-base vs. two-base mechanisms. Solvent protons (or deuterium) are denoted in red. E, enzyme; B, catalytic base.

isomerised product (but not into substrate) early in the reaction sequence (Gehmayr *et al.*, 2011; Heck *et al.*, 1996). The two-base mechanism is therefore consistent with the experimental results, whereas in a possible one-base mechanism both isomers are predicted to appear in their deuterated forms (albeit at distinct rates) from the beginning of the reaction.

Moreover, in D_2O, the reactions catalyzed by the spider as well as the frog isomerases were significantly retarded. This effect suggests that proton delivery to the α^2-carbon also significantly contributes to the reaction rate. Moreover, the observed equilibrium concentrations indicated that the symmetry of the reaction is shifted at the cost of the L→D reaction (frog enzyme). Apparently, the action of the bases is differentially impaired by the isotope effect.

2.1.2   Requirements for Substrate Binding and Substrate Specificity

While the previous chapters highlighted the similarities between the frog skin and the spider venom isomerases, and possibly also the isomerase from platypus venom, remarkable differences between them also exist. The frog and the platypus isomerase act exclusively on the second amino acid. Their substrate spectrum is largely defined by residues 1, 2 and 3 (Bansal *et al.*, 2008; Jilek *et al.*, 2012). As in the case of amino- and dipeptidylaminopeptidases, a free α-amino group is important for substrates of these isomerases. For the frog enzyme it has been shown that peptides with an acetylated amino group are not substrates (Jilek *et al.*, 2012). By contrast, in the case of the spider isomerase the site of stereo conversion is defined by the location of the strict consensus Leu-Ser-Phe-Ala (Ser may be replaced by Cys or Ala) within the sequence rather than by its distance from the COOH-terminus (Heck *et al.*, 1996). This indicates that substrate recognition is basically different in this enzyme.

The substrate spectrum of the enzyme from frog skin is largely defined by residues 1 and 3. Remarkably, in position 2, all tested amino acids reacted in the isomerization reaction. In peculiar peptides with Met, Phe, Leu and Trp in position 2 were good, some even excellent substrates. The peptide with Glu at position 2 was isomerised at a considerably lower reaction rate than a peptide with Asp in this position. An explanation might be an interference of the side chain carboxy group with the catalytic bases of the enzyme, leading to the possible formation of a six-membered ring by the γ-carboxy group of Glu (Glavas & Tanner, 1997; Lam et al., 1988). We also tested peptides with different amino acids in position 1. From these experiments, it can be deduced that the N-terminal residue of a good substrate is preferably hydrophobic or at least amphipathic (Trp, Lys). Exchanging the Gly in position 3 with amino acids with bulkier side chains yielded only relatively poor substrates. However, in spite of the large difference in size, the effect of a Phe in position 3 was comparable to that of an Ala.

The isomerase from platypus venom exerts a similar substrate selectivity (Bansal et al., 2008). The main differences are a higher tolerance of this enzyme towards substrates with bulky residues in position 3 and a substantial retarding effect of branched residues in position 2. However, it is an unexpected and somewhat puzzling finding that a peptide derived from the sequence of OvCNP has not been converted by the platypus enzyme.

2.2   Considerations on Analogue Design with Unnatural Amino Acids

In order to get further insight into the enzymatic reaction, a distinct functionality may be desired, which cannot be provided by the standard set of natural amino acids. In general, extraordinary steric arrangements or physicochemical properties may be required, or, in other cases, extended fluorescent properties (i.e., other than Trp or Tyr) for use as probes. Another important feature is the chemical behavior, which may result in the promotion of an alternative reaction pathway in an enzyme reaction. In our context, the presence of a good leaving group adjacent to the α-proton may favor a "promiscuous" (i.e., other than the naturally catalyzed isomerization) elimination reaction. Indeed, the above mentioned cofactor-independent amino acid racemases catalyze the elimination of HCl or HF from β-halo amino acids resulting in the transient formation of enamine species (Cardinale & Abeles, 1968; Glavas & Tanner, 1997; Lam et al., 1988; Liu et al., 2002; Neidhart et al., 1991; Rudnick & Abeles, 1975).

Compounds, which mimic the structure (and thus the geometry) of the transition state of an enzyme reaction and inhibit the catalysis, are appreciated and powerful means in elucidation of the reaction mechanism. The reactions catalyzed by the cofactor-independent amino acid racemases, for example, are well known to be inhibited by planar intermediate analogues: proline racemase is inhibited by the planar compound pyrrole-2-carboxylic acid, an unsaturated proline analogue (Rudnick & Abeles, 1975). Furthermore, planar enamine and imine species have been shown to serve as potent inhibitors of the enzymes diaminopimelate epimerase and glutamate racemase (Glavas & Tanner, 1997; Lam et al., 1988). These facts are consistent with the idea of planar transition states in these reactions.

In many cases, the synthesis of peptides containing such unusual residues can nevertheless be performed using standard protocols. tert-Butyloxycarbonyl (Boc)-protected amino acids can be added as terminal residue to standard fluorenylmethoxycarbonyl (Fmoc) solid phase chemistry or, alternatively, in solution via carbodiimide activation using the condensation reagent N,N'-Diisopropylcarbodiimid (DIC) and N-Hydroxysuccinimid (NHS) for formation of activated esters, i.e., the classical method for peptide synthesis with minor modifications as described by (Bour et al., 2005). If the protected amino acids were not commercially available, the introduction of the Boc-protective group was also performed using a standard protocol described by (Ponnusamy et al., 1986). α-hydroxyl groups, as present in phenyl-α-hydroxy-β-amino acid or phenyl-lactic acid (Pla), could be left unprotected, as these were not reactive under the reaction conditions.

In some cases, a strategy involving the derivatization of a solid phase synthesized precursor peptide can be successful; A peptide with an $\Delta^{2,3}$-Ala, for example, was synthesized with selenocysteine (Sec) in place of the desired dehydroalanine and subsequently oxidized under mild conditions (Okeley *et al.*, 2000). The synthesis of peptides containing such unusual residues can, however, require a completely different approach. The peptide with $\Delta^{2,3}$-Phe, for example, was synthesized through modified Erlenmeyer-Plöchl and Bergmann syntheses *via* the formation of an intramolecular azlactone (Dey *et al.*, 1996).

2.2.1   Substrates With Unusual Amino Acids and the Architecture of the Substrate Binding Site

The use of L-chloroalanine within a substrate peptide permitted a direct view into the reaction mechanism of the spider venom isomerase (Murkin & Tanner, 2002). When such a peptide was incubated with the isomerase, the formation of the dehydroalanine analogue could be demonstrated. The introduction of a good leaving group in place of the serine hydroxyl in the substrate promotes an elimination reaction that generates the dehydroalanine-containing species. Moreover, this finding provided a strong argument against a mechanism similar to the one in lanthionine formation, which involves the elimination of water from serine-46 to generate a dehydroalanine-46 and subsequent re-addition of water on the opposite face.

In order to investigate the role of a positively charged α-amino group in substrate recognition by the frog skin isomerase, we also replaced the α-amino with a hydroxyl group in two peptides with phenyl-lactic acid (Pla) instead of phenylalanine at position 1 (Jilek *et al.*, 2012). Peptide Pla-Ile-… did not yield a detectable amount of product; in the case of peptide Pla-Phe-…, however, product could clearly be detected albeit the isomerization reaction decreased by several orders of magnitude. Apparently, this difference reflects the proclivity of the enzyme for hydrophobic residues in position 2.

Kuchel *et al.* used a series of amino acids (alanine, R = CH$_3$; α-aminobutyric acid (Abu), R = CH$_2$-CH$_3$; norleucine (Nle), R = CH$_2$-CH$_2$-CH$_2$-CH$_3$) in order to evaluate the effects of chain length *versus* steric hindrance posed by β-substituents (methyl groups) in the second position within substrates on the reactivity of the Platypus venom isomerase. Apparently, good substrates needed to have long, unbranched side-chains in this position (Bansal *et al.*, 2008).

By contrast, the frog skin isomerase accepted longer side chain groups with and without heteroatoms in this position, as well as in the first position. These included an S-phenyl-cysteine in the first position (Figure 2) (Taucher & Jilek, unpublished) and, in the second position, an Nle and, most remarkably, a cysteine derivatized with the fluorophor Bodipy (Cs*). It is surprising that a residue with a rather bulky side chain is still a good substrate in the isomerization reaction.

Furthermore, we found that a peptide with phenylglycine (Phg) in the second position was an excellent substrate of this enzyme; in fact, the highest observed relative reaction rates were obtained with peptides containing either Phg or Met at position two. It is an intriguing finding that during the racemization of free amino acids the reactant side chain group also contributes to the stability of the enolate anion intermediate. Aryl side chain groups, such as in Phg, can stabilize an intermediate enolate anion primarily by resonance (Smith & Sivakua, 1983). In a similar manner, Met enhances the stability of the enolate by orbital overlap (Kovacs *et al.*, 1980).

2.2.2   Inhibition Experiments

Substances, which bind to the catalytic cleft, but cannot be processed, act as competitive inhibitors.

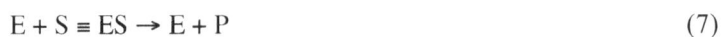

$$E + S \equiv ES \rightarrow E + P \tag{7}$$

$$E + S \overset{K_i}{\equiv} ES$$

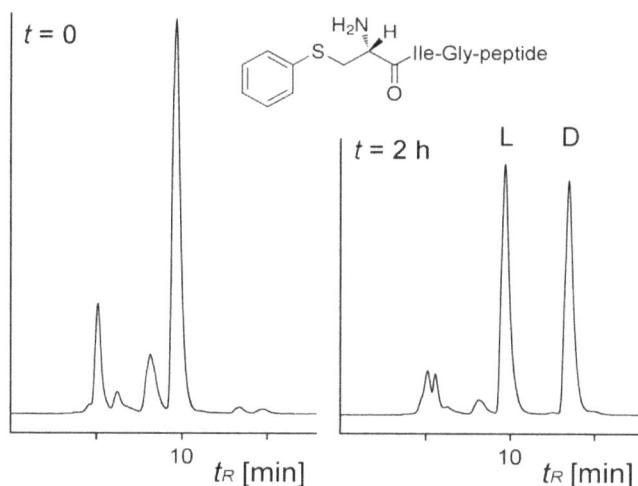

Figure 2: The HPLC-based enzyme assay: chromatograms of a reaction mixture with a substrate peptide containing S-phenyl-cysteine. Enzyme samples were added to substrate in 50 mM phosphate buffer, pH 6.5. Aliquots of the reaction mixture were injected onto a RP column immediately or after 2 hours of incubation and eluted with a gradient of acetonitrile. Fluorescence emission was recorded at 514 nm (excitation at 480 nm). Product with a D-Ile in position 2 is represented by D. peptide, Pro-Val-Leu-Cs*-amide.

For such a reaction scheme, the Michelis-Menten equation can be modified as follows:

$$v = v_{max} \, c_s / (c_s + K_M (1 + c_i / K_i)) \tag{8}$$

Competitive inhibitors usually share some structural similarity with the substrate. Moreover, they must have an affinity to the enzyme, which is similar to the substrate. From equation (8) it becomes evident that high substrate concentrations can restore enzymatic activity. This behavior is the characteristics of competitive inhibition. However, if the binding of the compound is very strong ("tight binding" situation), inhibitors act apparently irreversibly and inactivate a fraction of the enzyme according to the simple ligand-binding situation described by equation (2). Thus, the dissociation constants (K_D) can be derived from simple titration experiments assuming that the enzyme–inhibitor complex is catalytically inactive (Griffith, 1982). From a kinetic point of view, tight binding cannot easily be distinguished from a real irreversible inhibition where the compound acts by covalent binding. A textbook example for such an inhibitor is the serine protease inhibitor phenylmethylsulfonyl fluoride (PMSF), which acts as a so-called "suicide substrate" by formation of a stable covalent bond to the Ser in the catalytic triad, catalyzed by the enzyme itself (Walsh, 1984). In view of the similarity between the amino acid sequences of the spider isomerase and serine proteases, the inhibition of this isomerase by PMSF is an intriguing, yet mechanistically puzzling fact (Heck *et al.*, 1996).

Non-competitive as well as uncompetitive inhibition imply inhibitor binding at a site, which is different and sometimes even distant from the substrate binding site and can serve regulatory purposes of the enzyme activity. The kinetics of these types of inhibition, as well as exceptions from the described formalisms, are beyond the scope of this contribution and are reviewed elsewhere (Blat, 2010; Whiteley, 2000).

Suspecting a reaction mechanism similar to cofactor-independent racemases, one can expect an enolate ion reaction intermediate (9), which could be mimicked by an α,β-unsaturated amino acid (10):

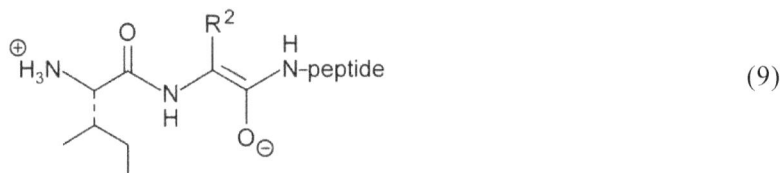

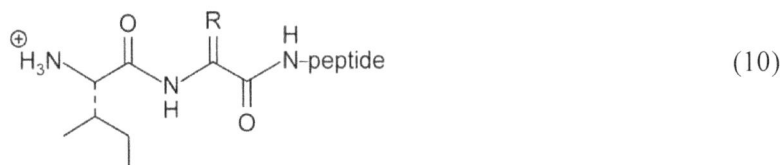

(9)

(10)

Therefore, substrate analogues with an α,β-unsaturated amino acid at the isomerization site were tested in the cases of the spider venom and frog skin isomerases (Gehmayr et al., 2011; Murkin & Tanner, 2002). Indeed, the peptide acetyl-Gly-Ile-$\Delta^{2,3}$-Ala-Phe-Ala was found to be a strong inhibitor of the spider enzyme. We tested the effect of the peptides Ile-$\Delta^{2,3}$-Ala-Gly-Pro-Val-Leu-amide (IΔA) and Ile-$\Delta^{2,3}$-Phe-Gly-Pro-Val-Leu-amide (IΔF) on the isomerization reaction catalyzed by the frog isomerase. The corresponding saturated peptides, IA and IF, are good substrates of the isomerase; however, their catalytic efficiencies differ significantly ($(k_{cat}/K_M)_{IF}/(k_{cat}/K_M)_{IA}=50$). The compounds IΔA and IΔF were found to be strong inhibitors independently of the direction of the enzymatic reaction, that is, either L→D or *vice versa*. α,β-unsaturated amino acid with a planar sp^2 hybridized α-carbon can therefore successfully mimic potential enolate anion intermediates or the planar transition states in an S$_N$2-type mechanism (concerted deprotonation/protonation).

Somehow unexpectedly, the inhibitors exerted a competitive mode of action. Neither enzymatic activity was restored by high substrate concentrations, nor any evidence of reactivation of partly inhibited enzyme was observed after 100-fold dilution into buffer. All these facts therefore indicated a tight, yet noncovalent binding of the inhibitors (Walsh, 1984). However, we cannot fully exclude the possibility that the $\Delta^{2,3}$-peptides could act as suicide substrates, because the determination of the release rates (off-rate) of the inhibitors from the enzyme was diffused by the rapid loss of the enzymatic activity in a diluted solution. It is possible, that a Michael-type addition of a nucleophilic group in the enzyme to the α,β-unsaturated carbonyl covalently inactivates the enzyme (Branneby et al., 2003; Jack & Jung, 2000). As discussed above for tight binding situations, the K_D was determined by titration experiments to be 0.94 µM for both compounds. Therefore, peptides IΔA and IΔF are apparently almost equally potent isomerase inhibitors, despite the fact that the corresponding saturated substrate peptides, Ile-Ala-… and Ile-Phe-… differ strongly in their catalytic efficiencies. It can be concluded that the side chain substituent at the second position contributes only little to the transition state binding.

A different effect was reported for amastatin and the related bestatin, two competitive aminopeptidase inhibitors, which carry either an aliphatic (amastatin) or an aromatic (bestatin) α-hydroxy-β-amino acid as an N-terminal residue. Interestingly, the platypus enzyme was shown to be inhibited by amastatin but not by bestatin (Torres et al., 2007; Torres et al., 2006). Therefore, it has been assumed that the different side chains are responsible to also determine the activity of the inhibitors and their binding to the active site (Torres *et al.*, 2007). On the other hand, both compounds have a similar, yet only relatively weak effect ($K_i > 10^{-4}$ M) on the reaction catalyzed by the frog isomerase (Gehmayr *et al.*, 2011). Apparently, these compounds with a β-amino acid most likely bind to the active site in a substrate-like manner, but cannot be processed, because the α^2-carbon is located in an improper position for catalysis. Therefore, these inhibitors do not provide a clue concerning the reaction mechanism. On the contrary, the unsaturated analogues, which bind to the transition state conformation of the enzyme, highlight the importance of geometry for catalysis.

3   Potential Further Applications

The previous chapters dealt mainly with mechanistic aspects of the isomerases. These concerned the elucidation of the reaction mechanism by inhibitor molecules, the determination of their binding strength, and the mapping of the binding site, which was then the basis for screening a data base for possible natural substrates (Jilek *et al.*, 2012). However, such inhibitors capable of interacting with an enzyme, which is in fact situated at a key position within a pathway, may yield interesting biological data and even become a valuable drug in the future. This is why the screening for inhibitor molecules is of peculiar interest to the pharmaceutical industry and a field of its own ("drug screening", currently about 200 reviews / year in PubMed). Meanwhile, the affinity between the enzyme and its substrates could nevertheless be used to solve more practical problems such as enzyme purification or specific labeling.

3.1   Exploiting Enzyme Affinity I

Preparative and analytical affinity chromatography, affinity capillary electrophoresis, or affinity gel electrophoresis are powerful methods in biochemistry, where substrate analogues could be conveniently integrated (Freitag, 1999). Most of these applications are performed in a heterogeneous setup, i.e., either the enzyme or the substrate is immobilized. However, attention has to be paid to the increased influence of mass transfer effects as a result of a limited diffusion due to the immobilization. In homogeneous enzyme reactions, where both reactants are in solution, mass transfer effects can usually be neglected, whereas these may become the rate-limiting step in heterogeneous reactions and must be counter-acted by appropriate measures. These include the introduction of a linker molecule between the immobilized agent and the resin. Further care has to be taken to prevent secondary non-specific interactions, i.e., with the stationary phase in gel filtration or the capillary wall in affinity capillary electrophoresis. Thereby, working at extreme pH or in the presence of certain buffer additives must be avoided, since they also influence the affinity interaction. Moreover, the inhibitor must fulfill some requirements for application in affinity chromatography. For example, besides a certain stability of the compound, it should also expose a functional group for a specific and well-defined covalent attachment to the linker. Moreover, the binding strength is an important parameter; the binding to a competitive inhibitor can be released simply by an excess of substrate, whereas a tight binding inhibitor is not desirable as harsh conditions are probably required for elution. Immobilized species of amastatin or bestatin could therefore be used in affinity chromatography setups involving the frog isomerase, although the affinity of these compounds to the enzyme was obviously weak ($K_i > 10^{-4}$ M). However, since those inhibitors with a β-amino acid likely bind to the active site in a substrate-like manner, it could be possible to design hybrid molecules with higher affinity based on the substrate specificity of the enzyme. As a first step, we synthesized a bestatin derivative, i.e., a peptide with sequence of bombinin H with the first residue replaced by α-hydroxy-β-amino-γphenylbutyric acid, and tested this compound as a possible inhibitor (Gehmayr & Jilek, unpublished). The preliminary results of these experiments were promising as we found K_i slightly decreased ($K_i \sim 10^{-4}$ M) (Figure 3). Currently we are investigating, whether these results could be further improved.

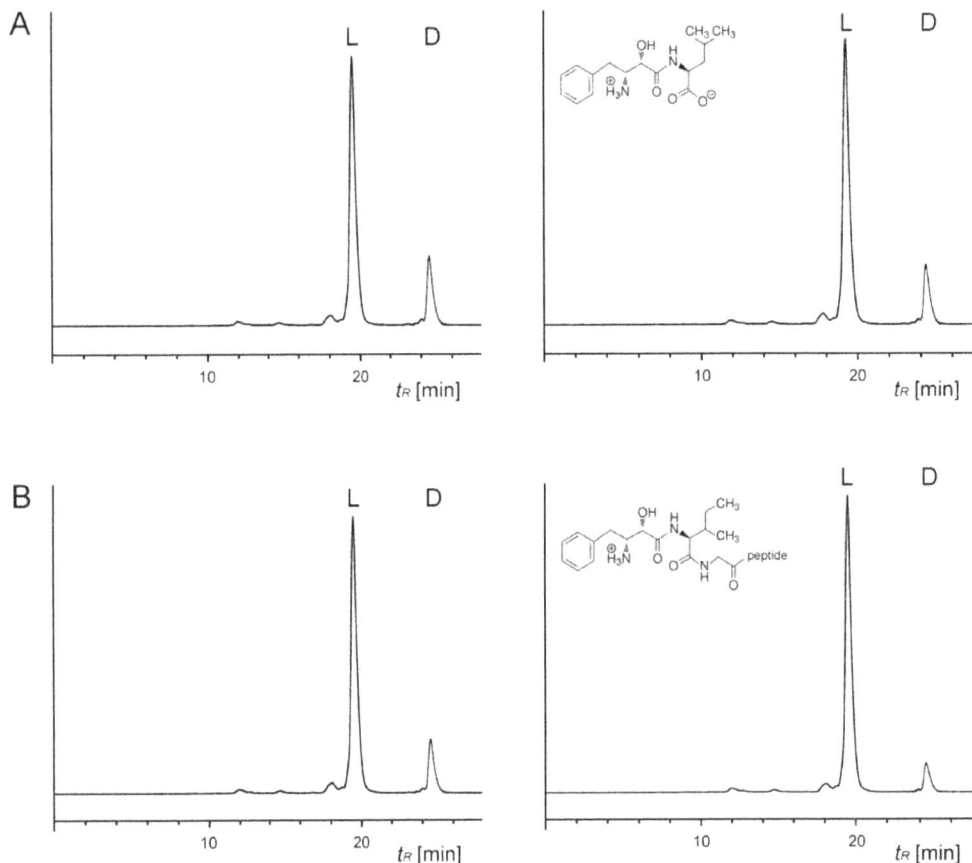

Figure 3: Effect of (A) bestatin and (B) bestatin-derivative on the enzyme reaction. HPLC chromatograms of reaction mixtures in presence (right panel) or absence (left panel) of inhibitor (100μM) is shown. Substrate was peptide Ile-Phe-Gly-Pro-Ser-Arg-Cs*-amide (100μM). Product is represented by D. Estimated $K_i \sim 10^{-4}$ M for bestatin-derivative.

3.2   Exploiting Enzyme Affinity II

Conversely, the properties of tight binding inhibitors can also be exploited in order to derive additional information. Titration experiments, for example, can be used not only to determine K_i, as already mentioned, but also to determine the concentration of active binding valencies of the enzyme and, in principle, to deduce the number of binding sites. A titration experiment with peptide IΔA is shown in Figure 4. Within experimental error, the calculated concentration of binding valencies of about 1 μM matches closely the enzyme concentration, which has been determined by UV absorption at 280 nm (based on a calculated extinction coefficient ε = 54445 $M^{-1}cm^{-1}$ by the ProtParam tool (http://expasy.org/tools/protparam.html) assuming that both Cys residues form cysteines). This fact can be interpreted in such a way that each enzyme molecule contains indeed one substrate-binding site. Moreover, other applications such as specific labeling can easily be envisioned.

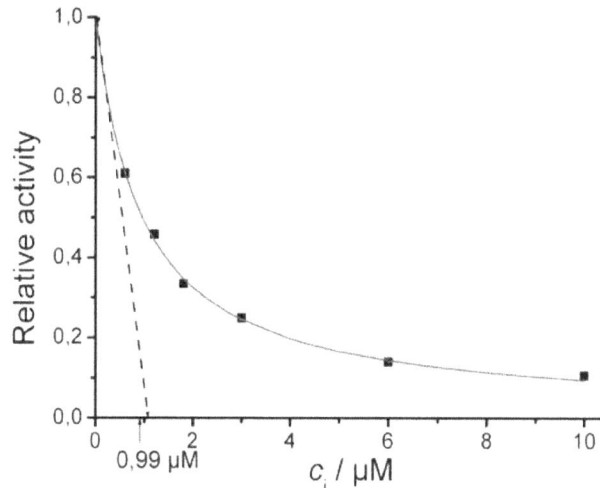

Figure 4: Titration experiment with peptide IΔA. Data from (Gehmayr *et al.*, 2011) are re-plotted in order to demonstrate the determination of the concentration of active binding sites. Enzyme concentration was 0.99 µM as determined by UV absorption at 280 nm.

4   Why D-Amino Acids in Peptide Linkage?

In dermorphins and deltorphins, the all L-forms lack opioid activity (Erspamer *et al.*, 1989; Kreil *et al.*, 1989; Montecucchi *et al.*, 1981; Mor *et al.*, 1989), and the D-residue is required for binding to the µ- and δ-opioid receptors, respectively. In fact, this observation has led to the discovery of the D-residues in frog opioids (Montecucchi *et al.*, 1981). There, the stereoinversion has apparently drastic consequences on peptide conformation and in turn on receptor interactions (Fraternali *et al.*, 1999). Later, it has been observed that these opioids are more resistant against degradation by neutral endopeptidase 24.11/CD10 than mammalian enkephalins (Stefano *et al.*, 1992). A higher stability against several other peptidases including amino peptidases has also been confirmed in several other cases (Dooley *et al.*, 1994; Heck *et al.*, 1996; Stefano *et al.*, 1992; Torres *et al.*, 2002).

More subtle differences between the two isomeric species have been reported for other cases. In particular, in bombinins H, antimicrobial peptides from the skin of fire-bellied toads, the D-residue substitution modulates the folding propensity under conditions, which promote self-aggregation (Bozzi *et al.*, 2008; Zangger *et al.*, 2008). Another example of an amyloid structure involved in innate immunity may be peptide aDrs from the skin of the Mexican tree frog (*Pachymedusa dacnicolor*), albeit the amyloid, assembled form is a deposit form rather than the active form (Gößler-Schöfberger *et al.*, 2009). The investigation of the effect of a predicted stereochemical modification in position 2 on aDrs aggregation has revealed interesting aspects of superstructural organization and polymorphism (Gößler-Schöfberger *et al.*, 2012). In fact, this modification results in a fundamental change in superstructural organization, which is particularly remarkable considering that the site of stereoinversion is not localized within the aggregation-prone sequence and, furthermore, this modification can be enzymatically introduced (Figure 5).

Therefore, D-amino acids could not only play a role in natural strategies to control protein aggregation in cases where amyloid with its unique properties is a functional, integrated component of the organism, but also in the pathogenesis of protein deposition disorders, i.e., certain neurodegenerative diseases or amyloidoses (Chiti & Dobson, 2006), where peptide turn-over, cross-seeding effects (Lundmark et al., 2005), and a differential toxicity of superstructure morphologies are important factors.

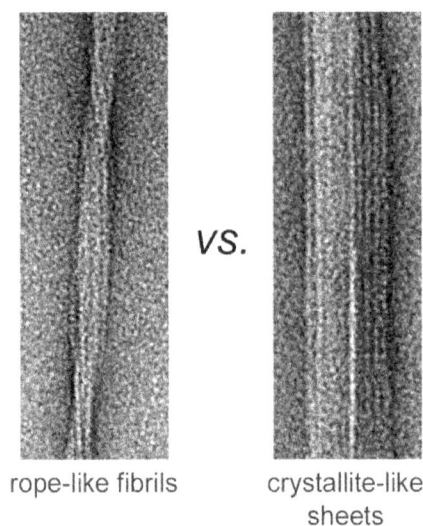

rope-like fibrils   vs.   crystallite-like sheets

Figure 5: Alternative amyloidous superstructures are preferentially formed from aDrs (rope-like fibrils) and its diastereomers [D-Leu2]-aDrs (crystalline-like sheets), respectively (Gößler-Schöfberger et al., 2012).

Acknowledgements

We wish to thank professors Günther Kreil and Heinz Falk for their substantial support over many years, and professor Christian Obinger for critically reading the manuscript. This work was supported by the Austrian Funding Agency FWF grant P22782 to A.J.

Appendix

Abu, α-aminobutyric acid; Boc, *tert*-butyloxycarbonyl; Cs*, cysteine derivatized with the fluorophor Bodipy Fl; DIC, N,N'-Diisopropylcarbodiimid; IΔA, Ile-$\Delta^{2,3}$-Ala-Gly-Pro-Val-Leu-amide; IΔF, Ile-$\Delta^{2,3}$-Phe-Gly-Pro-Val-Leu-amide; NHS, N-Hydroxysuccinimid; Nle, norleucine; Fmoc, fluorenyl methoxycarbonyl; Phg, phenylglycine; Pla, phenyl-lactic acid; PMSF, phenylmethylsulfonyl fluoride; Sec, selenocysteine;

Isomerase	Spider	Frog	Platypus
Sequence	serine protease-like	conserved domain	?
Catalytic bases	? (no Cys)	His (?)	His (?)
Dibase mechanism	yes	yes	?
Substrate requirements			
Isomerization site	C3-C5 (N46 in ω-agatoxin)	N2	N2
Consensus	Leu-<u>Ser</u>-Phe-Ala	very broad	broad
Residues isomerized	Ser, Cys, Ala	all tested (Ala, Ile, Leu, Nle, Phe, Phg, Met, Cs*, Trp, Lys, Thr, Gln, Asp, Glu)	Met, Nle, Phe
Free terminus required	no	yes	?
Kinetics			
Model substrate	Ac-Gly-Leu-<u>Ser</u>-Phe-Ala	Ile-<u>Phe</u>-Gly-Pro-Ser-Arg-Cs*-amide	Ile-(<u>D-Met</u>)-Phe-Phe-R
K_M	8mM	$700\mu M$	?
Inhibition			
ΔAla-analogue	IC_{50} = 0.5 μM	$K_i = 1\mu M$	-
ΔPhe-analogue	-	$K_i = 1\mu M$	-
Amastatin	-	$K_i > 100\mu M$	yes
Bestatin	-	$K_i > 100\mu M$	no
Bestatin-derivative	-	$K_i \sim 100\mu M$	-

Table 1: Compilation of various data on L/D-isomerases from different animals. R = 38 amino acids (β-DLP).

References

Arakawa, K., Koh, J. M., Crossett, B., Torres, A. M., & Kuchel, P. W. (2012). Detection of platypus-type L/D-peptide isomerase activity in aqueous extracts of papaya fruit. Biotechnol. Lett., 34(9), 1659-1665.

Bansal, P. S., Torres, A. M., Crossett, B., Wong, K. K., Koh, J. M., Geraghty, D. P., et al. (2008). Substrate specificity of platypus venom L-to-D-peptide isomerase. J Biol Chem, 283(14), 8969-8975.

Blat, Y. (2010). Non-competitive inhibition by active site binders. Chem Biol Drug Des, 75(6), 535-540.

Bour, P., Budesinsky, M., Spirko, V., Kapitan, J., Sebestik, J., & Sychrovsky, V. (2005). A complete set of NMR chemical shifts and spin-spin coupling constants for L-Alanyl-L-alanine zwitterion and analysis of its conformational behavior. J Am Chem Soc, 127(48), 17079-17089.

Bozzi, A., Mangoni, M. L., Rinaldi, A. C., Mignogna, G., & Aschi, M. (2008). Folding propensity and biological activity of peptides: the effect of a single stereochemical isomerization on the conformational properties of bombinins in aqueous solution. Biopolymers, 89(9), 769-778.

Branneby, C., Carlqvist, P., Magnusson, A., Hult, K., Brinck, T., & Berglund, P. (2003). Carbon-carbon bonds by hydrolytic enzymes. J Am Chem Soc, 125(4), 874-875.

Buczek, O., Yoshikami, D., Bulaj, G., Jimenez, E. C., & Olivera, B. M. (2005). Post-translational amino acid isomerization: a functionally important D-amino acid in an excitatory peptide. J Biol Chem, 280(6), 4247-4253.

Canaff, L., Bennett, H. P., & Hendy, G. N. (1999). Peptide hormone precursor processing: getting sorted? Mol Cell Endocrinol, 156(1-2), 1-6.

Cardinale, G. J., & Abeles, R. H. (1968). Purification and mechanism of action of proline racemase. Biochemistry, 7(11), 3970-3978.

Chiti, F., & Dobson, C. M. (2006). Protein misfolding, functional amyloid, and human disease. Annu Rev Biochem, 75, 333-366.

Cleland, W. W., Frey, P. A., & Gerlt, J. A. (1998). The low barrier hydrogen bond in enzymatic catalysis. J Biol Chem, 273(40), 25529-25532.

Dey, S., Mitra, S. N., & Singh, T. P. (1996). Design of peptides: synthesis, crystal structure and molecular conformation of N-Boc-L-Val-delta Phe-L-Ile-OCH3. Int J Pept Protein Res, 48(2), 123-128.

Dooley, C. T., Chung, N. N., Wilkes, B. C., Schiller, P. W., Bidlack, J. M., Pasternak, G. W., et al. (1994). An all D-amino acid opioid peptide with central analgesic activity from a combinatorial library. Science, 266(5193), 2019-2022.

Erspamer, V., Melchiorri, P., Falconieri-Erspamer, G., Negri, L., Corsi, R., Severini, C., et al. (1989). Deltorphins: a family of naturally occurring peptides with high affinity and selectivity for delta opioid binding sites. Proc Natl Acad Sci U S A, 86(13), 5188-5192.

Fraternali, F., Anselmi, C., & Temussi, P. A. (1999). Neurologically active plant compounds and peptide hormones: a chirality connection. FEBS Lett, 448(2-3), 217-220.

Freitag, R. (1999). Utilization of enzyme-substrate interactions in analytical chemistry. J Chromatogr B Biomed Sci Appl, 722(1-2), 279-301.

Fujisawa, Y., Ikeda, T., Nomoto, K., Yasuda-Kamatani, Y., Minakata, H., Kenny, P. T., et al. (1992). The FMRFamide-related decapeptide of Mytilus contains a D-amino acid residue. Comp Biochem Physiol C, 102(1), 91-95.

Gehmayr, V., Mollay, C., Reith, L., Müller, N., & Jilek, A. (2011). Tight binding of transition-state analogues to a peptidyl-aminoacyl-L/D-isomerase from frog skin. ChemBioChem 12, 1996-2000.

Glavas, S., & Tanner, M. E. (1997). The inhibition of glutamate racemase by D-N-hydroxyglutamate. Bioorg Med Chem Lett, 7(17), 2265-2270.

Gößler-Schöfberger, R., Hesser, G., Maria M. Reif, Friedmann, J., Duscher, B., Toca-Herrera, J. L., et al. (2012). A stereochemical switch in the aDrs model system, a candidate for a functional amyloid. Arch Biochem Biophys, in print.

Gößler-Schöfberger, R., Hesser, G., Muik, M., Wechselberger, C., & Jilek, A. (2009). An orphan dermaseptin from frog skin reversibly assembles to amyloid-like aggregates in a pH-dependent fashion. FEBS J, 276(20), 5849-5859.

Griffith, O. W. (1982). Mechanism of action, metabolism, and toxicity of buthionine sulfoximine and its higher homologs, potent inhibitors of glutathione synthesis. J Biol Chem, 257(22), 13704-13712.

Haldane, J. B. S. (1930). Enzymes. London: Longmans, Green and Co.

Han, Y., Huang, F., Jiang, H., Liu, L., Wang, Q., Wang, Y., et al. (2008). Purification and structural characterization of a D-amino acid-containing conopeptide, conomarphin, from Conus marmoreus. FEBS J, 275(9), 1976-1987.

Harada, N., Iijima, S., Kobayashi, K., Yoshida, T., Brown, W. R., Hibi, T., et al. (1997). Human IgGFc binding protein (FcgammaBP) in colonic epithelial cells exhibits mucin-like structure. J Biol Chem, 272(24), 15232-15241.

Heck, S. D., Faraci, W. S., Kelbaugh, P. R., Saccomano, N. A., Thadeio, P. F., & Volkmann, R. A. (1996). Posttranslational amino acid epimerization: enzyme-catalyzed isomerization of amino acid residues in peptide chains. Proc Natl Acad Sci U S A, 93(9), 4036-4039.

Heck, S. D., Siok, C. J., Krapcho, K. J., Kelbaugh, P. R., Thadeio, P. F., Welch, M. J., et al. (1994). Functional consequences of posttranslational isomerization of Ser46 in a calcium channel toxin. Science, 266(5187), 1065-1068.

Jack, R. W., & Jung, G. (2000). Lantibiotics and microcins: polypeptides with unusual chemical diversity. Curr Opin Chem Biol, 4(3), 310-317.

Jilek, A., Mollay, C., Lohner, K., & Kreil, G. (2012). Sustrate specificity of the L/D-isomerase from frog skin. Amino Acids, 42 (5), 1757-1764.

Jilek, A., Mollay, C., Tippelt, C., Grassi, J., Mignogna, G., Mullegger, J., et al. (2005). Biosynthesis of a D-amino acid in peptide linkage by an enzyme from frog skin secretions. Proc Natl Acad Sci U S A, 102(12), 4235-4239.

Jimenez, E. C., Olivera, B. M., Gray, W. R., & Cruz, L. J. (1996). Contryphan is a D-tryptophan-containing Conus peptide. J Biol Chem, 271(45), 28002-28005.

Koh, J. M., Chow, S. J., Crossett, B., & Kuchel, P. W. (2010). Mammalian peptide isomerase: platypus-type activity is present in mouse heart. Chem Biodivers, 7(6), 1603-1611.

Kovacs, J., Holleran, E. M., & Hui, K. Y. (1980). Kinetic studies in peptide chemistry. Coupling, racemization and evaluation of methods useful for shortening coupling time. The Journal of Organic Chemistry, 45 (6), 1060-1065.

Kreil, G. (1997). D-amino acids in animal peptides. Annu Rev Biochem, 66, 337-345.

Kreil, G., Barra, D., Simmaco, M., Erspamer, V., Erspamer, G. F., Negri, L., et al. (1989). Deltorphin, a novel amphibian skin peptide with high selectivity and affinity for delta opioid receptors. Eur J Pharmacol, 162(1), 123-128.

Lam, L. K., Arnold, L. D., Kalantar, T. H., Kelland, J. G., Lane-Bell, P. M., Palcic, M. M., et al. (1988). Analogs of diaminopimelic acid as inhibitors of meso-diaminopimelate dehydrogenase and LL-diaminopimelate epimerase. J Biol Chem, 263(24), 11814-11819.

Liu, L., Iwata, K., Kita, A., Kawarabayasi, Y., Yohda, M., & Miki, K. (2002). Crystal structure of aspartate racemase from Pyrococcus horikoshii OT3 and its implications for molecular mechanism of PLP-independent racemization. J Mol Biol, 319(2), 479-489.

Lundmark, K., Westermark, G. T., Olsen, A., & Westermark, P. (2005). Protein fibrils in nature can enhance amyloid protein A amyloidosis in mice: Cross-seeding as a disease mechanism. Proc Natl Acad Sci U S A, 102(17), 6098-6102.

Mangoni, M. L., Grovale, N., Giorgi, A., Mignogna, G., Simmaco, M., & Barra, D. (2000). Structure-function relationships in bombinins H, antimicrobial peptides from Bombina skin secretions. Peptides, 21(11), 1673-1679.

Mangoni, M. L., Papo, N., Saugar, J. M., Barra, D., Shai, Y., Simmaco, M., et al. (2006). Effect of natural L- to D-amino acid conversion on the organization, membrane binding, and biological function of the antimicrobial peptides bombinins H. Biochemistry, 45(13), 4266-4276.

Mignogna, G., Pascarella, S., Wechselberger, C., Hinterleitner, C., Mollay, C., Amiconi, G., et al. (1996). BSTI, a trypsin inhibitor from skin secretions of Bombina bombina related to protease inhibitors of nematodes. Protein Sci, 5(2), 357-362.

Mignogna, G., Simmaco, M., Kreil, G., & Barra, D. (1993). Antibacterial and haemolytic peptides containing D-alloisoleucine from the skin of Bombina variegata. EMBO J, 12(12), 4829-4832.

Montecucchi, P. C., de Castiglione, R., Piani, S., Gozzini, L., & Erspamer, V. (1981). Amino acid composition and sequence of dermorphin, a novel opiate-like peptide from the skin of Phyllomedusa sauvagei. Int J Pept Protein Res, 17(3), 275-283.

Mor, A., Delfour, A., Sagan, S., Amiche, M., Pradelles, P., Rossier, J., et al. (1989). Isolation of dermenkephalin from amphibian skin, a high-affinity delta-selective opioid heptapeptide containing a D-amino acid residue. FEBS Lett, 255(2), 269-274.

Murkin, A. S., & Tanner, M. E. (2002). Dehydroalanine-based inhibition of a peptide epimerase from spider venom. J Org Chem, 67(24), 8389-8394.

Neidhart, D. J., Howell, P. L., Petsko, G. A., Powers, V. M., Li, R. S., Kenyon, G. L., et al. (1991). Mechanism of the reaction catalyzed by mandelate racemase. 2. Crystal structure of mandelate racemase at 2.5-A resolution: identification of the active site and possible catalytic residues. Biochemistry, 30(38), 9264-9273.

Ohta, N., Kubota, I., Takao, T., Shimonishi, Y., Yasuda-Kamatani, Y., Minakata, H., et al. (1991). Fulicin, a novel neuropeptide containing a D-amino acid residue isolated from the ganglia of Achatina fulica. Biochem Biophys Res Commun, 178(2), 486-493.

Okeley, N. M., Zhu, Y., & van Der Donk, W. A. (2000). Facile chemoselective synthesis of dehydroalanine-containing peptides. Org Lett, 2(23), 3603-3606.

Ponnusamy, E., Fotadar, U., Spisni, A., & Fiat, D. (1986). A novel method for the rapid, non-aqueous t-Butoxycarbonylation of some 17O-labeled amino acids and 17O-NMR parametersof the products. Synthesis, 1, 48-49.

Richter, K., Egger, R., & Kreil, G. (1987). D-alanine in the frog skin peptide dermorphin is derived from L-alanine in the precursor. Science, 238(4824), 200-202.

Rudnick, G., & Abeles, R. H. (1975). Reaction mechanism and structure of the active site of proline racemase. Biochemistry, 14(20), 4515-4522.

Shikata, Y., Watanabe, T., Teramoto, T., Inoue, A., Kawakami, Y., Nishizawa, Y., et al. (1995). Isolation and characterization of a peptide isomerase from funnel web spider venom. J Biol Chem, 270(28), 16719-16723.

Simmaco, M., Barra, D., Chiarini, F., Noviello, L., Melchiorri, P., Kreil, G., et al. (1991). A family of bombinin-related peptides from the skin of Bombina variegata. Eur J Biochem, 199(1), 217-222.

Smith, G. G., & Sivakua, T. (1983). Mechanism of the racemization of amino acids. Kinetics of racemization of arylglycines. The Journal of Organic Chemistry, 48 (5), 627-634.

Soyez, D., Toullec, J. Y., Ollivaux, C., & Geraud, G. (2000). L to D amino acid isomerization in a peptide hormone is a late post-translational event occurring in specialized neurosecretory cells. J Biol Chem, 275(48), 37870-37875.

Stefano, G. B., Melchiorri, P., Negri, L., Hughes, T. K., Jr., & Scharrer, B. (1992). [D-Ala2]deltorphin I binding and pharmacological evidence for a special subtype of delta opioid receptor on human and invertebrate immune cells. Proc Natl Acad Sci U S A, 89(19), 9316-9320.

Torres, A. M., Menz, I., Alewood, P. F., Bansal, P., Lahnstein, J., Gallagher, C. H., et al. (2002). D-Amino acid residue in the C-type natriuretic peptide from the venom of the mammal, Ornithorhynchus anatinus, the Australian platypus. FEBS Lett, 524(1-3), 172-176.

Torres, A. M., Tsampazi, C., Geraghty, D. P., Bansal, P. S., Alewood, P. F., & Kuchel, P. W. (2005). D-amino acid residue in a defensin-like peptide from platypus venom: effect on structure and chromatographic properties. Biochem J, 391(Pt 2), 215-220.

Torres, A. M., Tsampazi, M., Kennett, E. C., Belov, K., Geraghty, D. P., Bansal, P. S., et al. (2007). Characterization and isolation of L-to-D-amino-acid-residue isomerase from platypus venom. Amino Acids, 32(1), 63-68.

Torres, A. M., Tsampazi, M., Tsampazi, C., Kennett, E. C., Belov, K., Geraghty, D. P., et al. (2006). Mammalian L-to-D-amino-acid-residue isomerase from platypus venom. FEBS Lett, 580(6), 1587-1591.

Walsh, C. T. (1984). Suicide substrates, mechanism-based enzyme inactivators: recent developments. Annu Rev Biochem, 53, 493-535.

Whiteley, C. G. (2000). Mechanistic and kinetic studies of inhibition of enzymes. Cell Biochem Biophys, 33(3), 217-225.

Zangger, K., Gößler, R., Khatai, L., Lohner, K., & Jilek, A. (2008). Structures of the glycine-rich diastereomeric peptides bombinin H2 and H4. Toxicon, 52(2), 246-254.

Effect of Pressure and Heat Treatment on Beef Proteins

Hanjun Ma
School of Food Science
Henan Institute of Science and Technology, China

Guanghong Zhou
College of Food Science and Technology
Nanjing Agricultural University, China

David A. Ledward
Department of Food Biosciences
University of Reading, UK

Xiaoling Yu
School of Food Science
Henan Institute of Science and Technology, China

Runshu Pan
School of Food Science
Henan Institute of Science and Technology, China

1   Introduction

High pressure processing is becoming increasingly used by the meat industry, as it can extend shelf life and improve the eating quality and functional properties of meat and meat products (Hugas, 2002; Torres & Velazquez, 2005; Marcos *et al.*, 2010). High pressure treatment can tenderize meat when applied pre-rigor, but it does not necessarily have such an effect on post-rigor meat at room temperature (20 ^{0}C) (Ma & Ledward, 2004). However, it is difficult for the industry to treat pre-rigor meat with high pressure (Cheftel & Culioli, 1997). Spores at ambient temperature can resist pressures up to 1000 MPa, but lower pressures (250 MPa) associated with mild temperatures (40 ^{0}C) can inactivate spores in a two stage process, pressure first inducing germination and then inactivating the baro-sensitive germinated spores (Lamballerie-Anton *et al.*, 2002), showing the benefits of combining high pressure technology with heat treatment. Therefore, high pressure technology can be applied in combination with heat treatment.

Pressure treatment can also bring about changes in the structure of meat, and affect functional properties such as color (Carlez *et al.*, 1995; Cheah and Ledward, 1997), texture (Angsupanich and Ledward, 1998; Angsupanich *et al.*, 1999; Ueno *et al.*, 1999; Suzuki *et al.*, 1993; Jung *et al.*, 2000; Beilken *et al.*, 1990; Bouton and Harris, 1972; Bouton *et al.*, 1977, 1980; Macfarlane, 1973), lipid oxidation (Cheah and Ledward, 1995, 1996, 1997) and flavour (Suzuki *et al.*, 1994). The components of muscle controlling toughness are the myofibrillar proteins and the connective tissue protein, collagen. As collagen is primarily stabilised by hydrogen bonds it is thought to be little affected by pressure, and the contractile myofibrillar proteins are thought to be primarily responsible for the change in textural properties observed when meat is subjected to high pressure.

Differential Scanning Calorimetry (DSC) is a powerful technique that has been used to study the structural and thermal properties of natural polymers such as proteins and it has been used to relate the denaturation of individual muscle proteins to the textural changes in meat caused by cooking (Martens *et al.*, 1982; Findlay *et al.*, 1986) and pressurization (Angsupanich & Ledward, 1998; Angsupanich *et al.*, 1999). The three major endothermic transitions seen in beef muscle, attributed to myosin, collagen and actin, have been associated with specific changes in beef texture.

Myofibrillar proteins have a significant relationship with meat functional properties, therefore it is important to understand the changes that happen to the myofibrillar proteins. Many previous investigations have shown that as a consequence of depolymerization, pressure induces increased solubilization of myofibrillar proteins. Macfarlane *et al.* reported that when ovine meat is pressurized at 150 MPa, a marked increase in the yield of solubilized myofibrillar proteins occurs, but the effects were dependent on pH, temperature, and salt type and concentration (Macfarlane *et al.*, 1974; Macfarlane & McKenzie, 1976). Similar observations were observed by Suzuki *et al.* in rabbit meat (Suzuki *et al.*, 1991). These authors found that proteins from the thin filament such as actin, tropomyosin, troponin C as well as M-protein were solubilized at 100 MPa, whereas solubilization of myosin heavy chains required higher pressures (300 MPa). McArthur and Wilding (2002) observed no solubilization of myosin heavy chains, even at 500 MPa, although myosin was shown to be partly denatured by differential scanning calorimetry.

The changes in myofibrillar proteins subjected to high pressures have been studied, but these studies were limited to ambient temperature. In the present study the effects of combined heat and pressure treatments on The objective was to further understand the relative effects of heat and pressure treatments on the myofibrillar proteins of beef muscle.

In the present study the effects of combined heat and pressure on whole beef muscle proteins and isolated myofibril solubility and protein electrophoretic pattern were investigated. The objective was to further understand the relative effects of heat and pressure treatments on the proteins of beef muscle.

2   Materials and Methods

2.1   Preparation of Sample

For the sequential studies the beef *Longissimus dorsi* was obtained from a supermarket in Nanjing, China. The meat was from two20 ~24 month old Luxi × Limousin crossbreeds; the weight of each side of the carcass was about 130 kg and had been kept at 4 ^{0}C for 3 days following slaughter. The beef sample was trimmed of all visible fat and cut into approximately 3 × 3 × 6 cm pieces with the fibers parallel to the longest axis, and packed in Multivac bags (Bosley International, London, UK), which were maintained at 4 °C for over 48 h until required (Ma & Ledward, 2007).

For the DSC studies, 4 kg of beef *Longissimus dorsi* (quality assured Scottish beef) was obtained from a local butcher. The animals were slaughtered conventionally at The University of Bristol abattoir and after storage at 2 ^{0}C for 8 days, the beef was trimmed of all visible fat and cut into portions weighing about 250g and subsequently stored at -18 ^{0}C. For each treatment samples were chosen at random and prior to use the frozen samples were left at 4 ^{0}C for 12 hours to thaw.

2.2   Myofibrillar Extraction

Myofibrils were extracted using the method of Busch *et al* (1972). Minced beef was homogenised for 20 s in a Waring blender with six volumes of extraction buffer (20mM Tris-HCl, pH 7.6, 5mM EDTA). After centifugation at 1,000 g for 10 min at 4 ^{0}C, the pellets were resuspended in the extraction buffer and the same operation was repeated five times. After the last centrifugation, the pellets were resuspended in five volumes of extraction buffer and homogenized in a Waring blender for 25 s. In order to remove the connective tissue, the homogenate was filtered through a 20 mesh nylon net, centrifuged at 1,000 g for 10 min and washed with the buffer. The pellets were resuspended in 100 mM KC1, centrifuged under the same conditions. Samples of 10 g were sealed in Multivac bags (Bosley, International, NL) for treatment.

2.3   Sample Treatments

For the DSC studies whole muscle samples, cut to about 2.5x2.5x6 cm with the fibres parallel to the longest axis were sealed in Mulivac bags (Bosley, International, NL). Samples were treated at 200 to 800 MP at room temperature, 40 ^{0}C, 60 ^{0}C and 70 ^{0}C for 20 min in a prototype Stansted Food lab high pressure rig (Stanstead Fluid Power Ltd, Stanstead, UK). Other samples were treated in sequence at 40 or 70 ^{0}C followed by pressure treatment at 200 or 600 MPa or vice versa. Myofibrillar protein samples (10 g) were sealed in Mulitvac bags (Bosley, International, NL) and treated under the same condition as the whole muscle samples. Some whole muscles and myofibrillar proteins were heated in water baths at 40 ^{0}C, 60 ^{0}C or 70 ^{0}C for 30 min (whole muscle) or 20 min (myofibrillar protein).

During pressurisation, the temperature in the high-pressure vessel gradually increased with pressure, rising to reach a maximum when the maximum pressure was attained, it then progressively decreased back to the originally set temperature. This is due to adiabatic compression of the fluid (20% Castor oil in ethanol) and causes a temperature increase of 2~3 ^{0}C per 100 MPa (Cheftel & Culioli, 1997).

The thermal profiles of the compression fluid during the measurements reported in this paper are shown in Figure 1.

For the sequential studies myofibrils were treated at 100 to 600 MPa at room temperature, 40 and 60 ^{0}C for 20 min in the high pressure rig (Kefa New Technology Food Machine, Ltd., Baotou, China). The pressure unit comprised a 3 L cylindrical pressure chamber fitted with a thermoregulated system. Room temperature was the control, 20 ^{0}C. Some myofibrillar samples were heated, in water baths at 40 ^{0}C and 60 ^{0}C for 20 min, as controls.

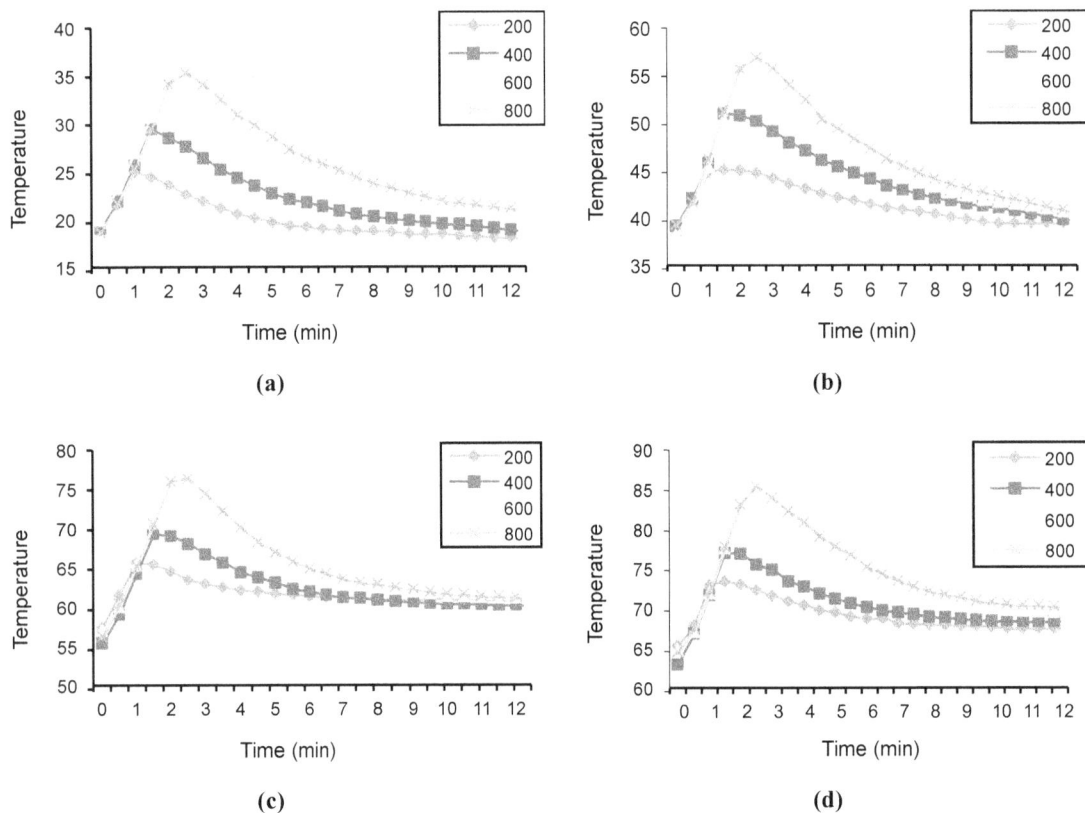

Figure 1: Temperature change during pressurization in "Food-Lab 900" at (a) 20 ^{0}C (b) 40 ^{0}C (c) 60 ^{0}C (d) 70 ^{0}C. 200, 400, 600, 800 represent different pressure value, respectively.

2.4 Differential Scanning Calorimetry (DSC)

A Perkin-Elmer DSC 7 Differential Scanning Calorimeter was used to study the thermal denaturation of the protein in the samples. The instrument was calibrated using Indium. 15-20mg of sample was weighed into an aluminium pan, sealed and heated at 10 ^{0}C min^{-1} over the range 30-100 ^{0}C. At least 3 runs per sample were carried out using an empty pan as a reference.

2.5   Assay of Protein Solubility

After pressure treatment, samples of myofibrils were centrifuged for 20 min at 14,000 g and 4 ^{0}C, supernatants and precipitates from each sample were collected. The protein concentration of the supernatant was determined by BCA kit (Pierce Biotechnology, Int., Rockford, IL, USA).

2.6   Electrophoretic Analysis

The SDS–PAGE analysis was conducted using a 12.5% acrylamide gradient separating gel and 4% acrylamide stacking gel, as in Laemmli (1970). Samples of supernatant and precipitate (mixed with 8 volumes of buffer) were mixed with SDS-PAGE sample buffer (4% SDS, 20% glycerol, 0.125 M Tris–HCl, 10% β-mercaptoethanol [pH 6.87]) in a 1:1 (v/v) ratio were heated in boiling water for 3 min. Aliquots of 20 μg of protein per lane were loaded onto the acrylamide gel. Electrophoresis was first run at 80 V for about 30 min, and then at 120 V for 3 h. Gel was stained in Coomassie brilliant blue R-250 (0.1% Coomassie brilliant blue R-250, 45% methanol, 10% acetic acid) for 2 h. Destaining was in 10% methanol, 10% acetic acid for 12 h.

2.7   Statistical Analysis

Data were analyzed by a two way analysis of variance. A confidence level of 5% was used to compare means ($P < 0.05$). When significance was detected between samples, the mean values were compared using Fisher's least significant difference (LSD) procedure.

3   Results and Discussion

3.1   Effect of Pressure and Heat on Beef Protein by DSC

3.1.1   Whole Muscle

Figure 2 shows the thermograms of intact beef muscle after treatment at pressures from 0.1 MP to 800 MPa at 20 ^{0}C for 20 min. The three major endothermic transitions seen have been attributed to myosin, collagen and actin (Martens et al., 1982) and the peak maxima in this study are seen at 54.6 ^{0}C (myosin), 67.1 ^{0}C (collagen) and 77.3 ^{0}C (actin). Treatment at 200 MPa decreased the myosin and actin peaks and at 400 MPa and higher, the actin peak is not seen. At the same time a new peak for myosin is seen around 50.1 ^{0}C as previously reported by Angupanich, Edde & Ledward (1999). The collagen peak is apparently not affected by pressure. This is in agreement with the work of Suzuki et al. (1993) who found that pressurization alone, without heat treatment, caused no significant changes in intramuscular collagen.

Figure 3 shows the thermograms when the samples are treated at 0.1 to 800 MPa at 40 ^{0}C for 20 min. At ambient pressure about 43% of the myosin, is denatured but there is no obvious effect on collagen and actin. At 200 MPa the myosin and collagen are merged into one broad peak with an onset temperature of 50.1 ^{0}C. At 400 MPa, the actin peak is not seen. When the pressure is increased to 600 MPa and 800 MPa, the new myosin peak and that of collagen are still discernible. This result is similar to that seen in turkey muscle (Angsupanich et al., 1999).

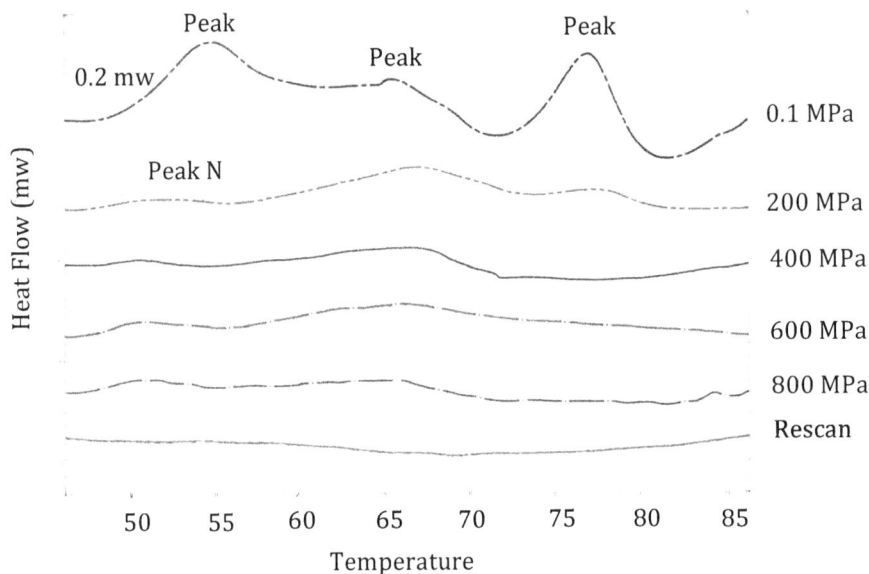

Figure 2: Thermograms of beef muscle, heated at 10 ^{0}C after treatment at difference pressure in air for 20 min at 20 ^{0}C, Peak 1, 2 and 3 correspond to myosin, collagen and actin, respectively. Peak N represents a structure produced after pressure treatment.

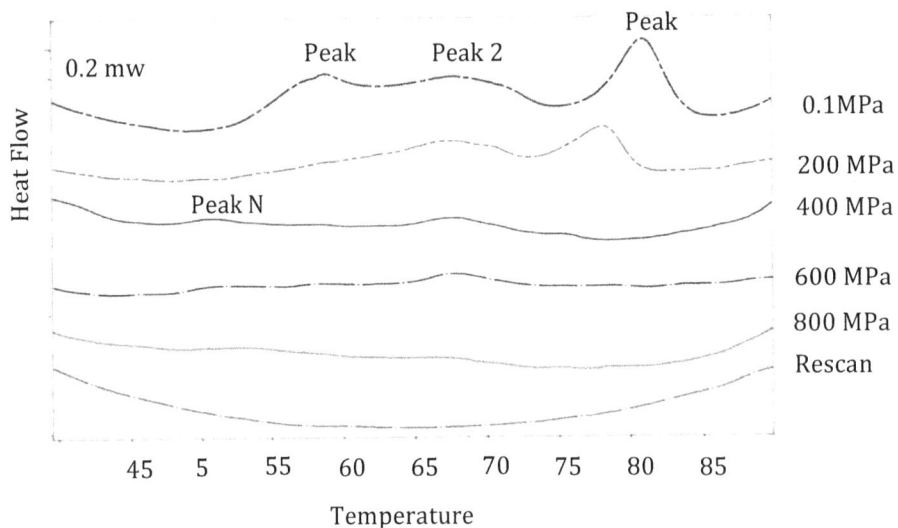

Figure 3: Thermograms of beef muscle, heated at 10 ^{0}C min-1 after treatment at different pressure in air for 20 min at 40 ^{0}C. Peaks 1, 2 and 3 correspond to myosin, collagen and actin, respectively. Peak N represents a structure produced after treatment.

The thermograms of samples treated at 0.1 MPa to 800 Mpa at 60 ^{0}C for 20 min are shown in Figure 4. At ambient pressure and 60 ^{0}C myosin is totally denatured but collagen and actin are not affected. This agrees with Martens *et al* (1982) who reported that myosin is labile to heat but collagen and actin are not. At 200 MPa and 60 ^{0}C only the collagen peak can be seen. When treated at 400 MPa, the peak temperature of collagen decreased from 67.5 ^{0}C to 65.3 ^{0}C and the net enthalpy decreased from 0.432 to 0.079 J/g (wet sample weight). At 600 MPa, the net enthalpy of the collagen increases slightly from 0.079 to 0.12J/g). At 800 MPa the myosin "new peak" and that of collagen can still be seen.

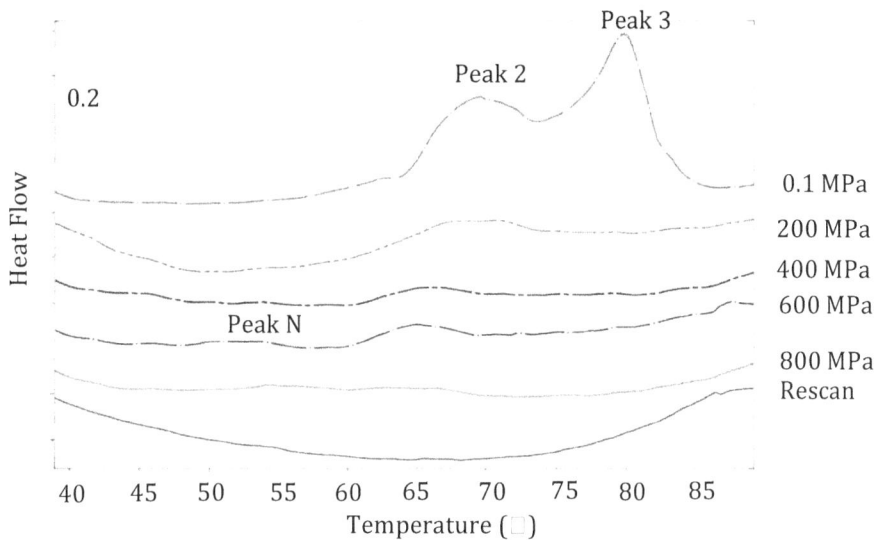

Figure 4: Thermograms of beef muscle, heated at 10 ^{0}C min-1 after treatment at different pressures in air for 20 min at 60 ^{0}C. Peak 2 and 3 correspond to collagen and actin, respectively. Peak N represents a structure produced after treatment.

3.1.2 Myofibrils

The thermograms of the untreated and pressure/heat treated beef myofibrillar proteins are shown in Figures 5 to 7. Two endothermic transitions at 58.3 and 69.7 ^{0}C are observed corresponding to myosin and actin denaturation. Compared to whole muscle, the endothermic transition temperature of the myosin in the extracted myofibrillar protein is higher (cf. 58.3 and 54.6 ^{0}C), but the actin in the extracted myofibrillar is denatured at a lower temperature (cf 69.7 and 77.3 ^{0}C), indicating purification changes the heat stability of the proteins. This result is a little different to that found by Angsupanich *et al.* (1999) on the extracted myofibrillar proteins of cod and turkey. These authors found that the extracted myofibrillar proteins from cod had denaturation peaks at lower temperatures than those of whole cod muscle, but in the turkey breast no marked decrease in stability was seen following extraction. When the extracted myofibrillar was subjected to pressure at ambient temperatures (Figure 5), 200 MPa led to some loss of both peaks, decreasing the peak denaturation temperatures (myosin from 58.3 to 55.5 ^{0}C and actin from 69.7 ^{0}C to 64.8 ^{0}C). Treatment at 400 MPa, caused a total loss of the actin peak and myosin was modified yielding a "new" structure with a peak temperature around 50 ^{0}C. From 400 MPa to 800 MPa no obvious changes are seen suggesting, as found by Angsupanich et al (1999) that the "new" structure is stable to pressure.

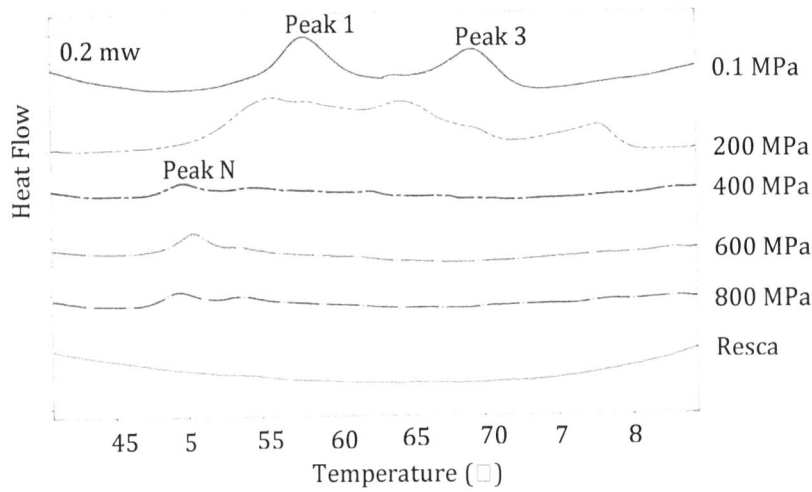

Figure 5: Thermograms of myofibrillar protein from beef muscle, heated at 10 ^{0}C min-1 after treatment at different pressures in air for 20 min at 20 ^{0}C. Peak 1 and 3 correspond to myosin and actin, respectively. Peak N resperents a structure produced after treatment.

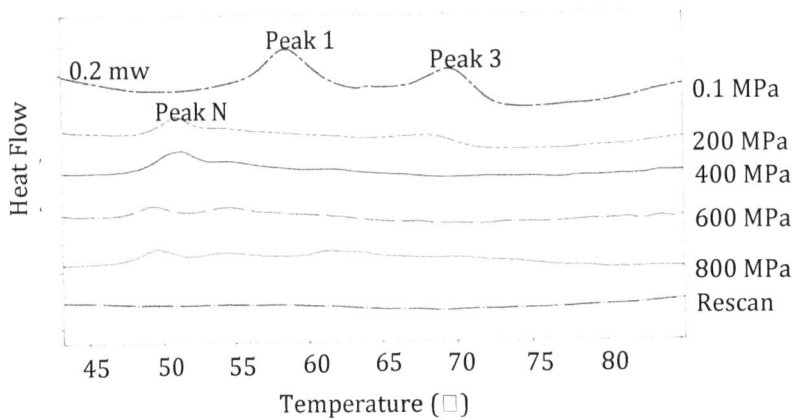

Figure 6: Thermograms of myofibrillar protein from beef muscle, heated at 10 ^{0}C min-1 after treatment at different pressures in air for 20 min at 40 ^{0}C. Peak 1 and 3 correspond to myosin and actin, respectively. Peak N resperents a structure produced after treatment.

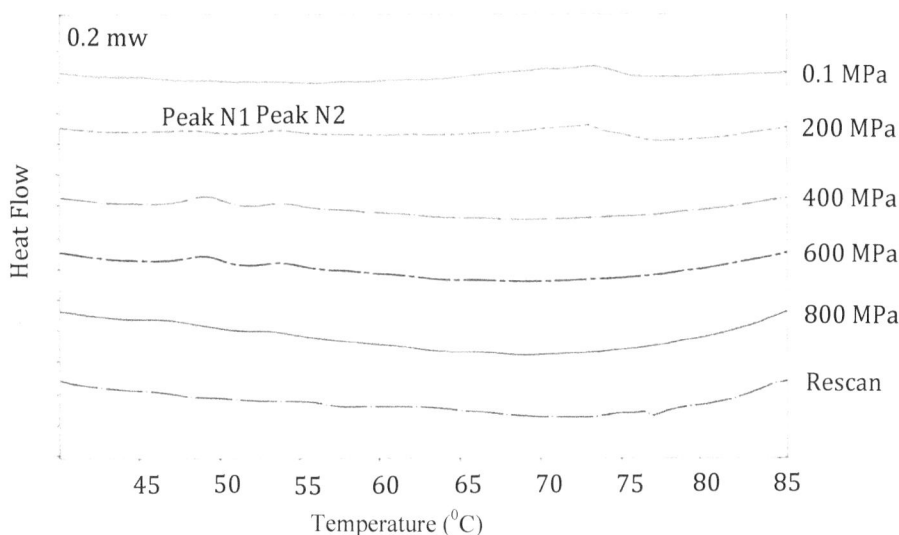

Figure 7 : Thermograms of myofibrillar protein from beef muscle, heated at 10 ^{0}C min-1 after treatment at different pressures in air for 20 min at 60 ^{0}C. Peak 1 and 3 correspond to myosin and actin, respectively. Peak N resperents a structure produced after treatment.

At 40 ^{0}C, heating caused no obvious changes in the myosin and actin and the results are similar to those seen at 20 ^{0}C (Figure 6). At 60 ^{0}C, almost all the protein is denatured (Figure 7). However when subjected to pressure, both at 40 ^{0}C and 60 ^{0}C, similar results are seen. Two new peaks are formed, (one with peak temperatures from 47.3 ^{0}C to 50.5 ^{0}C and another with peak temperatures from 53.4 ^{0}C to 54.3 ^{0}C), at all pressures up to 800 MPa. On rescanning the untreated samples and any pressure-heat treated ones, no peaks are seen indicating that the new or modified structure is destroyed by heat, suggesting that they are primarily stabilized by hydrogen bonds.

3.2   Effect of Pressure and Heat on the Solubilization of the Proteins

The effects of high pressure and temperature on the solubilization of myofibrillar proteins are presented in Figure 8.

On heat treatment at ambient pressure, the expected increase in the solubility of myofibrillar proteins with increasing temperature ($P < 0.05$), especially from 40 ^{0}C to 60 ^{0}C, was observed, where the concentration of soluble myofibrillar proteins increased from 0.273 mg/mL to 0.747 mg/mL.

At 20 °C, increasing pressure led to an increase in solubility of myofibrillar proteins, up to 400 MPa (1.403 mg/mL), the highest concentration for all treatments, after which a significant decrease with a further increase in pressure was observed. The pressure induced solubilization of beef myofibrillar proteins is similar to the results obtained for chicken (Yamamoto, *et al.,* 2002). Jung(2000), Lamballerie-Anton and Ghoul also found increases in soluble protein at 300 MPa compared to the control and treatment at 100 MPa, but there was no significant change when pressure was increased from 300 to 600 MPa (June *et al.,* 2000).

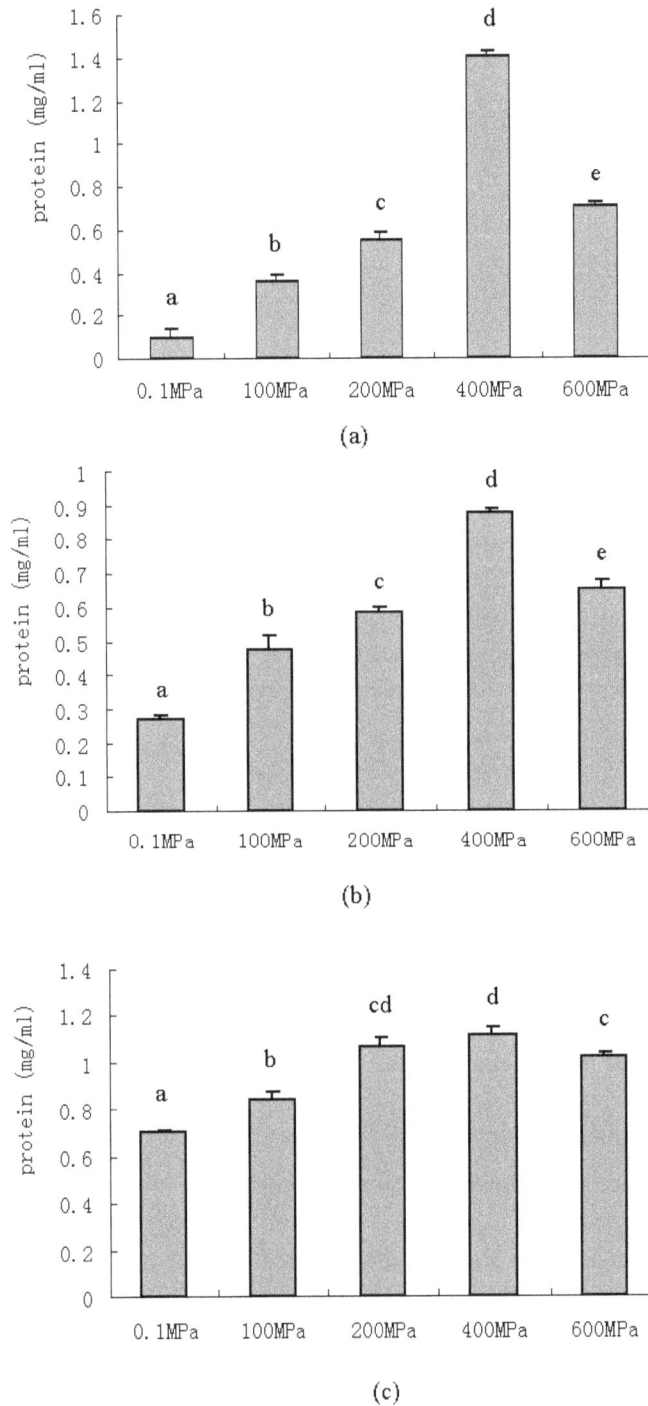

Figure 8: Changes in the concentration of myofibrillar protein in the supernatants after pressure treatment at (a) 20 ^{0}C (b) 40 ^{0}C (c) 60 ^{0}C. Means with different letters are significantly different (P < 0.05). The vertical bars represent the SD.

In comparison with the results obtained at 20 ^{0}C similar trends of protein solubilization were found when isolated myofibrils were subjected to pressure at 40 ^{0}C and 60 ^{0}C, an increase being observed with the increasing pressure up to 400 MPa, with a subsequent decrease at 600 MPa. Although similar trends of protein solubilization were found for pressure treatment at all temperatures, the extent and variability of the concentrations of soluble myofibrillar proteins differed at related pressures, which may be due to interactions between pressure and temperature.

3.3   Effect of Combined Pressure and Thermal Treatment on the Myofibrillar Proteins by SDS-PAGE Analysis

SDS-PAGE profiles from supernatants and precipitates of the myofibrils after pressure treatment at 20 ^{0}C are shown in Figure 9. From Figure 9(a) and the relative intensity of the bands (data not shown), it was found that proteins molecular weights over 41 kDa decreased in the supernatant, while proteins in the molecular weight range 35–16 kDa increased in both the supernatant and precipitate when samples were subjected to pressures over 100 MPa, due to depolymerization of the myofibrillar proteins treated at higher pressures.

Myosin heavy chain was observed in the supernatant from the control but was absent in the pressure treated samples. This is in agreement with Yamamoto *et al.* who found that the band of the myosin heavy chain was not observed in samples pressurized at 300 MPa for 10 to 30 min. This was attributed to the fact that the myosin heavy chain is not stable to pressurization and denatures to appear in the precipitate. The solubility of the myosin light chain increased with increasing pressure, as demonstrated by changes in the density of this band in the supernatant profiles.

α-Actinin is a component of the Z line of the myofibril. After treatment at 100 MPa, the density of this band in the supernatant was greater than in the control, but it disappeared gradually with increasing pressure, indicating that the solubility of α-actinin increased when subjected to 100 MPa at room temperature but decreased thereafter. Actin was observed in the supernatant of samples pressurized at 100 MPa for 20 min, but disappeared at pressures above 200 MPa. This result differs from Yamamoto *et al.* who observed actin in the supernatants after treatment at 300 and 400 MPa that was unchanged with increasing pressure (Yamamoto *et al.*, 2002). Troponin T, I/C and Tropomyosin, which are major components of thin filaments, were solubilized by pressure treatment, as the densities of these protein bands increased in the supernatants and decreased in the precipitates with increasing pressure. Thin filaments are sensitive to pressure and depolymerize into G-actin(Macfarlane & Morton, 1978) . June *et al.* also reported that the solubility of Troponin T, Tropomyosin and myosin light chains increased after pressure treatment (June *et al.*, 2000).

In the samples pressure treated at 40 ^{0}C and 60 ^{0}C, similar protein solubility changes were found (Figure 9(b) and Figure 9(c)). New banding patterns were observed. Lower molecular weight bands (below 35 KDa) increased with the pressure up to 200 or 400 MPa in the supernatants, but there were no significant changes in the precipitates. These results are similar to those of Sikes *et al.* who found that when the myofibrillar proteins of beef neck were treated at 200 MPa and 60 ^{0}C for 20 min a new type of structure between myosin and actin was formed and the myofibrillar proteins degraded to smaller molecules (Sikes, 2010). In the present study the band with the molecular weight of about 18 KDa (LC2) disappeared in the samples pressure treated at 40 ^{0}C and 60 ^{0}C, presumably due to the interactive effect of pressure and temperature treatment.

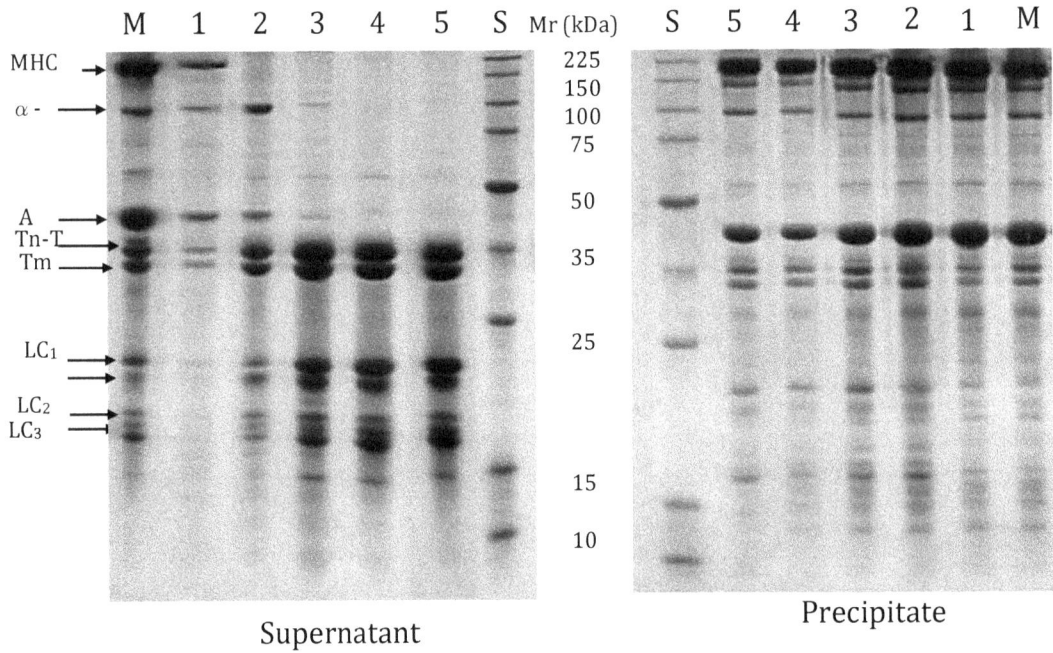

Supernatant   Precipitate

(a)

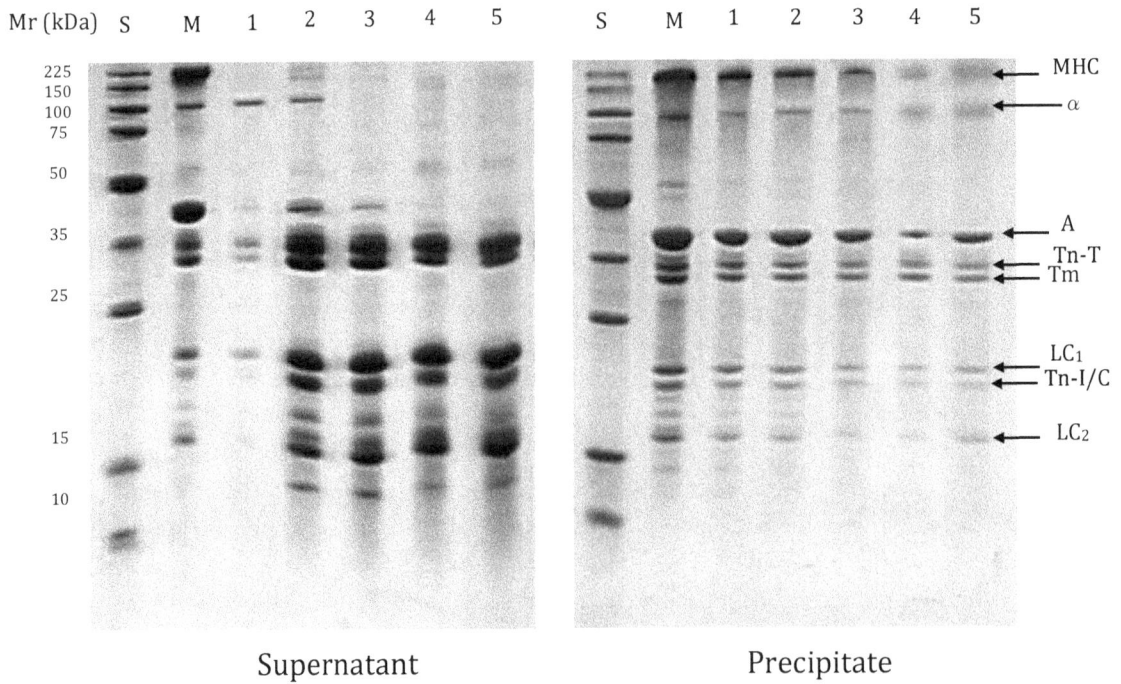

Supernatant   Precipitate

(b)

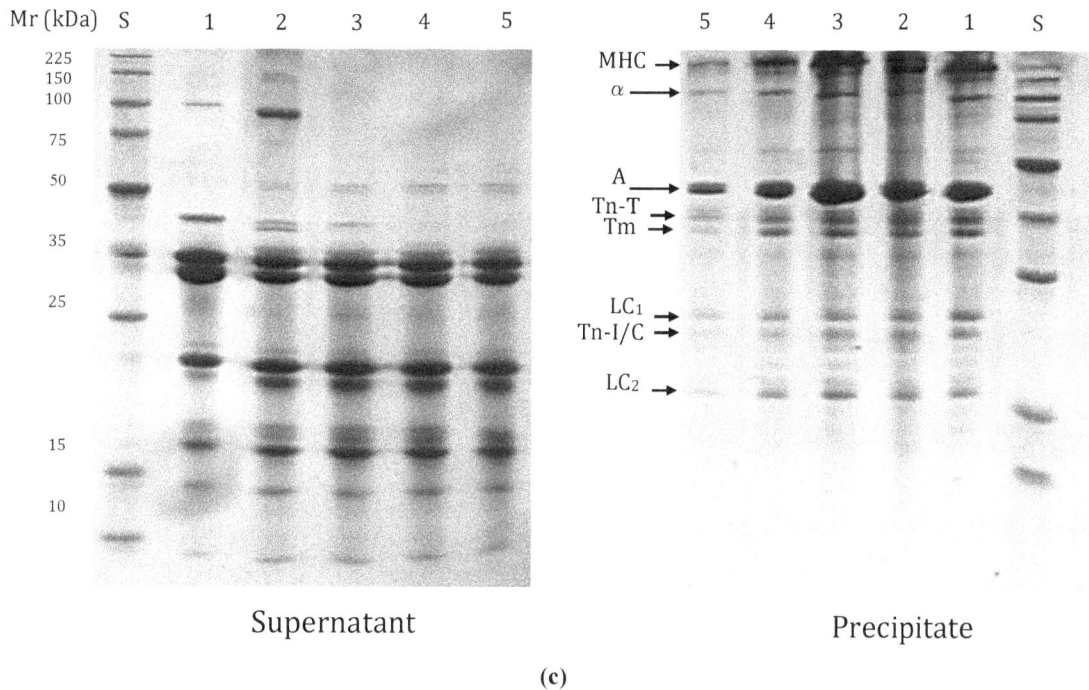

Figure 9: SDS-PAGE profiles from supernatants and precipitates of myofibrils after pressure treatment at(a) 20 ^{0}C (b) 40 ^{0}C (c)60 ^{0}C. M: myofibril; S: molecular weight standards;1, 2, 3, 4 and 5 represent control samples and samples after treatment at 100, 200, 400, 600MPa. MHC: myosin heavy chain; α: α-actinin; A: actin; Tn-T: troponin T; Tm: tropomyosin; Tn-I: troponin I; Tn-C: troponin C; LC1, 2, 3 represent myosin light chains 1, 2, 3, respectively.

4 Conclusion

The effects of pressure and heat treatment on beef proteins are rather complex, DSC shows myosin was relatively easily unfolded by both pressure and heat and when pressure denatured a new and modified structure was formed of low thermal stability, collagen was reasonably inert to pressure and only at temperatures of 60-70 ^{0}C was it denatured/unfolded. The solubility of myofibrillar proteins varied with pressure and temperature, but the highest solubility was induced by treatment at room temperature and 400 MPa. Myosin light chains and actin thin filaments were sensitive to pressure, and were released from myofibrils subjected to 100 MPa and higher pressures at the different temperatures tested.

It is a trend for applying of combined high pressure and temperature in meat processing, both for meat tenderization and sterilization. Although the mechanism is not clear, it is closely connected with the physical-chemical changes of proteins. In addition, high pressure and temperature treatment could result in the changes of functional properties of muscle, which can be attributed to the changes of structure, physical-chemical properties, intra- or intermolecular interactions of proteins. Therefore, researching work on the effect of high pressure and heat treatment on beef proteins will build up a foundation for application of high pressure processing in meat industry.

References

Angsupanich, K. and Ledward, D. A. (1998). High pressure treatment effects on cod (Gadus morhua) muscle. Food Chemistry, 63, 39-50.

Angsupanich, K., Edde, M. and Ledward, D. A. (1999). Effects of high pressure on the myofibrillar proteins of cod and turkey muscle. Journal of agricultural and food chemistry, 47, 92-99.

Beilken, S. L., Macfarlane, J. J. and Jones, P. N. (1990). Effect of high pressure during heat treatment on the warner-bratzler shear force values of selected beef muscles. Journal of Food Science, 55, 15-18.

Bouton, P. E., Ford, A. E., Harris, P. V., Macfarlane, J. J. and O'shea, J.M. (1977). Pressure-heat treatment of post-rigor muscle: Objective-subjective measurements. Journal of Food Science, 42, 857-859.

Bouton, P. E., Harris, P. V., and Macfarlane, J. J. (1980). Pressure-heat treatment of meat: Effect of prior aging treatments on shear properties. Journal of Food science. 45, 276-278.

Bouton, P.E. and Harris, P.V. (1972). The effects of cooking temperature and time on some mechanical properties of meat. Journal of Food science, 37, 140-143.

Busch, W. A., Stromer, M. H., Goll, D.E. and Suzuki, A. (1972). Ca^{2+} specific removal of Z lines from rabbit skeletal muscle. The Journal of Cell Biology, 52, 367-381.

Carlez, A., Veciana-Nogues, T. and Cheftel, J. C. (1995). Changs in colour and myoglobin of minced beef meat due to high pressure processing. Lebensm-wissu.- Technol., 28, 528-538.

Cheah, P. B. and Ledward, D. A. (1995). High pressure effects on lipid oxidation. Journal of American Oil Chemists Society, 72 (9), 1059-1063.

Cheah, P. B. and Ledward, D. A. (1996). High pressure effects on lipid oxidation in minced pork. Meat Science, 43, 2, 123-134.

Cheah, P. B. and Ledward, D. A. (1997). Catalytic mechanism of lipid oxidation following high pressure treatment in pork fat and meat. Journal of Food Science, 62, 1135-1138.

Cheftel, J.C.; Culioli, J. (1997). Effects of high pressure on meat: A review. Meat Sci., 46, 211–236.

Findlay, C. J. and Stanley, D. W. (1984). Differential scanning calorimetry of beef muscle: Influence of postmortem conditioning. Journal of Food Science, 49, 1513-516.

Hugas, M.; Garriga, M. Monfort, J.M. (2002). New mild technologies in meat processing: High pressure as a model technology. Meat Sci., 62, 359–371.

June, S.; Lamballerie-Anton, M.D.; Ghoul, M. (2000). Modification of ultrastructure and myofibrillar proteins of post-rigor beef treated by high pressure. Lebensm. Wiss. Technol. 33, 313–319.

Laemmli, U.K. (1970). Cleavage of structural proteins during the assembly of the head of bacteriophage T4. Nature. 227, 680–685.

Lamballerie-Anton, M.D.; ENITIAA, Taylor, R.G.; Culioli, J. (2002.). High pressure processing of meat. Meat processing: improving quality. Eds.; CRC Press: Cambridge, UK. 313-331.

Ma, H.J.; Ledward, D.A. (2004). High pressure/thermal treatment effects on the texture of beef muscle. Meat Sci. 68, 347–355.

Ma, H.J.; Ledward, D.A.; Zamri, A.I.; Frazier, R.A.; Zhou, G.H. (2007). Effects of high pressure/thermal treatment on lipid oxidation in beef and chicken muscle. Food Chem. 104, 1575–1579.

Macfarlane, J. J., (1973). Pre-rigor pressurization of muscle: Effects on pH, shear value and taste panel assessment. Journal of Food Science, 38, 294-298.

Macfarlane, J.J. (1974). Pressure-induced solubilization of meat proteins in saline solution. J. Food Sci. 39, 542–547.

Macfarlane, J.J.; McKenzie, I.J. (1976). Pressure-induced solubilization of myofibrillar proteins. J. Food Sci. 39, 1442–1446.

Macfarlane, J.J.; Morton, D.J. (1978). Effects of pressure treatment on the ultrastructure of striated muscle. Meat Sci. 2, 281–288.

Marcos, B.; Kerry, J.P.; Mullen, A.M. (2010). High pressure induced changes on sarcoplasmic protein fraction and quality indicators. Meat Sci. 85, 115–120.

Martens, H., Stabursvik, E. and Martens, M. (1982). During cooking related to thermal denaturation of muscle proteins. Journal of Texture Studies, 13, 291-309.

Mcarthur, A.J.; Wilding, P. (2002). High pressure effects on myofibrillar proteins. In High Pressure Bioscience and Biotechnology; Hayashi, R., Balny, C., Eds.; Elsevier: Amsterdam, The Netherlands, 323-356.

Sikes, A.; Tornberg, E.; Tume, R. (2010). A proposed mechanism of tenderising post-rigor beef using high pressure–heat treatment. Meat Sci. 84, 390–399.

Suzuki, A., Homma, N., Fukuda, A., Hirao, K., Uryu, T. and Ikeuchi, Y. (1994). Effects of high-pressure treatment on the flavor-related components in meat. Meat Science, 37 (3), 369-379.

Suzuki, A., Watanabe, M. and Ikeuchi, Y. (1993). Effects of high-pressure treatment on the ultrastructure and thermal behaviour of beef intramuscular collagen. Meat science, 35, 17-25.

Suzuki, A.; Suzuki, N.; Ikeuchi, Y.; Saito, M. (1991). Effects of high pressure treatment on the ultrastructure and solubilization of isolated myofibrils. Agr. Bio. Chem. 55, 2467–2473.

Torres, J.A.; Velazquez, G. (2005). Commercial opportunities and research challenges in the high pressure processing of foods. J. Food Engineer. 67, 95–112.

Ueno, Y., Ikeuchi, Y. and Suzuki, A. (1999). Effects of high pressure treatments on intramuscular connective tissure. Meat Science, 52, 143-150.

Yamamoto, K.; Yoshida, T.; Iwasaki, T. (2002). Hydrostatic pressure-induced solubilization and gelation of chicken myofibrils. In Trends in High Pressure Bioscience and Biotechnology; Hayashi, R., Ed.; Elsevier Science B.V: Amsterdam, The Netherlands; pp. 461-468.

The Normal Synovium

Malcolm D. Smith
Rheumatology Research Unit
Repatriation General Hospital, and Flinders University, Australia

Mihir D. Wechalekar
Rheumatology Research Unit
Repatriation General Hospital, and Flinders University , Australia

1   Introduction

The synovium is the soft tissue that lines diarthrodial joints, ensheaths tendons and forms the lining of bursae. The term is inclusive of a continuous layer of cells (intima) and the underlying tissue (subintima). Specialised macrophages and fibroblasts form the intima; the subintima contains resident fibroblasts, infiltrating cells and blood vessels in a scaffolding of extracellular matrix. Between the intimal surfaces is a small amount of fluid, usually rich in hyaluronan (hyaluronic acid). Taken together, this structure provides a non-adherent surface between tissue elements. The synovium is of ectodermal origin and bereft of basal lamina unlike other serosal surfaces that also have non-adherent properties. Recent evidence suggests that a mesenchymal cadherin, cadherin 11 (a member of the cadherin family which are usually calcium dependant integral membrane proteins responsible for tissue architecture and morphogenesis) is expressed on synovial fibroblasts and may be critical in the development of the synovial lining by facilitation of cellular organization, compaction, and matrix development to form a recognizable synovial lining. (Firestein, 2007; D. M. Lee *et al.*, 2007)

Despite the obvious importance of the absolute need to have extensive background knowledge of the normal synovium to appreciate synovial changes in disease states such as rheumatoid arthritis (RA) and the spondyloarthritidies (SpA), our knowledge of the normal synovial membrane architecture is surprisingly inadequate. The normal synovium is relatively acellular; it has a distinct 1-2 cell thick intimal lining and a sublining. The sublining is relatively acellular as well containing scattered blood vessels, adipocytes and fibroblasts with very few lymphocytes or macrophages. The intima is 20-40 μm thick in cross section in contrast to the areolar subintima, which can be up to 5 mm thick.

There can be considerable variations in the synovial membrane. At several sites, there is no distinct membrane, especially where subintima consists of fat pad or fibrous tissue. There can be considerable variation in the intima as well with some sites having absence of intimal cells. (Smith, 2011) Bursae have minimal or no hyluronan-rich fluid.(Canoso, Stack, & Brandt, 1983) Ganglia, despite containing hyaluronan-rich fluid are devoid of a typical intima; they do not occur at sites of shear and hence are not really synovial tissue. In contrast to the appearance of the synovium in health, in disease the synovium may lose recognisable lining structure and may only be definable by its relation to a joint; in inflammatory arthritis such as rheumatoid arthritis, the synovial thickness increases. The intimal layer becomes several layers thick owing to increased CD68+ macrophages; the subintima thickness increases because of cellular infiltration with T and B lymphocytes, macrophages and plasma cells, stromal oedema and blood vessel proliferation.

2   Structure

Structurally, the normal synovium can be divided into three types, with the subintimal structure forming the basis for these synovial subtypes: fibrous, areolar and adipose. (Key, 1932) (Figure 1 – 3). Of these, the areolar form (Figure 1) of synovium is the most specialised. It may have projections or villi, but more commonly it is crimped into folds that may disappear when stretched. A 2-3 cell deep (Singh, Arayssi, Duray, & Schumacher, 2004; Smith *et al.*, 2003) layer forms the surface; below are capillaries, and further below a plexus of small arterioles and venules (Davies, 1950; Wilkinson & Edwards, 1989) associated with mast cells. Lymphatic vessels- albeit infrequent in the fibrous form of synovium- are present in all types of synovial tissue. (Xu *et al.*, 2003) These vessels are usually found in the deep subintimal layers

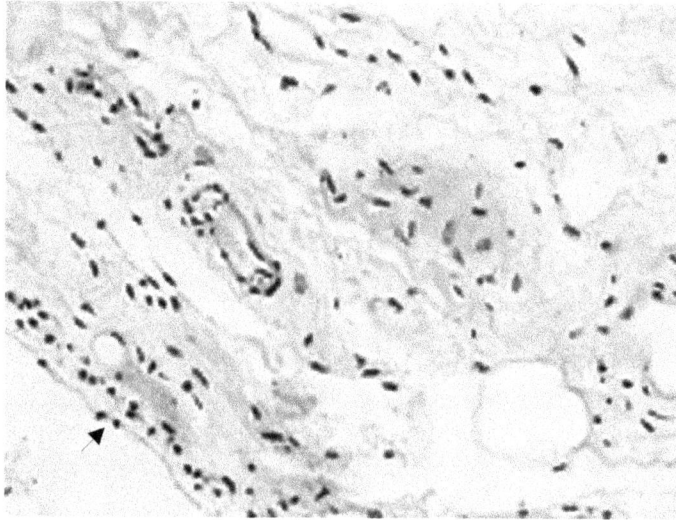

Figure 1: Areolar form of synovium with the synovial lining (arrow) and sublining

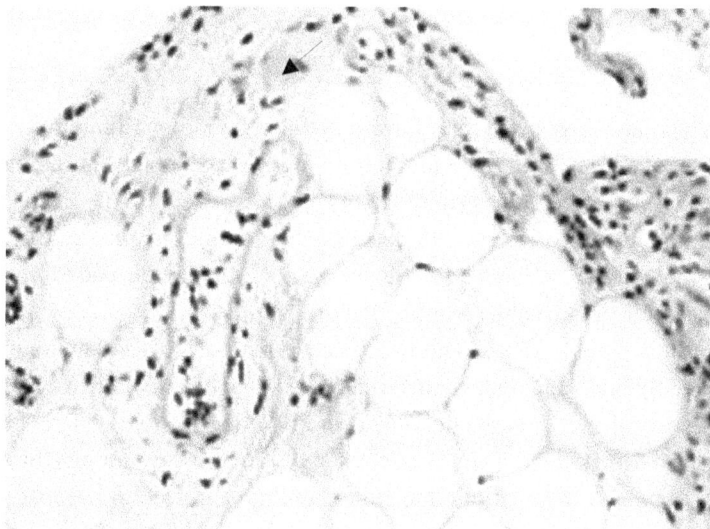

Figure 2: Adipose form of synovium (the arrow points to the lining); note the compact synovial lining and the abundance of adipose tissue in the sublining

of the normal synovium and in the presence of inflammatory arthritis such as RA, are found to be numerous and widespread. The synovium also has nerve fibres, usually present in association with blood vessels. (Mapp, 1995) The connective tissue matrix in the normal synovium consists of a fine fibrillar matrix with a few type I collagen fibres in the intima; what lies below is a layer relatively rich in type I collagen that forms the physical membrane. The loose connective tissue that lies deepest allows free movement of the synovial membrane. (Ghadially, 1978)

Adipose synovium (Figure 2) usually lies in relation to fat pads, but can be seen within villi; it has a complete intimal layer and a superficial network of capillaries. Villi usually have a central arteriole and

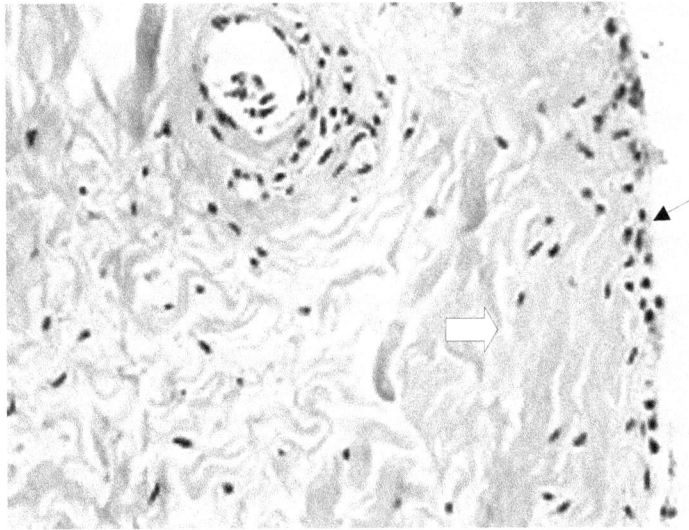

Figure 3: Fibrous form of synovium (the arrow points to the lining); note the fibrous sublining (block arrow)

venule but may be avascular. Adipocytes may form a bed for the intima, though there often is a collagen rich substratum with a deeper fat layer. The amount of fat is variable and increasing age reflects as decreased fat and increased fibrous content. (Smith, 2011)

Fibrous synovium (Figure 3) is easier to describe than define; it consists of fibrous tissue such as ligament or tendon on which lies an intermittent layer of cells. In annular pads found in finger joints, fibrous synovium may be indistinguishable. (Smith, 2011)

The synovial intima consists of synovial lining cells or synoviocytes that are of two microscopically, immunohistochemically and functionally differing types. This distinction was first proposed by Barland *et al.* ((Barland, Novikoff, & Hamerman, 1962) who reported the two distinct cell types on the basis of differences on electron microscopy. Type A synoviocytes are more numerous, have a prominent Golgi apparatus, numerous vacuoles, many filopodia, mitochondria, intracellular fibrils, micropinocytic like vesicles and manifest surface markers of the macrophage lineage. Type B synoviocytes contain large amounts of granular endoplasmic reticulum with fewer large vacuoles, micropinocytic vesicles and mitochondria; these cells show fibroblast lineage surface markers. (Barland, et al., 1962) Evidences from several elegant immunohistochemical animal studies and other lines of evidence point to intimal macrophages as being true macrophages, derived from bone marrow derived precursors (though it is not certain if differentiation occurs *in situ* or prior to arrival), whereas the intimal fibroblasts are locally derived. (Barland, *et al.*, 1962; Bartok & Firestein, 2010; J. C. Edwards, 1994; J. C. Edwards & Willoughby, 1982; Henderson, Revell, & Edwards, 1988) Fibroblasts are the dominant cell type in the normal synovium, and in most disease states including RA, the increase in synovial intimal cells reflects a rise in intimal macrophages secondary to influx from the vascular compartment orchestrated by cytokines and cell adhesion molecules. (Henderson, *et al.*, 1988; Smith, *et al.*, 2003; Smith & Walker, 2010) Immunohistochemistry, as opposed to electron microscopy, is now the preferred method for cellular identification. Intimal macrophages show expression of surface markers such as CD68 (a macrophage marker related to lysosomal glycoprotein (Holness & Simmons, 1993)), CD163 (a monocyte/ macrophage lineage marker), CD45 (common haematopoietic antigen) and non-specific esterase (NSE) activity; intimal fibroblasts reveal intense activity of the enzyme uridine diphosphoglucose dehydrogenase (UDPGD, an enzyme involved in hyaluronan synthesis and a specific marker of this cell type) (Wilkinson, Pitsillides, Worrall, & Edwards, 1992) and prominent expression of vascular cell adhesion molecule 1 (VCAM-1, a cell adhesion molecule) and CD55 [complement decay-accelerating factor (DAF)].

2.1 Synovial Macrophages

Synovial macrophages (Figure 4) are present in both the intimal and subintimal layers in the normal synovium. They bear typical macrophage lineage markers and show strong CD68 and CD163 positivity but less so for CD14 (a membrane protein that normally functions as a pattern recognition receptor). A subset of intimal (but not subintimal) macrophages show strong FcγRIIIa expression; interestingly, this corresponds closely to sites of macrophage activation in rheumatoid disease: synovial, alveolar, serosal, scleral, salivary gland, lymphoid and bone marrow macrophages, and Kupffer cells. (Bhatia, Blades, Cambridge, & Edwards, 1998) Z39Ig, a recently described inducible cell surface receptor linked to the classic complement pathway, is also expressed by synovial macrophages. Expression of this receptor can occur during macrophage differentiation and induce activation of the transcription factor NF- κB and production of the matrix degrading enzyme matrix metalloproteinase 9 (MMP-9). (Kim *et al.*, 2005; M. Y. Lee *et al.*, 2006; Poulter & Janossy, 1985; Walker, 2002)

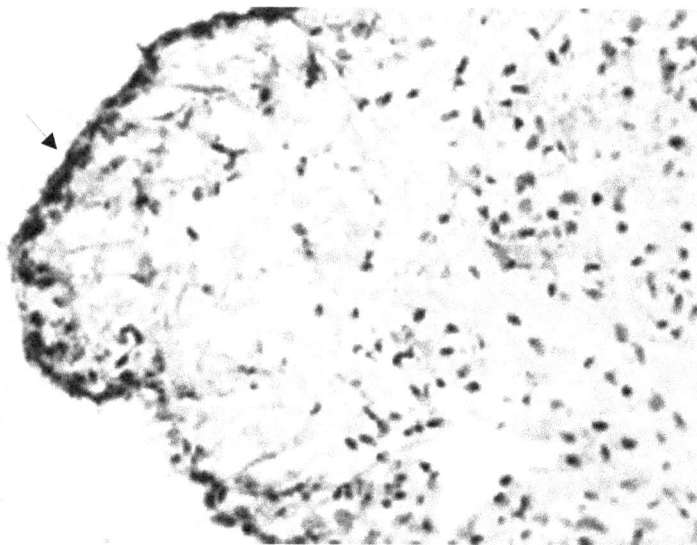

Figure 4: Synovial macrophages (normal synovium, x200 magnification), stained for CD68

Macrophages normally make up a minority of cells in the normal intima in contrast to that in inflammatory arthritis in which macrophage numbers increase dramatically (Figure 5). In RA synovium macrophages can account for up to 80% of the intimal layer, with the usual pattern being that of a superficial layer of macrophages with an intimal phenotype below which lie a layer of intimal fibroblasts. The subintima may have a zone of NSE-weak, strongly CD14+ FcγRI+ macrophages in association with venules.

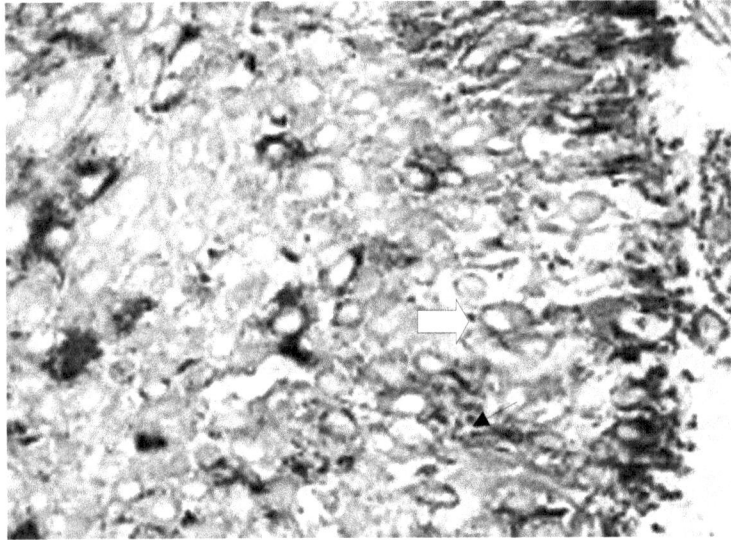

Figure 5: Synovium in rheumatoid arthritis (x400 magnification). Note the thickened intimal layer containing mainly CD68+ macrophages (red; arrow) on the surface and weakly CD55+ synovial fibroblast cells (blue; block arrow) beneath.

A small number of antigen presenting dendritic cells are also present in the normal synovium; these significantly increase in numbers in the diseased synovium, though in this state identification is difficult because of increased overlap of identifying markers. (Poulter & Janossy, 1985; Wilkinson, Worrall, Sinclair, & Edwards, 1990) Available evidence indicates that both intimal and subintimal macrophages derive from the bone marrow via circulating monocytes, many of which probably arrive via subintimal venules and migrate to the intima; this migration is supported by several mediators including CD11/18, Very Late Antigen-4 (CD49d/CD29), Very Late Antigen-5 (CD49e/CD29), and Vascular Cell Adhesion Molecule-1 (CD106). (J. C. Edwards, 1994; J. C. Edwards & Willoughby, 1982; Shang, Lang, & Issekutz, 1998; Smith, 2011)

2.2   Synovial Fibroblasts

Synovial fibroblasts (Figure 6) are thought to derive from division within synovium although the exact site remains uncertain. While it is possible that intimal fibroblasts might have their origin from a different lineage as opposed to subintimal fibroblasts, the current view supports a single origin that can take on an intimal phenotype in response to local stimuli (J. C. Edwards, 2000); the alternative hypothesis relates to mesenchymal origin for these cells. (Bartok & Firestein, 2010) Rates of cell division within the intima are very low, even in disease, as shown by thymidine labelled studies. (Mohr, Beneke, & Mohing, 1975) Following arthroplasty or synovectomy intimal cells reappear and express CD55, UDPGD, and VCAM-1; these may arise from intimal rests but it is probable that they are replaced from the subintima.

Synovial fibroblasts are adapted to hyaluronan production, with UDPGD activity being a specific marker of this cell type. This enzyme converts UDP-glucose into UDP-glucoronate, which is one of the two substrates required by hyaluronan synthase for assembly of the hyaluronan polymer. (Wilkinson, *et al.*, 1992) Disease states led to reduced UDPGD activity in synovial fibroblasts. CD55 expression by synovial fibroblasts is used to distinguish these from synovial macrophages. When cell suspensions generated from inflamed synovium are grown in tissue culture, cells showing fibroblast characteristics and ramifying processes with production of high levels of metalloproteinases are seen. (Krane, Goldring, & Dayer, 1982)

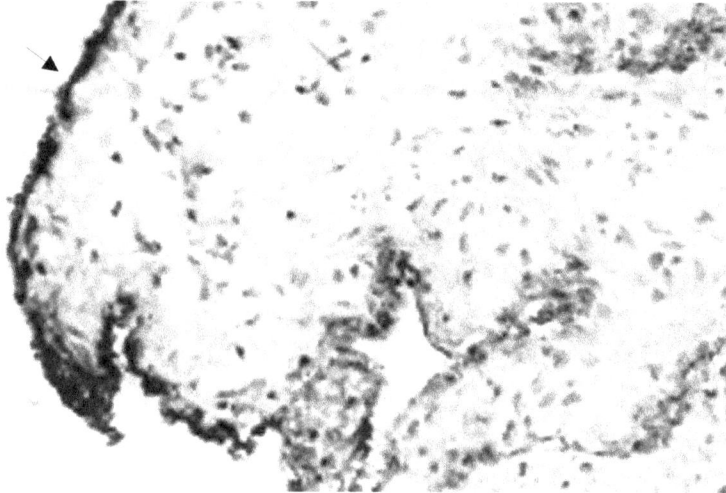

Figure 6: Synovial fibroblasts (arrow) in the normal synovium (x200 magnification) stained for CD55.

Synovial fibroblasts express several adhesion molecules including VCAM-1, intercellular adhesion molecule (ICAM)-1, CD44, β_1 and β_3 integrins. (Connolly, Veale, & Fearon, 2011; J. C. Edwards, 1995; Smith, *et al.,* 2003) The expression of VCAM-1 is intriguing and unusual as it is absent in most other fibroblast populations, though CD44 and β_1 integrins can be expressed in low levels on normal fibroblasts. (J. C. Edwards, 1995; Smith, *et al.,* 2003) VCAM-1 in this context may be important in cellular trafficking; its ligand $\alpha_4\beta_1$ integrin is present on mononuclear leukocytes but not granulocytes. VCAM-1 on synovial fibroblasts may allow transmigration of polymorphs into synovial fluid and potentially trap macrophages and lymphocytes within the synovial membrane in disease states such as RA. Disaggregated and cultured synovial fibroblasts lose VCAM-1 and DAF expression but readily reacquire these markers following cytokine stimulation. In culture, fibroblasts can be induced to express complement receptor-2 (CR2, CD21), though this receptor is not usually expressed on synovial fibroblasts in the normal synovium. (Leigh, Cambridge, & Edwards, 1996) This receptor, along with DAF and VCAM-1 is involved in B lymphocyte survival as is a bone marrow stromal cell marker, BST-1, reported to be expressed on fibroblasts in rheumatoid (but not normal) intima. (B. O. Lee *et al.*, 1996) Synovial fibroblasts can be induced to express several other molecules including the chemokine SDF-1 and bone morphogenetic proteins and their receptors (Fowler *et al.*, 1998; Marinova-Mutafchieva, Taylor, Funa, Maini, & Zvaifler, 2000; Seki, Selby, Haupl, & Winchester, 1998) under various conditions. In addition, lubricin, a glycoprotein found in synovium and the superficial zone of articular cartilage,(Jay, Britt, & Cha, 2000) derives from the same gene as megakaryocyte stimulating factor. A defect of this gene leads to the Camptodactyly- Arthropathy- Coxa vara- Pericarditis (CACP) syndrome.(Marcelino *et al.*, 1999)

In addition to lubricin, synovial fibroblasts synthesize several normal matrix components including laminin, collagens, fibronectin, proteoglycans among other proteins. In inflammatory arthritis, transformed fibroblasts have enormous capacity to produce cytokines, adhesion molecules and metalloprotein-ases. (Bartok & Firestein, 2010)

The presence of both clusterin (a glycoprotein involved in recycling and apoptosis) and podoplanin (a membrane glycoprotein with diverse functions) has recently been reported in normal synovial fibro-blasts. Of interest, podoplanin (which in context of neoplasia is associated with poor prognosis and meta-static disease) has been shown to be highly expressed in RA synovial fibroblasts, known to have migrato-ry and invasive potential. (Boland, Folpe, Hornick, & Grogg, 2009; Ekwall *et al.*, 2011)

The synovium is also a source of mesenchymal stem cells. These cells have the ability to self re-new and differentiate; they compare favourably to bone marrow derived MSCs in terms of their ability to differentiate into bone, cartilage and adipose tissue. (Arufe, De la Fuente, Fuentes-Boquete, De Toro, & Blanco, 2009; Arufe, De la Fuente, Fuentes, de Toro, & Blanco, 2010; De Bari, Dell'Accio, Tylzanowski, & Luyten, 2001; Sakaguchi, Sekiya, Yagishita, & Muneta, 2005)

2.3   Other Sub-intimal Cell Populations

Other cells including CD3+ T cells, (including CD4+ and CD8+ cells), with some having a memory T cell phenotype, B cells and plasma cells can be found within the normal synovial tissue.(Singh, et al., 2004; Smith, 2004) It is possible that some of these cells may simply be trafficking through the normal synovium, but their role, if any, in the homeostasis of synovial tissue remains unknown. (Smith, 2011)

2.4   Inflammatory Cytokine Production within the Normal Synovium

Inflammatory cytokine production, including that of interleukin (IL)-1, IL-6, and tumor necrosis factor alpha (TNF-α) can be seen within the normal synovium,(Smith, *et al.*, 2003) it is far less than that seen in inflammatory states such as RA, and in normal tissue is outweighed by the amount of anti-inflammatory cytokine production, at least in the case of IL-1 receptor antagonist (the naturally occurring inhibitor of IL-1). Similarly, receptor activator of nuclear factor kappa-B ligand (RANKL, an essential factor for the development of osteoclasts) seen in normal synovial tissue is low (Smith, *et al.*, 2003) and easily out-weighed by osteoprotegerin (Figure 7), its naturally occurring decoy receptor, thus effectively suppress-ing osteoclast function.

2.5   The Intimal Matrix

The intimal matrix has an amorphous or fine fibrillar ultrastructure, containing collagens III, IV, V and VI with minimal type I collagen. Despite the presence of several basement membrane components in-cluding laminin, fibronectin and chondroitin-6- sulfate-rich proteoglycan in the intimal matrix, the base-ment membrane is conspicuous by its absence. (Ashhurst, Bland, & Levick, 1991; Revell, al-Saffar, Fish, & Osei, 1995) This may be due to the absence of entactin, which normally links other components in basement membrane together. Intimal microfibrils include fibrillin-1 microfibrils that form a basketwork around cells and collagen VI microfibrils that form a uniform mesh. Hyaluronan is prominent mainly in the intimal and superficial subintimal layers of the normal synovium but fades in the deeper sublining layer possibly indicating diffusion of hyaluronan (HA) from the surface towards clearing lymphatics.

2.6   The Vascular Net

Just beneath the synovial surface lies a rich microvascular network. The synovial vascular supply stems from multiple feeding small vessels which communicate and branch freely in the deeper layers of the

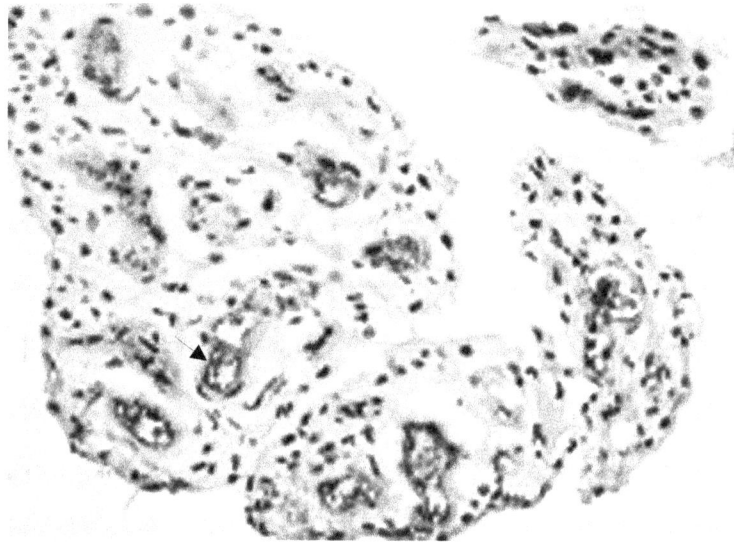

Figure 7: Normal synovium (x200 magnification) stained with an antibody against osteoprotegerin (arrow)

synovium; as they become more superficial they form multiple branches to contribute to the capillary network. These capillaries become less prominent with age; some capillaries are fenestrated and fenestrae tend to face the tissue surface.(Suter & Majno, 1964) Apart from fenestration of superficial capillary endothelial cells, there is little evidence of specialization in synovial endothelium. 50 to 100 μm beneath the surface, small venules are prominent. An anastomosing quadrilateral array is formed 200 μm beneath the surface with larger venules, arterioles and lymphatics (Figure 10).(Xu, *et al.*, 2003)

In disease states such as RA in which increased turnover of hyaluronic acid and leukocyte trafficking is seen, vessels with lymphatic staining (can be immunohistochemically stained with LYV-1 antibody) characteristics are prominent. It has been proposed that failure of lymphatic drainage of synovial fluid may be a cause of villous proliferation in RA synovial tissue. If correct, this may reflect overloading of existing lymphatic channels with HA-rich extracellular fluid and leukocytes rather than a lack of lymphatic channels.(Xu, *et al.*, 2003)

Physiologically, synovial fluid flow is increased by heat and exercise and reduced by immobilization. In the presence of knee effusion, even modest elevations in intra-synovial pressures of up to 45mmHg in the context of daily activities were associated with synovial blood flow compromise and hypoxia; (James, Cleland, Rofe, & Leslie, 1990) in the context of RA, hypoxia is thought to be a key regulator of synovial angiogenesis and inflammation. (Konisti, Kiriakidis, & Paleolog, 2012)

2.7 The Nerve Supply

The synovium has a rich nerve supply, (Mapp, 1995; Pereira da Silva & Carmo-Fonseca, 1990) including from the sympathetic nervous system (Widenfalk, 1991) with most of the nerve supply being perivascularly located and some extending into the intimal layers. In RA synovium, reduced nerve supply is seen, especially in the more superficial intimal regions.

3   Function of the Normal Synovium

The functions of synovial tissue are thought to be self-evident, but precisely defining them is difficult.(J. C. W. Edwards, 1987) The synovial lining provides a deformable packing that enables movement between adjacent, relatively non-deformable tissues; in addition, areolar synovium may also have specialized viscoelastic properties for coping with the stretching, rolling, and folding it undergoes during joint movement. Furthermore the synovium maintains an intact non-adherent tissue surface, provides cartilage lubrication and nutrition and regulates synovial fluid volume and composition.

3.1   Maintenance of Tissue Surface

To allow continued movement, synovial surfaces must be non-adherent; hyaluronan production by intimal fibroblasts may play an important role in this regard. Plasminogen activator and DAF from intimal fibroblasts may inhibit fibrin formation and scarring. Synovial fluid retention requires the allowance by the intimal matrix for free exchange of crystalloids and proteins but inhibit rapid transit of the viscous hyaluronan solution. These functions are probably subserved by the intimal macrophages and fibroblasts. The vasculature is probably important in both intimal cell nutrition and recruitment of new cells. Blood monocytes will replenish macrophages while perivascular fibroblasts may provide the main pool of intimal fibroblast precursors.

3.2   Lubrication

Synovial fluid probably lubricates cartilage because of the presence of a glycoprotein, especially a glycoprotein known both as 'lubricin' and 'superficial zone protein' because of its localization to the surface of both synovium and cartilage. (Jay, *et al.*, 2000) Hyaluronan is probably responsible for retaining a constant synovial fluid volume during exercise (Levick & McDonald, 1995) and in maintaining a film of lubricant on the cartilage surfaces but does not appear to contribute to the ability of synovial fluid to lubricate cartilage. This ability of hyaluronan to maintain a constant synovial fluid volume during exercise is probably important as a cushion for synovial tissue and as a reservoir of lubricant for cartilage. It is likely that the rate of hyaluronan synthesis and its export into the joint cavity are dependent on the mechanical stimulation of intimal fibroblasts and influenced by the effectiveness of the synovial fluid cushion.

Joint effusions are created by two, probably interrelated mechanisms. (Pelletier, Martel-Pelletier, & Abramson, 2001) Mechanical irritation of the synovium by bone and cartilage leads to an effusion with reasonably normal composition (frictional force induced hyaluronan production retains plasma dialysate in the joint cavity). In addition, a low grade inflammatory immune reaction to bone and cartilage products may contribute to an effusion. Recent proteomic evidence suggests that the increased vascular permeability of inflammation may be related not only to increase in inter endothelial gaps, but also to glycocalyceal damage and aquaporin upregulation. (Shahrara, Volin, Connors, Haines, & Koch, 2002)

3.3   Chondrocyte Nutrition

The synovium provides the major route for chondrocytes nutrition. In a normal joint, a surprisingly large proportion of hyaline cartilage lies within 50μm of a synovial surface with only a small proportion of cartilage apposed to the other articular surface in any one position; the synovium packs most of the space between less congruent areas. In immature but not adult joints the incomplete subchondral plate may contribute to nutrition and hence cartilage nutrition especially in areas that do not come into close contact with synovium must be by an indirect route. In this case, nutrition may occur by indirect routes through cartilage matrix and the apposed articular cartilage may be more important. Although synovial blood vessels potentially provide the most direct route for cartilage nutrition, there is little evidence of structural adaptation for this function. Diarthrodial joints have high levels of transforming growth factor β (TGF β) in cartilage and the synovium. TGF β is known to exist in two forms: a latent form that can be activated in vivo and vitro, and an active form that interacts with cell surface receptors. (Albro *et al.*, 2012; Fava, Olsen, Keski-Oja, Moses, & Pincus, 1989). In the latent form, TGF β is linked non-covalently to a 70 kDa latency associated peptide; this complex is called the large latent complex. TGF β must undergo activation to be able to bind to receptors and induce a biological response. Recent in vivo experiments suggest that shearing of synovial fluid as a result of physiologic joint motion may play an important role in TGF β activation, which may be essential to maintain the biochemical content and structural integrity of healthy cartilage. (Albro, *et al.*, 2012; Fava, *et al.*, 1989; Miossec, Naviliat, Dupuy d'Angeac, Sany, & Banchereau, 1990)

4   The Synovium as a Site of Pathology in Inflammatory Arthritis

Synovitis or inflammation of the synovial membrane is a consequence of a multitude of immunological and inflammatory disorders, including RA, systemic lupus erythematosus and spondyloarthritis. The knowledge of normal synovium including its considerable normal variation is critical to understand relevant changes in synovial tissue architecture and immunopathology in disease states. Despite this variation, there are general consistencies across the broad spectrum of normal, which can be contrasted with that seen in the chronically inflamed synovial tissue. An example is the marked increase in synovial lining layer thickness, with a reverse of normal ratio of type A to type B synoviocytes, favoring type B cells in normal synovium and types A cells in RA. Other examples include changes in subintimal cell content, cytokine and chemokine production, vascular and lymphatic changes as well as production of metalloproteinases and stimulators of osteoclast formation. It is important to understand these synovial changes of chronic inflammation and contrast them with those seen in the normal synovium, to identify suitable therapeutic targets at various stages in the evolution of a chronic inflammatory arthritis.

The identification of TNF, IL-1, IL-6 and IL-17 as four likely therapeutic targets is an example of how such a strategy can lead to useful therapeutic interventions being introduced into the management of several chronic inflammatory arthritides including RA, psoriatic arthritis and ankylosing spondylitis. Recent work on a mouse model of arthritis has also raised the possibility of cadherin-11 expression on synovial fibroblasts as a potential therapeutic target in the treatment of RA.(D. M. Lee, *et al.*, 2007)(Firestein, 2007) Inhibition of cadherin-11 interactions in this model interfered with both the synovial inflammation and the cartilage invasion by pannus, without any effect on bone erosion, which is predominantly dependent on osteoclast function. Inflammation in this model could be substantially ameliorated by antibodies to cadherin-11 or a cadherin-Fc fusion protein. In further studies, cadherin 11 expression (Figure 8) has been found to promote invasive behavior of fibroblasts and is increased by IL-17 and tumour necrosis factor α (TNF α), cytokines very relevant in RA pathophysiology. (Kiener *et al.*, 2009; Park *et al.*, 2011; Vandooren *et al.*, 2008)

There is still much to be learned about the immunological microenvironment of articular tissues, particularly the normal synovium.

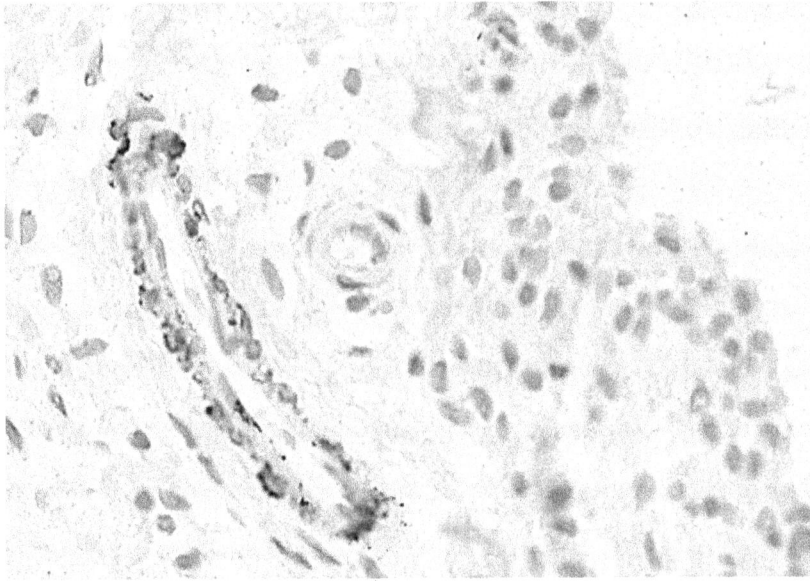

Figure 8: Cadherin 11 expression in the normal synovium (x400 magnification).

5   Summary

In summary, the normal synovium consists of the intima and subintima, and is essential for normal articular homeostasis. There is a considerable morphological and immunological variation in the cytokine, cellular and vascular content in health and disease, which highlights the importance of having an understanding of the normal synovium prior to appreciating changes in pathological states such as the inflammatory arthritides. Knowledge of the architecture of the normal synovium is surprisingly limited.

References

Albro, M. B., Cigan, A. D., Nims, R. J., Yeroushalmi, K. J., Oungoulian, S. R., Hung, C. T., & Ateshian, G. A. (2012). Shearing of synovial fluid activates latent TGF-beta. Osteoarthritis Cartilage, http://dx.doi.org/10.1016/j.joca.2012.07.006. doi: 10.1016/j.joca.2012.07.006

Arufe, M. C., De la Fuente, A., Fuentes-Boquete, I., De Toro, F. J., & Blanco, F. J. (2009). Differentiation of synovial CD-105(+) human mesenchymal stem cells into chondrocyte-like cells through spheroid formation. J Cell Biochem, 108(1), 145-155. doi: 10.1002/jcb.22238

Arufe, M. C., De la Fuente, A., Fuentes, I., de Toro, F. J., & Blanco, F. J. (2010). Chondrogenic potential of subpopulations of cells expressing mesenchymal stem cell markers derived from human synovial membranes. J Cell Biochem, 111(4), 834-845. doi: 10.1002/jcb.22768

Ashhurst, D. E., Bland, Y. S., & Levick, J. R. (1991). An immunohistochemical study of the collagens of rabbit synovial interstitium. J Rheumatol, 18(11), 1669-1672.

Barland, P., Novikoff, A. B., & Hamerman, D. (1962). Electron microscopy of the human synovial membrane. J Cell Biol, 14, 207-220.

Bartok, B., & Firestein, G. S. (2010). Fibroblast-like synoviocytes: key effector cells in rheumatoid arthritis. Immunol Rev, 233(1), 233-255. doi: 10.1111/j.0105-2896.2009.00859.x

Bhatia, A., Blades, S., Cambridge, G., & Edwards, J. C. (1998). *Differential distribution of Fc gamma RIIIa in normal human tissues and co-localization with DAF and fibrillin-1: implications for immunological microenvironments.* Immunology, 94(1), 56-63.

Boland, J. M., Folpe, A. L., Hornick, J. L., & Grogg, K. L. (2009). *Clusterin is expressed in normal synoviocytes and in tenosynovial giant cell tumors of localized and diffuse types: diagnostic and histogenetic implications.* Am J Surg Pathol, 33(8), 1225-1229. doi: 10.1097/PAS.0b013e3181a6d86f

Canoso, J. J., Stack, M. T., & Brandt, K. D. (1983). *Hyaluronic acid content of deep and subcutaneous bursae of man.* Ann Rheum Dis, 42(2), 171-175.

Connolly, M., Veale, D. J., & Fearon, U. (2011). *Acute serum amyloid A regulates cytoskeletal rearrangement, cell matrix interactions and promotes cell migration in rheumatoid arthritis.* Ann Rheum Dis, 70(7), 1296-1303. doi: 10.1136/ard.2010.142240

Davies, D. V. (1950). *The structure and functions of the synovial membrane.* Br Med J, 1(4645), 92-95.

De Bari, C., Dell'Accio, F., Tylzanowski, P., & Luyten, F. P. (2001). *Multipotent mesenchymal stem cells from adult human synovial membrane.* Arthritis Rheum, 44(8), 1928-1942. doi: 10.1002/1529-0131(200108)44:8<1928::aid-art331>3.0.co;2-p

Edwards, J. C. (1994). *The nature and origins of synovium: experimental approaches to the study of synoviocyte differentiation.* J Anat, 184 (Pt 3), 493-501.

Edwards, J. C. (1995). *Synovial intimal fibroblasts.* Ann Rheum Dis, 54(5), 395-397.

Edwards, J. C. (2000). *Fibroblast biology. Development and differentiation of synovial fibroblasts in arthritis.* Arthritis Res, 2(5), 344-347.

Edwards, J. C., & Willoughby, D. A. (1982). *Demonstration of bone marrow derived cells in synovial lining by means of giant intracellular granules as genetic markers.* Ann Rheum Dis, 41(2), 177-182.

Edwards, J. C. W. (1987). *Functions of synovial lining. In B. Henderson & J. C. W. Edwards (Eds.), The synovial lining in health and disease (pp. 41-74).* London: Chapman & Hall.

Ekwall, A. K., Eisler, T., Anderberg, C., Jin, C., Karlsson, N., Brisslert, M., & Bokarewa, M. I. (2011). *The tumour-associated glycoprotein podoplanin is expressed in fibroblast-like synoviocytes of the hyperplastic synovial lining layer in rheumatoid arthritis.* Arthritis Res Ther, 13(2), R40. doi: 10.1186/ar3274

Fava, R., Olsen, N., Keski-Oja, J., Moses, H., & Pincus, T. (1989). *Active and latent forms of transforming growth factor beta activity in synovial effusions.* J Exp Med, 169(1), 291-296.

Firestein, G. S. (2007). *Every joint has a silver lining.* Science, 315(5814), 952-953. doi: 10.1126/science.1139574

Fowler, M. J., Jr., Neff, M. S., Borghaei, R. C., Pease, E. A., Mochan, E., & Thornton, R. D. (1998). *Induction of bone morphogenetic protein-2 by interleukin-1 in human fibroblasts.* Biochem Biophys Res Commun, 248(3), 450-453. doi: 10.1006/bbrc.1998.8988

Ghadially, F. N. (1978). *Fine structure of joints. In L. Sokoloff (Ed.), The joints and synovial fluid (pp. 105-176).* New York: Academic Press.

Henderson, B., Revell, P. A., & Edwards, J. C. (1988). *Synovial lining cell hyperplasia in rheumatoid arthritis: dogma and fact.* Ann Rheum Dis, 47(4), 348-349.

Holness, C. L., & Simmons, D. L. (1993). *Molecular cloning of CD68, a human macrophage marker related to lysosomal glycoproteins.* Blood, 81(6), 1607-1613.

James, M. J., Cleland, L. G., Rofe, A. M., & Leslie, A. L. (1990). *Intraarticular pressure and the relationship between synovial perfusion and metabolic demand.* J Rheumatol, 17(4), 521-527.

Jay, G. D., Britt, D. E., & Cha, C. J. (2000). *Lubricin is a product of megakaryocyte stimulating factor gene expression by human synovial fibroblasts.* J Rheumatol, 27(3), 594-600.

Key, J. A. (1932). The synovial membrane of joints and bursae. Special cytology. New York: PB Hoeber.

Kiener, H. P., Niederreiter, B., Lee, D. M., Jimenez-Boj, E., Smolen, J. S., & Brenner, M. B. (2009). Cadherin 11 promotes invasive behavior of fibroblast-like synoviocytes. Arthritis Rheum, 60(5), 1305-1310. doi: 10.1002/art.24453

Kim, J. K., Choi, E. M., Shin, H. I., Kim, C. H., Hwang, S. H., Kim, S. M., & Kwon, B. S. (2005). Characterization of monoclonal antibody specific to the Z39Ig protein, a member of immunoglobulin superfamily. Immunol Lett, 99(2), 153-161. doi: 10.1016/j.imlet.2005.02.012

Konisti, S., Kiriakidis, S., & Paleolog, E. M. (2012). Hypoxia--a key regulator of angiogenesis and inflammation in rheumatoid arthritis. Nat Rev Rheumatol, 8(3), 153-162. doi: 10.1038/nrrheum.2011.205

Krane, S. M., Goldring, S. R., & Dayer, J. M. (1982). Interactions among lymphocytes, monocytes and other synovial cells in the rheumatoid synovium. Lymphokines, 7, 75-87.

Lee, B. O., Ishihara, K., Denno, K., Kobune, Y., Itoh, M., Muraoka, O., . . . Hirano, T. (1996). Elevated levels of the soluble form of bone marrow stromal cell antigen 1 in the sera of patients with severe rheumatoid arthritis. Arthritis Rheum, 39(4), 629-637.

Lee, D. M., Kiener, H. P., Agarwal, S. K., Noss, E. H., Watts, G. F., Chisaka, O., . . . Brenner, M. B. (2007). Cadherin-11 in synovial lining formation and pathology in arthritis. Science, 315(5814), 1006-1010. doi: 10.1126/science.1137306

Lee, M. Y., Kim, W. J., Kang, Y. J., Jung, Y. M., Kang, Y. M., Suk, K., . . . Lee, W. H. (2006). Z39Ig is expressed on macrophages and may mediate inflammatory reactions in arthritis and atherosclerosis. J Leukoc Biol, 80(4), 922-928. doi: 10.1189/jlb.0306160

Leigh, R. D., Cambridge, G., & Edwards, J. C. W. (1996). Expression of B-cell survival cofactors on synovial fibroblasts. Br J Rheumatol, 1 (suppl), 110.

Levick, J. R., & McDonald, J. N. (1995). Fluid movement across synovium in healthy joints: role of synovial fluid macromolecules. Ann Rheum Dis, 54(5), 417-423.

Mapp, P. I. (1995). Innervation of the synovium. Ann Rheum Dis, 54(5), 398-403.

Marcelino, J., Carpten, J. D., Suwairi, W. M., Gutierrez, O. M., Schwartz, S., Robbins, C., . . . Warman, M. L. (1999). CACP, encoding a secreted proteoglycan, is mutated in camptodactyly-arthropathy-coxa vara-pericarditis syndrome. Nat Genet, 23(3), 319-322. doi: 10.1038/15496

Marinova-Mutafchieva, L., Taylor, P., Funa, K., Maini, R. N., & Zvaifler, N. J. (2000). Mesenchymal cells expressing bone morphogenetic protein receptors are present in the rheumatoid arthritis joint. Arthritis Rheum, 43(9), 2046-2055. doi: 10.1002/1529-0131(200009)43:9<2046::aid-anr16>3.0.co;2-8

Miossec, P., Naviliat, M., Dupuy d'Angeac, A., Sany, J., & Banchereau, J. (1990). Low levels of interleukin-4 and high levels of transforming growth factor beta in rheumatoid synovitis. Arthritis Rheum, 33(8), 1180-1187.

Mohr, W., Beneke, G., & Mohing, W. (1975). Proliferation of synovial lining cells and fibroblasts. Ann Rheum Dis, 34(3), 219-224.

Park, Y. E., Woo, Y. J., Park, S. H., Moon, Y. M., Oh, H. J., Kim, J. I., . . . Kim, S. I. (2011). IL-17 increases cadherin-11 expression in a model of autoimmune experimental arthritis and in rheumatoid arthritis. Immunol Lett, 140(1-2), 97-103. doi: 10.1016/j.imlet.2011.07.003

Pelletier, J. P., Martel-Pelletier, J., & Abramson, S. B. (2001). Osteoarthritis, an inflammatory disease: potential implication for the selection of new therapeutic targets. Arthritis Rheum, 44(6), 1237-1247. doi: 10.1002/1529-0131(200106)44:6<1237::aid-art214>3.0.co;2-f

Pereira da Silva, J. A., & Carmo-Fonseca, M. (1990). Peptide containing nerves in human synovium: immunohistochemical evidence for decreased innervation in rheumatoid arthritis. J Rheumatol, 17(12), 1592-1599.

Poulter, L. W., & Janossy, G. (1985). The involvement of dendritic cells in chronic inflammatory disease. Scand J Immunol, 21(5), 401-407.

Revell, P. A., al-Saffar, N., Fish, S., & Osei, D. (1995). Extracellular matrix of the synovial intimal cell layer. Ann Rheum Dis, 54(5), 404-407.

Sakaguchi, Y., Sekiya, I., Yagishita, K., & Muneta, T. (2005). Comparison of human stem cells derived from various mesenchymal tissues: superiority of synovium as a cell source. Arthritis Rheum, 52(8), 2521-2529. doi: 10.1002/art.21212

Seki, T., Selby, J., Haupl, T., & Winchester, R. (1998). Use of differential subtraction method to identify genes that characterize the phenotype of cultured rheumatoid arthritis synoviocytes. Arthritis Rheum, 41(8), 1356-1364. doi: 10.1002/1529-0131(199808)41:8<1356::aid-art4>3.0.co;2-x

Shahrara, S., Volin, M. V., Connors, M. A., Haines, G. K., & Koch, A. E. (2002). Differential expression of the angiogenic Tie receptor family in arthritic and normal synovial tissue. Arthritis Res, 4(3), 201-208.

Shang, X.-z., Lang, B. J., & Issekutz, A. C. (1998). Adhesion Molecule Mechanisms Mediating Monocyte Migration Through Synovial Fibroblast and Endothelium Barriers: Role for CD11/CD18, Very Late Antigen-4 (CD49d/CD29), Very Late Antigen-5 (CD49e/CD29), and Vascular Cell Adhesion Molecule-1 (CD106). The Journal of Immunology, 160(1), 467-474.

Singh, J. A., Arayssi, T., Duray, P., & Schumacher, H. R. (2004). Immunohistochemistry of normal human knee synovium: a quantitative study. Ann Rheum Dis, 63(7), 785-790. doi: 10.1136/ard.2003.013383

Smith, M. D. (2004). Immunohistochemistry of normal synovium. Ann Rheum Dis, 63(11), 1532-1533; author reply 1533. doi: 63/11/1532 [pii]

Smith, M. D. (2011). The Normal Synovium. Open Rheumatol J, 5, 100-106. doi: 10.2174/1874312901105010100

Smith, M. D., Barg, E., Weedon, H., Papengelis, V., Smeets, T., Tak, P. P., . . . Ahern, M. J. (2003). Microarchitecture and protective mechanisms in synovial tissue from clinically and arthroscopically normal knee joints. Ann Rheum Dis, 62(4), 303-307.

Smith, M. D., & Walker, J. G. (2010). The Normal Synovium. In M. C. Hochberg, A. J. Silman, J. S. Smolen, M. E. Weinblatt & M. H. Weisman (Eds.), Rheumatology (5th ed., Vol. 1, pp. 51-56). Philadelphia: Mosby.

Suter, E. R., & Majno, G. (1964). Ultrastructure of the joint capsule in the rat: presence of two kinds of capillaries Nature, 202, 920-921.

Vandooren, B., Cantaert, T., ter Borg, M., Noordenbos, T., Kuhlman, R., Gerlag, D., . . . Baeten, D. (2008). Tumor necrosis factor alpha drives cadherin 11 expression in rheumatoid inflammation. Arthritis Rheum, 58(10), 3051-3062. doi: 10.1002/art.23886

Walker, M. G. (2002). Z39Ig is co-expressed with activated macrophage genes. Biochim Biophys Acta, 1574(3), 387-390.

Widenfalk, B. (1991). Sympathetic innervation of normal and rheumatoid synovial tissue. Scand J Plast Reconstr Surg Hand Surg, 25(1), 31-33.

Wilkinson, L. S., & Edwards, J. C. (1989). Microvascular distribution in normal human synovium. J Anat, 167, 129-136.

Wilkinson, L. S., Pitsillides, A. A., Worrall, J. G., & Edwards, J. C. (1992). Light microscopic characterization of the fibroblast-like synovial intimal cell (synoviocyte). Arthritis Rheum, 35(10), 1179-1184.

Wilkinson, L. S., Worrall, J. G., Sinclair, H. D., & Edwards, J. C. (1990). Immunohistological reassessment of accessory cell populations in normal and diseased human synovium. Br J Rheumatol, 29(4), 259-263.

Xu, H., Edwards, J., Banerji, S., Prevo, R., Jackson, D. G., & Athanasou, N. A. (2003). Distribution of lymphatic vessels in normal and arthritic human synovial tissues. Ann Rheum Dis, 62(12), 1227-1229.

www.ingramcontent.com/pod-product-compliance
Lightning Source LLC
Chambersburg PA
CBHW061420210326
41598CB00035B/6278